American Diabetes Association Guide to Medical Nutrition Therapy for Diabetes

Clinical Education Series

American Diabetes Association Guide to Medical Nutrition Therapy for Diabetes

Marion J. Franz, MS, RD, LD, CDE,
and John P. Bantle, MD, Editors

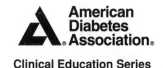

American Diabetes Association®

Clinical Education Series

Book Acquisitions	Robert J. Anthony
Editor	Aime M. Ballard
Production Director	Carolyn R. Segree
Production Coordinator	Peggy M. Rote
Composition	Harlowe Typography, Inc.
Text and Cover Design	Wickham & Associates, Inc.

Printed in Canada

1 3 5 7 9 10 8 6 4 2

The suggestions and information contained in this publication are generally consistent with the *Clinical Practice Recommendations* and other policies of the American Diabetes Association, but they do not represent the policy or position of the Association or any of its boards or committees. Reasonable steps have been taken to ensure the accuracy of the information presented. However, the American Diabetes Association cannot ensure the safety or efficacy of any product or service described in this publication. Individuals are advised to consult a physician or other appropriate health care professional before undertaking any diet or exercise program or taking any medication referred to in this publication. Professionals must use and apply their own professional judgment, experience, and training and should not rely solely on the information contained in this publication before prescribing any diet, exercise, or medication. The American Diabetes Association—its officers, directors, employees, volunteers, and members—assumes no responsibility or liability for personal or other injury, loss, or damage that may result from the suggestions or information in this publication.

ADA titles may be purchased for business or promotional use or for special sales. For information, please write to: Lee M. Romano, Special Sales & Promotions, at the address below.

American Diabetes Association
1660 Duke Street
Alexandria, Virginia 22314

Library of Congress Cataloging-in-Publication Data

American Diabetes Association's guide to medical nutrition therapy for
    diabetes / Marion J. Franz and John P. Bantle, editors.
        p.   cm. — (Clinical education series)
    Includes bibliographical references and index.
    ISBN 1-58040-006-X (pbk.)
    1. Diabetes—Diet therapy. 2. Diabetes—Nutritional aspects.
I. Franz, Marion J. II. Bantle, John P., 1947-   . III. American
Diabetes Association. IV. Title: Guide to medical nutrition therapy
for diabetes. V. Series.
    [DNLM: 1. Diabetes Mellitus—diet therapy. WK 818 A512 1999 / WK
818 A512 1999]
RC662.A435   1999
616.4'620654—dc21
DNLM/DLC
for Library of Congress   98-47839
                                                                                            CIP

Contents

Nutrition Issues of Special Populations

Medical Nutrition Therapy and Diabetes Complications

Acknowledgments

It has been a pleasure to edit this book. We are indebted to the chapter authors for the excellence and thoughtfulness given to the preparation of their chapters. They truly represent the breadth of nutrition expertise in the U.S.—from seasoned and well-respected researchers to caring and committed clinicians. We are grateful to them for their willingness to share their knowledge, expertise, and experiences with you, the reader of this book. A special thanks to Aime Ballard for her determination to keep the whole process moving and for her thorough and careful editing. And, of course, thanks to the American Diabetes Association for its dedication to providing professionals with the latest and most accurate information available.

Integrating Nutrition Therapy into Diabetes Management

1. A Dietitian's Perspective on Medical Nutrition Therapy for Diabetes

MARION J. FRANZ, MS, RD, LD, CDE

Highlights

- Although research has focused on a search for the ideal percentage of calories from carbohydrate, protein, and fat, glycemic control can be attained with varying percentages of macronutrients. Therefore, medical nutrition therapy must begin with the goals of therapy and the nutrition-related strategies to achieve these goals.
- The dietitian should determine the nutrition prescription based on the food/nutrition assessment of what the individual with diabetes is currently eating. Eating patterns are modified based on treatment goals and changes an individual with diabetes agrees to incorporate into his/her lifestyle.
- Successful nutrition therapy is based on assessment and on setting goals, choosing appropriate educational materials, facilitating behavior change, evaluating outcomes, and working with a diabetes health care team.
- Hospitals and long-term care facilities should consider implementing a consistent-carbohydrate diabetes meal planning system in place of the traditional standardized calorie-level meal patterns based on exchange lists.

INTRODUCTION

Historically, diet or nutrition therapy has been viewed as the cornerstone of therapy for management of diabetes (1). However, even today controversy exists as to what is the ideal diet, and research is still needed to confirm or refute many of the nutrition recommendations given to

3

people with diabetes. What is clear is that to achieve the level of metabolic control that is desired today (2), it is essential that people with diabetes pay some attention to lifestyle changes. In the Diabetes Control and Complications Trial, individuals in the intensive therapy group who reported following their meal plan ~90% of the time had HbA_{1c} levels 1% lower than those individuals who reported following their meal plan only 40% of the time (3). In a study of nutrition practice guidelines for type 2 diabetes, intensive nutrition therapy lowered HbA_{1c} ~1% (8.3 ± 1.8% to 7.4 ± 1.3%) in contrast to a comparison group who had no nutrition intervention and whose HbA_{1c} remained stable (4). Although additional outcome studies are needed, those that have been published have supported the importance of nutrition therapy in diabetes management (4–7).

Most of the research done in the past has addressed the issue of ideal macronutrient percentages in the diet for people with diabetes. However, glycemic control can be achieved with varying percentages of macronutrients (8). Therefore, medical nutrition therapy (MNT) for diabetes should instead begin with the goals of therapy and the lifestyle strategies that lead to achievement of these goals. Just as there is no longer one insulin regimen that can be applied to all people with diabetes who need insulin, there is no longer one nutrition prescription based on ideal macronutrient percentages that applies to everyone with diabetes.

CHANGING THE EMPHASIS OF NUTRITION THERAPY

The emphasis of MNT for diabetes has thus shifted from determining the ideal percentages of carbohydrate, protein, and fat for all people with diabetes to determining goals and nutrition-related strategies to achieve these goals. The first goal of MNT is to assist an individual in achieving and maintaining as near-normal blood glucose control as possible. In the clinical trials for nutrition practice guidelines for type 2 and type 1 diabetes, when dietitians implemented practice guideline care, there was an increased emphasis on changes in lifestyle that improved blood glucose control (4,7). Unfortunately, historically, a nutrition prescription was determined, usually by a physician, based on theoretical caloric needs and ideal percentages of macronutrients with no knowledge of what individuals with diabetes were currently eating and/or any changes they were willing and able to make in their habits. It is not surprising that much of this was wasted effort because many individuals with diabetes found it impossible to maintain in the long term the type of lifestyle changes that this approach required (9). Today, the approach is to individualize treatment, basing the nutrition prescription on the food/nutrition assessment and focusing on metabolic and quality-of-life goals (10). By changing the emphasis, dietitians can help people with diabetes make feasible lifestyle changes that improve glycemic control.

Other nutrition-related goals are to assist people with diabetes to achieve optimal lipid levels, to achieve and maintain a reasonable body weight in adults, to provide for the nutritional needs for normal growth and development in children and teens with diabetes, and to improve health with optimal nutrition and increased physical activity (11,12). To meet these goals, nutrition-related strategies must first be prioritized. Furthermore, dietitians must have a clear understanding of diabetes management and have the skills and ability to implement effective counseling strategies (13). To be an effective counselor, a dietitian must use motivational strategies, such as determining readiness to change, setting goals, involving the client in decision making, using behavior modification, and providing follow-up and support.

NUTRITION STRATEGIES FOR TYPE 1 DIABETES

To help people receiving insulin therapy achieve target blood glucose goals, it is essential that insulin regimens be integrated into usual eating and exercise habits. Unfortunately, individuals are often asked to change long-standing eating and exercise habits to coincide with insulin regimens, making it difficult for individuals to comply (Table 1.1). Chapter 3 covers this process in more detail.

Table 1.1   Integrating Insulin Therapy into Lifestyle Habits

1. An individualized meal plan is developed by a registered dietitian based on an assessment of usual eating and exercise habits. Lifestyle habits and meal plan are communicated to the team member responsible for determining insulin therapy.

2. An insulin regimen is planned that will integrate insulin therapy into usual lifestyle habits.

3. Individuals with diabetes are asked to eat consistently and to monitor blood glucose levels.

4. Insulin doses, regimen (or meal plan), or both are adjusted based on blood glucose patterns.

5. After basic insulin doses are determined, algorithms for adjustments in premeal regular or lispro insulin can be added for deviations from the meal plan and to correct blood glucose levels that are not in the target goal range.

From Franz MJ: Lifestyle modifications for diabetes management. *Endocrinol Metab Clin North Am* 26:500, 1997.

To make this system work, the nutrition prescription must be based on the assessment of what individuals are currently doing, what needs to be changed to improve glycemic control or for a healthier lifestyle, and what the individual is willing and able to do. The American Diabetes Association (ADA) standards of medical care (2) recommend that every person with diabetes have an individualized consultation with a registered dietitian to tailor a food/meal plan to his or her lifestyle and health needs. The registered dietitian is the medical team member who should plan, implement, and evaluate nutrition therapy. The minimum referral data needed to begin the process are outlined in Table 1.2 (14).

Using the food history and the food/nutrition assessment information, the dietitian can determine a preliminary nutrition prescription for a meal plan and share it with the provider who is determining the insulin regimen so that insulin therapy can be integrated. The meal plan can be evaluated by asking the following questions: *1*) Does the individual with diabetes believe it is feasible to implement? *2*) Is it appropriate for diabetes management? *3*) Are the calories appropriate? *4*) Does it encourage healthful eating? Both short- and long-term medical and behavioral goals should be mutually identified by the individual with diabetes and the nutrition professional. An appropriate meal planning approach is selected, and strategies for behavior change that enhance motivation and adherence to necessary lifestyle changes are identified. Sample menus can also be discussed.

At follow-up visits, food and blood glucose monitoring records can be used to determine whether blood glucose values outside target ranges can be corrected by adjustments in the meal plan or whether it would be more appropriate and easier for the individual to make insulin or other medication adjustments. Finally, documentation is essential for communication and reimbursement.

Table 1.2 Minimum Referral Data Needed by Dietitians to Provide Nutrition Therapy for Individuals with Diabetes

- Diabetes treatment regimen
- Laboratory data: HbA_{1c}, cholesterol and fractionations, blood pressure, microalbumin (when appropriate)
- Team goals for patient care: target blood glucose ranges and frequency of blood glucose monitoring
- Medical history: dyslipidemia, hypertension, renal disease, autonomic neuropathy, especially gastrointestinal
- Medications that affect nutrition therapy
- Medical clearance and/or limitations for exercise

From Monk et al. (14).

Table 1.3 Nutrition-Related Strategies for Improved Glycemic Control in People with Type 2 Diabetes

- Moderate weight loss of 4.5–9 kg (10–20 lb)
- Hypocaloric diet—even if this does not result in weight loss, it may assist with blood glucose control
- Better food choices, especially to reduce fat intake, because a high-fat diet may aggravate insulin resistance
- Food intake spread throughout the day (five to six small meals and snacks rather than only two or three meals)
- Increased physical activity
- Monitoring of blood glucose levels to determine whether medications need to be added or adjusted

From Franz MJ: Lifestyle modifications for diabetes management. *Endocrinol Metab Clin North Am* 26:500, 1997.

NUTRITION STRATEGIES FOR TYPE 2 DIABETES

The traditional dietary advice for people with type 2 diabetes has been to avoid sugar and lose weight. However, individuals with diabetes usually have found this advice difficult, if not impossible, to follow and have therefore abandoned all attempts at making lifestyle changes. Although moderate weight loss is desirable, the fact remains that individuals may lose weight, but the majority are unable to maintain long-term weight loss. Although a large percentage of the American population, especially women, report being on a diet and an enormous amount of money is spent on this effort, long-term success rates have been dismal. One year after completion of a weight-loss program, participants had regained one-third of the lost weight, with a return to baseline weight after 3–5 years (15). Variables associated with successful weight loss have been studied in populations with and without diabetes. In both groups, sex (male) was the primary variable associated with success (16,17).

Because maintaining weight loss may be difficult, if not impossible, for many individuals with type 2 diabetes on currently available therapies, the focus needs to be on other lifestyle strategies (Table 1.3) that can contribute to improvements in metabolic control. There is no clear answer as to which of these strategies should be the first priority. Monitoring blood glucose levels is essential to determine whether target blood glucose goals have been met or whether medications need to be added or doses adjusted. In the field trial of nutrition practice guidelines for type 2 diabetes, the results of lifestyle changes were evident by 6 weeks to 3 months, and that is when decisions as to the success of MNT or the need to change therapy should be made (4).

Both moderate weight loss—10–20% of body weight or as little as 5–20 lb (18,19)—and energy restriction per se (20,21) have been shown to lead to improved glycemic control. Marked improvements in glycemia disproportionate to weight loss after short periods of energy restriction as well as improvements in insulin sensitivity in obesity and mild type 2 diabetes have been reported. Markovic et al. (22) reported that early improvements in glycemia with energy restriction were related to changes in macronutrient intakes, i.e., reduced carbohydrate intake, whereas later changes in glycemia and insulin sensitivity were related to changes in abdominal fat. Modest weight loss was also correlated with a less atherogenic lipid profile associated with a reduction in central abdominal fat (23).

Two problems are often associated with nutrition therapy for type 2 diabetes. The first relates to the nutrition prescription. Frequently, patients are instructed on diets with unrealistically low calorie levels, with little likelihood they will be followed long term. This may be because calorie levels are usually determined by subtracting 500 to 1,000 calories from some predetermined calorie need. Instead, as stated earlier, the nutrition prescription should begin with an assessment of how many calories an individual has been eating on a daily basis and, more importantly, by collaborating with the patient to modify his or her intake based on his or her willingness and ability to do so. It is unrealistic to ask someone who has been eating 3,000 calories a day to eat 1,200 calories a day, when in reality, if this person can decrease his or her intake to 2,500 calories a day, it may lead to major improvements in metabolic control.

The second problem is that all too often the outcomes from nutrition therapy and/or increased physical activity are not evaluated. Individuals who need therapy changes often go months or years before it is determined whether medication adjustments need to be added to lifestyle changes. In the clinical trial of nutrition practice guidelines for type 2 diabetes, dietitians examined the outcomes from nutrition therapy at 6 weeks (or at the third visit) to determine whether changes in therapy were needed (4). Some individuals could reduce or eliminate oral glucose-lowering medications, and others had not achieved glycemic goals. The physician was then notified so that medications could be changed or added. As a result, intensive nutrition therapy, involving a series of visits to the dietitian instead of just one session, became cost-effective. The savings from individuals' receiving proper medication were greater than the costs of the dietitian visits (24).

Motivational techniques must also be used. In a survey of dietitians, the top five strategies considered to affect adherence were "Tailor the diet to the client's lifestyle," "Involve client in decision making," "Promote exercise," "Promote self–blood glucose monitoring," and "Identify areas client is willing to change." Those strategies not considered to be effective were "Provide list of good and bad foods," "Promote urine glucose monitoring," "Use computer-assisted management," and "Constructive confrontation" (25).

CARBOHYDRATE EMPHASIS—TOTAL NOT SOURCE

There is no ideal percentage of calories from carbohydrate that applies to all people with diabetes. Some individuals prefer a higher carbohydrate intake, whereas others may benefit from a more moderate intake. The level of carbohydrate intake is determined by the food history and treatment goals. For people with type 1 diabetes, adequate insulin must be given to cover the carbohydrate intake. For people with type 2 diabetes, in line with reducing total calories, carbohydrate and fat intakes will both need to be reduced.

Although differing carbohydrates do have varying glycemic indexes, as pointed out by Nuttall and Gannon in chapter 6, the glycemic response is not well-defined today. Furthermore, just as people with diabetes cannot eat unlimited portions of "sugar-free" foods, they cannot eat unlimited portions of foods with low glycemic indexes. First priority needs to be given to portion sizes; carbohydrate counting or taking into account the total amount of carbohydrate, not the source of the carbohydrate in foods, has been shown to be helpful for many individuals with either type 1 or type 2 diabetes (26,27). Individuals need the flexibility to incorporate many foods into their meal plans and not to be limited to a few foods with low glycemic indexes. In a number of studies comparing carbohydrates without sucrose to equal amounts of carbohydrates incorporating sucrose, no differences were noted in postmeal glycemic responses (28–30). In fact, meals with sugars have been reported to have the lowest glycemic response (31). It should also be remembered that other factors, such as the level of premeal blood glucose, will also influence the postmeal response. For example, gastric emptying is inhibited in hyperglycemia and enhanced in hypoglycemia (32,33).

QUESTIONS ABOUT PROTEIN

Although from a clinical standpoint, carbohydrate has been quite well studied, the effects of protein and fat on glycemia and insulin response remain largely unstudied. As reviewed by Gannon and Nuttall in chapter 7, protein from foods has minimal effects on blood glucose levels despite evidence that gluconeogenesis occurs. The question why remains to be answered: Does it happen so gradually throughout a 24-h period that the effect is never noticed? Is the glucose from gluconeogenesis stored as liver or muscle glycogen and released as glucose when blood glucose levels are low or glucagon levels are elevated? Or does less than 50–60% of protein go through the process of gluconeogenesis?

Individuals with diabetes are frequently advised that because half of protein is converted to glucose, protein will have half the effect on blood glucose levels compared with carbohydrate. Or they may be told to add protein to a snack, especially a bedtime snack, either to slow the absorption of carbohydrate or to prevent late-onset hypoglycemia. However, in a study by Peters and Davidson (34), 5 h after adding 200 calories from either protein or fat to a standard lunch, there were minimal differences in blood glucose levels. Adding protein to the treatment of hypoglycemia using 15 g carbohydrate had no effect on treatment response, and subsequent hypoglycemia occurred at identical times, despite the addition of protein to treatment. Again, the question why remains to be answered. The authors concluded that adding protein to the treatment of hypoglycemia only added often unneeded and unwanted calories. The same may be true regarding the advice to add protein (meat) to snacks.

Protein appears to stimulate the release of more insulin in subjects with mild type 2 diabetes than in subjects without diabetes after a carbohydrate load (35). It is unknown whether this is beneficial in controlling postprandial glycemia or is of concern because of the potential to contribute to hyperinsulinemia. Other concerns include increases in the protein content of the diet in individuals with undiagnosed nephropathy and the palatability of protein foods without fat.

Adding protein may be beneficial, especially in people with type 1 diabetes, because it may provide additional food to eat (if individuals are still hungry after eating their carbohydrate choices) with minimal effects on blood glucose levels, but not because it slows absorption of carbohydrate or provides glucose later for the prevention of hypoglycemia—both statements frequently made to individuals with diabetes. Protein does, however, require insulin, so it is assumed that some background insulin, such as NPH, ultralente, or endogenous insulin, is used for protein metabolism.

FAT INTAKE AND TREATMENT GOALS

As pointed out in chapter 8 by Purnell and Brunzell, benefits from both low-fat, high-carbohydrate diets and diets high in monounsaturated fats have been demonstrated. However, whatever approach is selected, it remains important that saturated fat intake be limited. The concern with any diet high in fat, regardless of the type of fat, is the potential for unwanted added calories. If the monounsaturated fat intake is increased, some other nutrient (usually carbohydrate) must be decreased. Unfortunately, the type of fat that most patients want to eat is not of the monounsaturated variety. They often find it difficult to lower both saturated fat and carbohydrate intake at the same time. In counseling patients, the nutrition professional must determine easily understood priorities. Patients often find it easier to understand the concept of reducing total fat, and this may be an appropriate starting point. However, patients also need to be reminded that because foods are fat-free does not necessarily mean they are also calorie-free.

Regardless of the emphasis on the type and amount of fat, visceral obesity should be monitored. For weight management, a moderate reduction in fat is usually prudent, and for some individuals a low fat intake may make watching total calories easier. This approach usually allows for foods that have greater bulk and satiety values than do foods containing monounsaturated fats, such as olive and canola oils, peanuts, avocados, and olives.

The role and mechanism of dietary fat in insulin resistance also requires study. Furthermore, is total fat more important, or do differing types of fatty acids have differing effects on insulin resistance?

OTHER RESEARCH NEEDS

Although Fagen, McLaughlin, and Sharp have contributed excellent chapters, it is evident that nutrition recommendations for pregnancy and diabetes, especially gestational diabetes, for the elderly, and for children and adolescents have limited research and are usually based on clinical expertise. Additional research is also needed related to nutrition therapy and the complications of diabetes: amount and type of fats for the treatment of lipid abnormalities; amount of protein, type of protein, and when to recommend changes in protein intake for nephropathy; recommendations for gastroparesis and other gastrointestinal problems; and so forth.

Although studies are underway to determine whether type 2 diabetes can be prevented or delayed, the role of foods, nutrients, and weight for prevention remains unclear. As noted by Wing, making small lifestyle changes, such as increasing physical activity and losing a moderate amount of weight, may help. However, what is necessary to prevent a disease may not be the same as the treatment once a disease develops. For example, weight loss or weight maintenance may be important for prevention of chronic diseases, including type 2 diabetes, but if an individual has a chronic disease, treatment goals need to focus on abnormal metabolic parameters associated with the disease. Nutrition therapy that will contribute to the return and maintenance of normal metabolic factors, such as glucose, lipids, and blood pressure, should be emphasized.

Although research determines the direction nutrition recommendations should take, we need to be constantly reminded that it is the person with diabetes who ultimately decides what she or he will eat and how much physical activity he or she will do. In her chapter, Maryniuk eloquently reminds us that changing behaviors first requires commitment of the person with diabetes to make changes. The best advice based on the best research is worthless if it cannot be implemented in the world in which people with diabetes live. The practice—or art—of nutrition therapy is the individualized application of scientific knowledge (36). This should be the unique skill the dietitian brings to the health care team.

TRANSLATING NUTRITION RECOMMENDATIONS INTO HOSPITALS AND LONG-TERM CARE FACILITIES

The ADA recommendations are primarily intended to be implemented in an outpatient setting and apply to people living at home. However, many dietitians are involved in making decisions for the nutritional care of hospitalized patients with diabetes or for people living in long-term care facilities. Central to the nutrition recommendations are the needs to individualize therapy, to integrate nutrition into the overall diabetes management plan, and to use an interdisciplinary team approach (11). These also apply to nutritional care in institutions.

Standardized calorie-level meal patterns based on the exchange lists have traditionally been used to plan meals for hospitalized patients. However, it has been recommended that hospitals consider alternative meal planning approaches (37,38). Today, because hospitalized patients are generally quite ill, what is served in the hospital setting is not as important as it once was. Instead, whatever time is available should be used in helping the patient and/or his or her family better understand what needs to be done after the patient leaves the hospital. Therefore, it has been suggested that hospitals consider a system termed the "consistent-carbohydrate diabetes meal plan." This system uses menus without a specific calorie level and incorporates a consistent carbohydrate content from day to day at the morning, midday, and evening meals. The amount of carbohydrate in each meal in a given day is not necessarily comparable, e.g., the carbohydrate content may be less in the morning meal than in the midday meal. This plan also incorporates fat modifications and consistent timing of meals and snacks.

Providing adequate nutrition is the primary concern of dietitians working with residents of long-term care facilities. It is appropriate to serve regular (unrestricted) menus with consistent amounts of carbohydrate at meals. Regular menus in long-term care facilities are generally between 1,800 and 2,000 calories. They generally are consistent in calories, are served at consistent times, and contain small portions of food. If desserts are served, the portions are usually small. As pointed out by McLaughlin in her chapter on nutrition therapy for the older adult with diabetes, fat restriction often is not indicated for this population because of the risk of malnutrition. Increased quality of life, heightened satisfaction, improved nutritional status, and decreased feelings of isolation in residents are potential benefits of this approach (37,38).

Nutrition prescriptions such as no concentrated sweets, no sugar added, low sugar, and liberal diabetic diet are no longer appropriate. These diets do not reflect the ADA nutrition recommendations and unnecessarily restrict sucrose. In long-term care facilities, problems attaining adequate glycemia are usually a function of the need for change in medications rather than the need for change in food intake (37,38).

SUMMARY

Facilitating behavior change takes time and requires a system of care that allows for evaluation of outcomes and for ongoing education and support. Information and strategies for needed changes must be provided for individuals over a period of time: nutrition self-management is a continual process of care. Education begins with initial survival skills and expands until the individual with diabetes can integrate and use nutrition information and strategies to manage his or her diabetes better. Nutrition self-management education provides the skills that allow for flexibility, optimal control of diabetes, and improved quality of life.

To date, true outcomes-based research that supports the benefits of MNT and diabetes education has been limited. Of the studies that have occurred, only a few have been prospective, randomized, clinical trials. In today's health care environment, the future will depend on documenting medical, clinical, and quality-of-life outcomes from both MNT and diabetes education.

REFERENCES

1. West KM: Diet therapy of diabetes: an analysis of failure. *Ann Intern Med* 79:425–434, 1973

2. American Diabetes Association: Standards of medical care for patients with diabetes mellitus (Position Statement). *Diabetes Care* (Suppl. 1):S23–S31, 1998

3. Delahanty LM, Halford BN: The role of diet behaviors in achieving improved glycemic control in intensively treated patients in the Diabetes Control and Complications Trial. *Diabetes Care* 16:1453–1458, 1993

4. Franz MJ, Monk A, Barry B, McLain K, Weaver T, Cooper N, Upham P, Bergenstal R, Mazze RS: Effectiveness of medical nutri-

tion therapy provided by dietitians in the management of non-insulin-dependent diabetes mellitus: a randomized, controlled clinical trial. *J Am Diet Assoc* 95:1009–1017, 1995

5. Johnson EQ, Valera S: Medical nutrition therapy in non-insulin dependent diabetes mellitus improves clinical outcomes. *J Am Diet Assoc* 95:700–701, 1995

6. Brown SA: Studies of educational interventions and outcomes in diabetic adults: a meta-analysis revisited. *Patient Educ Couns* 16:189–215, 1990

7. Kulkarni K, Castle G, Gregory R, Holmes A, Leontos C, Powers M, Snetselaar L, Splett P, Wylie-Rosett J: Nutrition practice guidelines for type 1 diabetes mellitus positively affect dietitian practices and patient outcomes. *J Am Diet Assoc* 98:62–70, 1998

8. Milne RM, Mann JI, Chisolm AW, William SM: Long-time comparison of three dietary prescriptions in the treatment of NIDDM. *Diabetes Care* 17:74–80, 1994

9. Arnold MS, Stepien CJ, Hess GE, Hiss RG: Guidelines vs. practice in the delivery of diabetes nutrition care. *J Am Diet Assoc* 93:34–39, 1993

10. Tinker LF, Heins JM, Holler HJ: Commentary and translation: 1994 nutrition recommendations for diabetes. *J Am Diet Assoc* 94:507–511, 1994

11. American Diabetes Association: Nutrition recommendations and principles for people with diabetes mellitus (Position Statement). *Diabetes Care* 21 (Suppl. 1):S32–S35, 1998

12. Franz MJ, Horton ES, Bantle JP, Beebe CA, Brunzell JD, Coulston AM, Henry RR, Hoogwerf BJ, Stacpoole PW: Nutrition principles for the management of diabetes and related complications (Technical Review). *Diabetes Care* 17:490–518, 1994

13. Schlundt DG, Rea MR, Kline SS, Prichert JW: Situational obstacles to dietary adherence for adults with diabetes. *J Am Diet Assoc* 94:874–879, 1994

14. Monk A, Barry B, McClain K, Weaver T, Cooper N, Franz MJ: Practice guidelines for medical nutrition therapy by dietitians for persons with non-insulin-dependent diabetes mellitus. *J Am Diet Assoc* 95:999–1008, 1995

15. Foreyt JP: Evidence for success of behavior modification in weight loss control. *Ann Intern Med* 119:698–701, 1993

16. Lavery MA, Loewy JW: Identifying predictive variables for long-term weight change after participation in a weight loss program. *J Am Diet Assoc* 93:1017–1024, 1993

17. Wing RR, Shoemaker M, Marcus MD, McDermott M, Gooding W: Variables associated with weight loss and improvements in glycemic control in type II diabetic patients in behavioral weight control programs. *Int J Obesity* 14:495–503, 1990

18. Watts NB, Spanheimer RG, DiGirolamo M, Gebhart SSP, Musey VC, Siddiq K, Phillips LS: Prediction of glucose response to weight loss in patients with non-insulin-dependent diabetes mellitus. *Arch Intern Med* 150:803–806, 1990

19. Wing RR, Koeske R, Epstein LH, Nowalk MP, Gooding W, Becker D: Long-term effects of modest weight loss in type II diabetic patients. *Arch Intern Med* 147:1749–1753, 1987

20. Kelley DE, Wing R, Buonocore C, Sturis J, Polonsky K, Fitzsimmons M: Relative effects of caloric restriction and weight loss in non-insulin-dependent diabetes mellitus. *J Clin Endocrinol Metab* 77:1287–1293, 1993

21. Wing RR, Blair EH, Bononi P, Marcus MD, Watanabe R, Bergman RN: Caloric restriction per se is a significant factor in improvements in glycemic control and insulin sensitivity during weight loss in obese NIDDM patients. *Diabetes Care* 17:30–36, 1994

22. Markovic TP, Jenkins AB, Campbell LV, Furler SM, Kraegen EW, Chisholm DJ: The determinants of glycemic responses to diet restriction and weight loss in obesity and NIDDM. *Diabetes Care* 21:687–694, 1998

23. Markovic TP, Campbell LV, Balasubramanian S, Jenkins AB, Fleury AC, Simons LA, Chisholm DJ: Beneficial effect on average lipid levels from energy restriction and fat loss in obese individuals with or without type 2 diabetes. *Diabetes Care* 21:695–700, 1998

24. Franz MJ, Splett P, Monk A, Barry B, McClain K, Weaver T, Upham P, Bergenstal R, Mazze RS: Cost-effectiveness of medical nutrition therapy by dietitians for persons with non-insulin-dependent diabetes mellitus. *J Am Diet Assoc* 95:1018–1024, 1995

25. Hauenstein DJ, Schiller MR, Hurley RS: Motivational techniques of dietitians counseling patients with type II diabetes. *J Am Diet Assoc* 87:37–42, 1987

26. The DCCT Research Group: Nutrition interventions for intensive therapy in the Diabetes Control and Complications Trial. *J Am Diet Assoc* 93:768–772, 1993

27. Gillespie S, Kulkarni K, Daly A: Using carbohydrate counting in diabetes clinical practice. *J Am Diet Assoc* 98:897–905, 1998

28. Peterson DB, Lambert J, Gerring S, Darling P, Carter RD, Jelfs R, Mann JI: Sucrose in the diet of diabetic patients—just another carbohydrate? *Diabetologia* 29:216–220, 1986

29. Bantle JP, Swanson JE, Thomas JW, Laine DC: Metabolic effects of dietary sucrose in type II diabetic subjects. *Diabetes Care* 16:1301–1305, 1992

30. Loghmani E, Rickard K, Washburne L, Vandagriff H, Fineberg N, Golden M: Glycemic response to sucrose-containing mixed meals in diets of children with insulin-dependent diabetes mellitus. *J Pediatrics* 119:531–537, 1991

31. Wolever TMS, Nguyen P-M, Chiasson J-L: Determinants of diet glycemic index calculated retrospectively from diet records of 342 individuals with non-insulin-dependent diabetes mellitus. *Am J Clin Nutr* 59:1265–1269, 1994

32. Fraser RJ, Horowitz M, Maddox AF, Harding PE, Chatterton BE, Dent J: Hyperglycaemia slows gastric emptying in type I (insulin-dependent) diabetes mellitus. *Diabetologia* 33:675–680, 1990

33. Schvarcz E, Palmer M, Aman J, Lindkvist B, Beckman K-W: Hypoglycaemia increases the gastric emptying rate in patients with type 1 diabetes mellitus. *Diabetic Med* 10:660–663, 1993

34. Peters AL, Davidson MB: Protein and fat effects on glucose response and insulin requirements in subjects with insulin-dependent diabetes mellitus. *Am J Clin Nutr* 58:555–560, 1993

35. Nuttall FQ, Mooradian AD, Gannon MC, Billington C, Krezowski P: Effect of protein ingestion on the glucose and insulin response to a standardized oral glucose load. *Diabetes Care* 7:465–470, 1984

36. Wheeler ML: The art of nutrition: multiple aspects of diabetes medical nutrition therapy. *Diabetes Spectrum* 9:97–98, 1996

37. Schafer R, Bohannon B, Franz MJ, Freeman J, Holmes A, McLaughlin S, Haas L, Kruger D, Lorenz R, McMahon M: Translation of the diabetes nutrition recommendations for health care facilities (Technical Review). *Diabetes Care* 20:96–105, 1997

38. American Diabetes Association: Translation of the diabetes nutrition recommendations for health care institutions (Position Statement). *Diabetes Care* 21 (Suppl. 1):S66–S68, 1998

Ms. Franz is Director of Nutrition and Professional Education at the International Diabetes Center, Institute for Research and Education, HealthSystem Minnesota, Minneapolis, MN.

2. A Physician's Perspective on Medical Nutrition Therapy for Diabetes

JOHN P. BANTLE, MD

Highlights

- For a variety of reasons, nutrition therapy is difficult to implement successfully. Health care providers should keep this in mind.
- Nutrition recommendations should be based on scientific evidence. If no evidence exists, recommendations should be made with caution, if at all.
- All patients with diabetes should restrict saturated fat intake to <10% of total calories and cholesterol intake to <300 mg daily. Patients with established nephropathy should restrict protein intake.
- Patients with type 1 diabetes should learn how to estimate carbohydrate and caloric intake for the purpose of adjusting premeal insulin.
- For patients with type 2 diabetes, effective weight loss strategies remain to be defined. The optimal distribution of macronutrients also remains to be determined and may vary depending on the specific situation.

INTRODUCTION

The fundamental treatments for diabetes are nutrition therapy, exercise, and hypoglycemic medication. Of these three treatments, nutrition therapy is probably the most difficult to implement successfully (1). Twenty-five years ago, West documented "the rarity with which diabetics understand and follow their diet prescriptions" (2). Although we have learned much about the dietary treatment of diabetes in the intervening 25 years, it is still probably true that most patients with diabetes have difficulty understanding and adhering to the nutritional component of their treatment. This, of course, compromises the level of control they are able to achieve.

Possible reasons why nutrition therapy is difficult for patients are listed in Table 2.1. First, and not to be underestimated, nutrition recommendations have changed over time, often in contradictory ways. This has created confusion and doubt. These contradictions have usually been the result of recommendations made in the absence of supporting scientific data. When data do become available, the data have often dictated that the current recommendations be changed. This creates confusion and erodes public confidence in the recommendations.

Second, many physicians treating patients with diabetes do not understand the principles of nutrition therapy and do not emphasize the importance of strategies to help achieve food-related goals. These physicians do their patients a disservice. One way to help physicians learn more about nutrition therapy would be to have each physician, with the help of a knowledgeable dietitian, design a diabetic meal plan for him or herself and attempt to follow it for at least 1 week. This would also help physicians understand some of the difficulties inherent to implementing a meal plan. Those physicians who do not wish to learn about nutrition therapy should, at the very least, enthusiastically refer their patients to a knowledgeable dietitian and emphasize the importance of attempting to follow the recommendations they receive.

A third reason that nutrition therapy is difficult is that adherence to any diet is difficult if it differs from that of the general population. For instance, it is often difficult to follow a meal plan when eating in a restaurant or in a friend's home simply because appropriate food choices may not be available. It is also difficult for a family member to follow a meal

---

Table 2.1   Reasons It Is Difficult to Implement Nutrition Therapy Effectively

1. Nutrition recommendations for diabetes have changed over time, often in contradictory ways.
2. Many physicians do not understand and do not emphasize nutrition/food principles and strategies.
3. Adherence to any diet that differs from that of the general population is difficult.
4. In our society, food has many purposes in addition to meeting nutritional needs.
5. Energy intake, energy expenditure, and thereby energy balance appear to be closely regulated by the central nervous system.

plan when other members of his or her family are not following the same meal plan. Finally, even the most motivated and competent of individuals with diabetes is likely to develop a sense of deprivation if he or she must avoid foods that others are eating and enjoying.

Fourth, in our society, food has many purposes in addition to meeting nutritional needs (1). Food is often the focus of social activities. Moreover, food is frequently used as a reward, as a means of expressing affection, and as a means of helping cope with anxiety. We are constantly bombarded with appealing advertisements for food that exploit these factors. Even the most motivated patient can be expected to intermittently succumb to these influences.

Fifth, and perhaps most important, it now appears that energy intake, energy expenditure, and thereby energy balance are closely regulated by the central nervous system. (This is discussed in more detail in chapter 5.) Thus, when we ask our overweight patients to diet and lose weight, we may be asking them to override by force of will a powerful biological control system. This is something most people simply cannot do and may help explain why, when someone is hungry and gazing into the refrigerator, it is so difficult to do the right thing.

Although nutritional treatment of diabetes is difficult and there are multiple barriers that must be overcome for it to be successful, we should do all we can to help our patients achieve success. Proper diet is a key element in establishing control of glycemia and lipemia and in the maintenance of health.

THE NEED FOR A SCIENTIFIC BASIS TO NUTRITION RECOMMENDATIONS

It would be desirable to provide people with diabetes with a comprehensive set of nutrition recommendations. However, it is important that such recommendations be based on scientific data documenting efficacy. Although well intended, recommendations based on assumptions, inferences, or clinical experience can create both public and professional confusion if scientific evidence later proves them to be wrong. The need to revise a recommendation, particularly if the new recommendation contradicts the old one, erodes general confidence in the recommendation.

Several examples of ill-fated recommendations can be cited. As recently as 1979, the Committee on Food and Nutrition of the American Diabetes Association (ADA) recommended restriction of sucrose in the diabetic diet (3). This recommendation was consistent with the widely held belief that people with diabetes should avoid "sugar." The origin of this belief is uncertain, but it may be related to statements made by Allen in the 1920s describing sugar as a dangerous food for people with diabetes (4). It was thought that dietary sugars, such as sucrose, were more rapidly digested and absorbed than dietary starches and that they thereby aggravated hyperglycemia. However, as was recently summarized in an ADA technical review, research studies comparing sucrose to starch demonstrated that sucrose did not adversely affect glycemia (5). The 1994 ADA nutrition recommendations acknowledged this and lifted the restriction on sucrose for people with diabetes (6). Nonetheless, many people with diabetes continue to believe that elimination of sucrose from their diet is important in the management of their diabetes. Focus on this belief interferes with their ability to implement beneficial dietary changes and needlessly decreases opportunities to enjoy life.

Another example of recommendations without scientific support that have created confusion are the recommendations about the macronutrient distribution of the diabetic diet. The changing recommendations are nicely summarized in the 1994 ADA nutrition recommendations (6). Although from the 1920s to the present the amount of protein recommended has remained relatively constant at 10–20% of total calories, the amount of carbohydrate recommended has varied from 20 to 60% of total calories and the amount of fat from 70% to <30% of total calories. The 1994 recommendations are probably the first recommendations that are scientifically defensible. These recommendations make it clear that we do not yet know the optimal distribution of carbohydrate and fat in the diabetic diet, and thus, calories from fat and carbohydrate should be individualized based on the nutrition assessment and treatment goals.

THE MOST IMPORTANT NUTRITION ISSUES FOR ALL PEOPLE WITH DIABETES

Diabetes is a potent independent risk factor for cardiovascular disease. Thus, all people with diabetes should attempt to limit their intake of dietary saturated fat and cholesterol. The 1994 ADA nutrition recommendations suggest that <10% of daily calories be derived from saturated fat and that daily cholesterol intake not exceed 300 mg (6). The same suggestions are made for the general U.S. population, so they do not create a special situation for people with diabetes. Data are available that demonstrate that diabetic patients who reduce their intake of saturated fat are likely to experience a decrease in serum LDL cholesterol (7). This issue is discussed in more detail in chapter 8.

Patients with diabetes and established nephropathy should be encouraged to restrict dietary protein. In diabetic subjects, a low-protein diet has been demonstrated to retard the increase in urinary albumin excretion and the decline in glomerular filtration rate (8). There is, however, some uncertainty about how much protein intake should be reduced to retard nephropathy without causing protein malnutrition. These issues are discussed further in chapter 17.

THE MOST IMPORTANT NUTRITION ISSUES
FOR PEOPLE WITH TYPE 1 DIABETES

Optimal treatment of type 1 diabetes requires that insulin administration and food intake be coordinated such that insulin increases in the postprandial period, when blood glucose is rising, and decreases in the postabsorptive period so that hypoglycemia is avoided. With conventional insulin therapy, patients were given one or two constant daily doses of insulin and an effort was made to maintain constant daily carbohydrate and caloric intake. Exchange lists have been used commonly as the tool for helping the person with diabetes eat in a consistent way from day to day. However, exchange lists may be considered complicated and difficult to use. Moreover, the need to be consistent with food intake limits flexibility and spontaneity for people with diabetes. Fortunately, publication of the results of the Diabetes Control and Complications Trial (9) has made conventional therapy obsolete.

For all willing patients with type 1 diabetes, conventional therapy has been replaced by intensive therapy. Patients receiving intensive therapy use either an insulin infusion pump or multiple (three or more) daily injections of insulin. Insulin administration is adjusted to match food intake in an effort to simulate normal endogenous insulin production. The amount of insulin administered before each meal is adjusted on the basis of carbohydrate and caloric intake. Thus, insulin can be reduced for a small meal and increased for a large meal or a meal that includes dessert.

To make such a system work effectively, the person with diabetes must, when taking premeal insulin, consider current blood glucose, recent and future activity, and anticipated carbohydrate and caloric intake. A system for estimating carbohydrate intake that is currently in wide use is carbohydrate counting. Carbohydrate counting and other nutrition strategies for type 1 diabetes are summarized in chapter 3. It is also possible for a person with type 1 diabetes to learn through trial and error how to effectively adjust insulin for specific foods. Since most people eat a limited number of foods on a regular basis, it is possible to learn how much insulin to take for meals in which the principal foods might be, for instance, pizza, spaghetti and bread, hamburger and french fries, or chow mein and rice. With practice, it is also possible to administer insulin effectively before a spontaneously eaten food, such as an ice cream cone. Patients, of course, need to factor in portion sizes.

Since there are no direct comparisons between trial-and-error methods and carbohydrate counting or other more formal systems, it is not clear which system of estimating carbohydrate and caloric intake works best. Potentially, different systems will work better for different people. Almost certainly, any system will work better if a supportive physician and a knowledgeable dietitian are involved in its implementation.

THE MOST IMPORTANT NUTRITION ISSUES FOR PEOPLE WITH TYPE 2 DIABETES

Most people with type 2 diabetes are overweight, and weight loss is thus an important treatment goal. Nutrition strategies for weight loss are summarized in chapter 4. Unfortunately, traditional strategies usually have not been effective in achieving long-term weight loss. Experimental treatments, such as gastric-reduction surgery and weight-loss drugs, are summarized in chapter 5. The use of these treatments is considered experimental because no long-term data on efficacy and safety are available.

A second important issue for people with diabetes pertains to the macronutrient composition of their diets. In an effort to reduce intake of saturated fat and cholesterol, it has been recommended that the diet contain 30% or fewer calories from total fat. Such a diet necessarily derives 50 or 60% of calories from carbohydrate. In conflict with this idea are several recent studies that suggest that a high-carbohydrate diet may not be optimal for people with type 2 diabetes (10–12). These studies demonstrated that when saturated fat intake was kept low but a portion of the carbohydrate in the diet was replaced by monounsaturated fat, diabetic subjects experienced reductions in glycemia, insulinemia, and triglyceridemia. There were no differences between high–monounsaturated fat diets and high-carbohydrate diets in fasting total and LDL cholesterol because both diets were low in saturated fats. These studies suggest that diets relatively high in monounsaturated fat and low in carbohydrate may have metabolic benefits for people with type 2 diabetes. However, there is evidence that high-fat diets increase energy intake (13) and may thereby cause weight gain. Therefore, it has not been established whether a high-carbohydrate diet or a high–monounsaturated fat diet is preferable for patients with type 2 diabetes. If weight loss is the primary issue, a diet low in fat may be preferable, whereas if hyperglycemia and hypertriglyceridemia are the issues, a diet high in monounsaturated fat may be preferable. These issues are discussed in detail in chapters 6 and 8.

SUMMARY

Only a limited number of dietary modifications have documented efficacy in the treatment of diabetes. Vigorous attempts should be made to implement them. However, dietary modifications that do not have documented efficacy should be implemented with caution, if at all. To ask a person with diabetes to eat in a way that is different from that of his or her family or cultural group is to ask a great deal. This should be done only if the benefit is worth the price paid to achieve the benefit. Additional outcome-based research is necessary to define beneficial nutrition therapies.

REFERENCES

1. Bantle JP: Thoughts on the dietary treatment of diabetes mellitus. *Diabetes Care* 15:1821–1823, 1992

2. West KM: Diet therapy of diabetes: an analysis of failure. *Ann Intern Med* 79:425–434, 1973

3. Committee on Food and Nutrition of the American Diabetes Association: Principles of nutrition and dietary recommendations for individuals with diabetes mellitus: 1979. *J Am Diet Assoc* 75:527–530, 1979

4. Allen FM: Experimental studies on diabetes: effects of carbohydrate diets. *J Exp Med* 31:381–402, 1920

5. Franz, MJ, Horton ES, Bantle JP, Beebe CA, Brunzell JD, Coulston AM, Henry RR, Hoogwerf BJ, Stacpoole PW: Nutrition principles for the management of diabetes and related complications. *Diabetes Care* 17:490–518, 1994

6. American Diabetes Association: Nutrition recommendations and principles for people with diabetes mellitus (Position Statement). *Diabetes Care* 17:519–522, 1994

7. Abbottt WGH, Boyce VL, Grundy SM, Howard BV: Effects of replacing saturated fat with complex carbohydrate in diets of subjects with NIDDM. *Diabetes Care* 12:102–107, 1989

8. Pedrini MT, Levey AS, Lau J, Chalmers TC, Wang PH: The effect of dietary protein restriction on the progression of diabetic and nondiabetic renal diseases: a meta-analysis. *Ann Intern Med* 124:632–628, 1996

9. The Diabetes Control and Complications Trial Research Group: The effect of intensive treatment of diabetes on the development and progression of long-term complications of insulin-dependent diabetes mellitus. *N Engl J Med* 329:977–986, 1993

10. Garg A, Bonanome A, Grundy SM, Hnang Z-J, Unger RH: Comparison of a high-carbohydrate diet with a high-monounsaturated-fat diet in patients with non-insulin-dependent diabetes mellitus. *N Engl J Med* 319:829–834, 1988

11. Coulston AM, Hollenbeck CB, Swislocki ALM, Reaven GM: Persistence of hypertriglyceridemic effect of low-fat high-carbohydrate diets in NIDDM patients. *Diabetes Care* 12:94–101, 1989

12. Garg A, Bantle JP, Henry RR, Coulston AM, Griver KA, Raatz SK, Brinkley L, Chen Y-DI, Grundy SM, Huet BA, Reaven GM: Effects of varying carbohydrate content of diet in patients with non-insulin-dependent diabetes mellitus. *JAMA* 271:1421–1428, 1994

13. Lissner L, Levitsky DA, Strupp BJ, Kalkwarf HJ, Roe DA: Dietary fat and the regulation of energy intake in human subjects. *Am J Clin Nutr* 46:886–892, 1987

Dr. Bantle is Professor of Medicine, Division of Endocrinology and Diabetes, at the University of Minnesota Medical School, Minneapolis, MN.

3. Nutrition Therapy for Type 1 Diabetes

KARMEEN KULKARNI, MS, RD, CDE, AND MARION J. FRANZ, MS, RD, LD, CDE

Highlights

- A meal or food plan based on an individual's food preferences and usual mealtimes should be agreed on by the person with diabetes and the dietitian. Either a conventional (standard) or an intensive insulin regimen can then be integrated into the person's lifestyle.
- The meal planning approach selected should be one that the individual with diabetes can understand and use to plan appropriate food and meal choices. Carbohydrate counting is a well-received system and is based on the concept that carbohydrate is the major macronutrient influencing postprandial glucose levels. However, total caloric intake cannot be ignored because with improved glycemic control, weight gain can become a concern.
- People with diabetes should be taught prevention and appropriate treatment of hypo- and hyperglycemia, and how and when to increase carbohydrate and/or decrease insulin with exercise.
- Nutrition practice guidelines for type 1 diabetes describe responsibilities within the scope of practice for qualified dietetics professionals, guide practice decisions, promote self-management education of patients, facilitate self-management by patients, and define state-of-the-art nutrition therapy based on available scientific evidence and experience of experts.

INTRODUCTION

Medical nutrition therapy (MNT) is integral to the care and management of type 1 diabetes. In the Diabetes Control and Complications Trial

(DCCT), MNT was essential to achieving optimal glycemic control (1). When the food/meal plan is developed first, the insulin regimen can be integrated into usual eating and exercise habits (2,3). Individuals receiving conventional or standard insulin therapy (two injections of mixed insulin) must be more consistent in the timing and the amount of food they eat, whereas people receiving intensive insulin therapy (multiple daily injections [MDIs] or insulin pumps) have more flexibility in when and what they eat.

Optimal management can only be accomplished by evaluating blood glucose monitoring records, modifying food and exercise behaviors, and recommending insulin adjustments. This approach must be individualized and requires effective nutrition self-management education. This chapter will review *1*) insulin regimens, *2*) nutrition-related strategies for conventional and intensive insulin therapies, *3*) use of carbohydrate counting and other meal planning approaches, *4*) prevention of weight gain associated with improved metabolic control and appropriate treatment of hypoglycemia, *5*) nutrition and/or insulin adjustments for acute illnesses and exercise, and *6*) the role of nutrition practice guidelines for type 1 diabetes.

INSULIN REGIMENS

Insulin regimens are adjusted to match food intake and to duplicate endogenous insulin in a person without diabetes. This requires the use of background (sometimes also called basal) insulins, such as NPH, lente, or ultralente, and rapid- or short-acting (sometimes called bolus) insulins, such as lispro (Humalog) or regular. The rapid- or short-acting insulin is used to cover the rise in blood glucose after eating and may also be used to correct blood glucose levels that are not in the goal range, especially before meals, quickly.

The type and timing of insulin regimens should be individualized, based on eating and exercise habits and blood glucose levels. A single dose of insulin is seldom effective for optimal blood glucose control in type 1 diabetes. A commonly used regimen or conventional insulin therapy combines short- and intermediate-acting insulins (such as NPH or lente) given before breakfast and the evening meal. Another common regimen combines short- and intermediate-acting insulins before breakfast, short-acting insulin before the evening meal, and intermediate-acting insulin (such as NPH) at bedtime. The intermediate-acting insulin is moved to bedtime to control the early morning surge in blood glucose levels (dawn phenomenon).

Intensive insulin regimens consist of MDIs of insulin or insulin pump therapy. With MDI regimens, a background insulin is given once or twice a day and a rapid- or short-acting insulin is given before meals to provide bolus insulin. These types of insulin regimens allow more flexibility in the type and timing of meals. The amount of rapid- or short-acting insulin can be adjusted based on the composition of the meal and/or its carbohydrate content. Continuous subcutaneous insulin infusion (CSII) using an insulin pump is another popular option. Insulin pump therapy provides basal rapid- or short-acting insulin pumped continuously by a mechanical device in micro-amounts through a subcutaneous catheter that is monitored 24 h a day. Boluses of the rapid- or short-acting insulin are then given before meals (4).

To achieve desirable blood glucose goals (5), the majority of people with type 1 diabetes generally require some form of intensive insulin therapy. This was clearly demonstrated by the DCCT (6). At diagnosis, some individuals with type 1 diabetes may achieve adequate glycemic control with standard insulin regimens, but this is rarely the case as the duration of diabetes increases.

Premeal Short-Acting Insulin

Short-acting (regular) insulin begins to have some effect on blood glucose levels 30–45 min after injection, peaks in 2–3 h, and has a duration of ~4–6 h. It also has a slow onset of activity and controls postmeal blood glucose levels better if given 30–45 min before the meal. As the dose increases, the action peak is later and the action duration longer. Because of its erratic absorption, it acts most consistently when the site used is most consistent (7). Furthermore, because its peak is later than that of most postprandial glucose levels, snacks between meals are usually required.

Premeal Rapid-Acting Insulin

In contrast to human regular insulin, human lispro insulin begins to have some effect in 5–15 min, peaks at 30–75 minutes, and has a duration of ~2–3 h. Because lispro begins to act quickly, it should be given at the start of a meal. Its hypoglycemic effect peaks more than two times higher and in less than half the time of human regular insulin. When given immediately before the meal or within 15 min after the start of a meal, it provides excellent control of postmeal hyperglycemia. However, to achieve more ideal overall glycemic control, it may be necessary to modify the background insulin dosage. In general, background insulin using currently available insulins should be given twice a day to provide a relatively uniform level of insulin during fasting. The dosage of lispro is regulated by assessing 2-h postprandial glucose levels, and premeal glucose values, i.e., fasting and pre–evening meal levels, are used for the adjustment of the background insulin (8,9).

In comparison with regular insulin, lispro has less variability and no shift in time to peak action. There is also less change in duration as dose is increased, and the injection site does not affect onset of action (10). Lispro has been shown to reduce nocturnal hypoglycemic episodes (midnight to 6:00 A.M.) (11), and in well-controlled type 1 patients, insulin lispro has reduced the incidence of severe hypoglycemia and coma (12).

Lispro insulin appears to work better with meals containing carbohydrate. In type 1 patients, postprandial blood glucose excursions after a carbohydrate-rich meal (140 g carbohydrate) were reduced after premeal injection of lispro in comparison with regular human insulin (13). For meals with a high carbohydrate content, the optimal time for the injection of lispro is premeal. In contrast, for meals with a high fat content, postprandial injection of lispro may be preferable (14). Snacks are usually not needed, and additional lispro is generally required for snacks containing more than 15–30 g carbohydrate.

Hypoglycemia is more likely to be a concern if exercise is within 2 h after injection of premeal lispro rather than premeal regular insulin. In contrast, if exercise is performed >2 h after injection of lispro, there is less hypoglycemia than with premeal injections of regular insulin. Therefore, if individuals take premeal lispro and exercise immediately after the meal, the lispro dose will need to be reduced. However, exercising 2 h after the premeal lispro and the meal can help control increases in blood glucose levels 3–4 h after the meal and insulin (15).

NUTRITION-RELATED STRATEGIES FOR INSULIN THERAPY

Conventional or Standard Insulin Therapy

A meal or food plan based on an individual's food preferences and usual mealtimes should be agreed upon by the individual with diabetes and the dietitian. When this information is shared with other team members, insulin regimens can be integrated into the person's lifestyle. If the individual is using conventional insulin therapy, such as twice daily injections of short- and intermediate-acting insulins before breakfast and the evening meal, the timing of food intake should be synchronized with the administration of insulin. However, even using conventional insulin therapy, individuals can use blood glucose monitoring results and, on the basis of blood glucose patterns, make adjustments in insulin to cover usual meal amounts. It is generally easier to adjust an insulin dose than to change long-standing eating patterns. Individuals need to be consistent in the timing and quantity of their food intake and to understand the onset, peak, and duration of their insulin dose in relation to their meals and snacks.

Nutrition goals are based on the individual's overall diabetes management goals. Each person with diabetes needs to know target glycemic goals, and nutrition-related behaviors that affect these goals should be emphasized. Fat modification recommendations for the achievement of optimal lipid levels are similar to those for the general public, but dependent on lipid values, there may be more focus on types and amounts of fat.

Intensive Insulin Therapy

Intensive therapy provides flexibility for the individual with diabetes: it can be adapted to many lifestyles because of the many insulin options available. MDIs of insulin or insulin pumps are used for intensive therapy.

It is still essential to integrate the insulin regimen into the individual's lifestyle. Individuals need to know their basic insulin doses for both background and meal insulins. They can then adjust the rapid- or short-acting insulin dose when they deviate from their usual meal plans and/or exercise programs. Even with the increased flexibility, overall management tends to be easier with consistency in eating and exercise habits.

Delahanty and Halford (1) surveyed DCCT participants in the intensive therapy group and identified the following four nutrition-related behaviors that were associated with maintenance of lower glycated hemoglobin (HbA$_{1c}$) levels:

1. Decreased food variations that require insulin adjustments—people who reported following their prescribed meal plan >90% of the time had mean HbA$_{1c}$ values ~1% lower than did those who followed their meal plan <40% of the time.
2. Prompt treatment of hyperglycemia—lower HbA$_{1c}$ levels were associated with adjustments in insulin, food, or both in response to hyperglycemia.
3. Eating the prescribed evening snack more consistently.
4. Appropriate treatment of hypoglycemia—higher HbA$_{1c}$ levels were associated with overtreating hypoglycemia and consuming extra snacks beyond the meal plan.

Studies such as this are important because they help professionals focus on behaviors that lead to improved metabolic control.

Patient selection for intensive insulin therapy is important. This type of therapy may not be appropriate or may require modified blood glucose goals for people with hypoglycemia unawareness, advanced complications, or psychological limitations (16). Other contraindications for intensive therapy, especially food-related ones, include *1*) fear of weight gain, *2*) eating disorders, *3*) history of severe hypoglycemia and/or overtreatment of hypoglycemia, *4*) psychological problems, especially those related to eating patterns, i.e., binge eating, severe dieting, dysfunctional eating, and so forth, and 5) age, i.e., very young or elderly (17).

Furthermore, it is essential that patients have detailed information about food, exercise, and insulins; know how to use blood glucose monitoring records to adjust insulin doses; and know appropriate treatment of hypoglycemia. Patients must evaluate glycemic control and blood glucose patterns and have an action plan to implement for improved control when needed. Ongoing contact with the entire health care team is essential.

Before initiating intensive insulin therapy, the individual needs 1) a consistent eating pattern or food plan adjusted to lifestyle and calorie requirements, 2) a successful basic insulin regimen that covers the usual food plan, 3) the ability to identify portions and macronutrient content of food items and/or to read labels to determine carbohydrate content, and 4) a willingness to test blood glucose levels four or five times a day with occasional 3:00 A.M. testing to determine success of adjustments (17).

The health care team (physician, dietitian, nurse, and/or other team members) should establish target blood glucose goals in conjunction with each person with diabetes. Using blood glucose monitoring patterns, changes in insulin doses can be made to meet identified goals. If the individual is willing and able, changes in the timing and the amount of food eaten may lead to improved control.

Patients need to be reminded that out-of-target blood glucose results are not always caused by food. Stress, illness, changes in exercise, unpredictable insulin absorption, and inappropriate insulin regimens also contribute.

MEAL PLANNING APPROACHES

Carbohydrate Counting

Carbohydrate counting was one of four meal planning approaches used in the DCCT, and because of the success using this approach, it has received increasing attention (18). The basic concept of this system is that the carbohydrate found in foods is the major macronutrient influencing postprandial glucose excursions (19) and that it affects premeal insulin requirements more than the amount of protein and fat in the meal (20). This meal planning approach focuses on the total amount of carbohydrate, not the source of the carbohydrate, eaten at meals and for snacks. Careful attention to carbohydrate quantity and distribution can improve metabolic control, and a consistent carbohydrate intake facilitates insulin adjustments and minimizes blood glucose variability secondary to variable food intake. Carbohydrate counting assumes that background insulins (i.e., NPH, lente, and ultralente) cover noncarbohydrate needs for insulin, such as for the metabolism of protein and fat.

Carbohydrate counting can be a simpler meal planning approach because the initial focus is on one macronutrient and because it can provide greater precision in estimating carbohydrate intake than can other systems of meal planning. Emphasis is placed on eating consistent amounts of carbohydrate at meals and snacks. Foods can basically be divided into three categories: carbohydrate, meat and meat substitutes, and fat. Food carbohydrate sources are starches, fruits, milks, and sweets. Vegetables (except the starchy vegetables), unless eaten in servings >15 g, do not need to be counted. Individuals either count carbohydrate choices—one carbohydrate choice is based on the amount of food that contains 15 g carbohydrate—or count actual grams of carbohydrate in a meal and/or snack. Individuals with diabetes, like all people, do not always eat nutritionally balanced meals, and by counting the amount of carbohydrate eaten, regardless of the source, they can improve or maintain glycemic control. However, meats and fats cannot be completely ignored because of their calorie and fat content; if attention is not given to their intake, weight gain and/or lipid abnormalities can result.

Carbohydrate counting empowers individuals with diabetes to learn the relationships among food, insulin, physical activity, and blood glucose level and to make appropriate adjustments in their diabetes management plan (21).

Three levels of carbohydrate counting have been identified: *1*) level one, or basic, carbohydrate counting skills; *2*) level two, or intermediate, skills; and *3*) level three, or advanced, skills (22–24). Basic skills include knowing about food carbohydrate sources, how to count grams of carbohydrate in food, and the relationship between portion size and carbohydrate content. Individuals with diabetes record their usual carbohydrate intake and with the dietitian determine the target amount of carbohydrate for meals and, if desired or needed, snacks.

Intermediate skills include pattern management, which is used to identify blood glucose patterns that are impacted by food, insulin, and physical activity. Individuals with diabetes identify and interpret patterns to make adjustments in their diabetes regimens. Rapid- and/or short-acting insulins are matched to the carbohydrate content of the usual meals, and insulin doses can be adjusted when deviations from the usual carbohydrate content are made. In general, for every 15–20 g carbohydrate added or subtracted from a meal, an adjustment of 1–2 U of rapid- or short-acting insulin is typically suggested (25). However, because insulin requirements can vary dramatically with body weight and activity, each person's requirement should be individualized.

Individuals on intensive insulin therapy use the skills of advanced carbohydrate counting. Insulin can be adjusted on the basis of a ratio of grams of carbohydrate intake to doses of rapid- or short-acting insulin. By eating meals that are consistent in carbohydrate and adjusting insulin doses to achieve target blood glucose levels, a carbohydrate-to-insulin ratio can be determined and individualized. The dietitian assists the person with diabetes in calculating the carbohydrate-to-insulin ratio for each meal using food, insulin, and blood glucose monitoring records. Ratios may vary from meal to meal, from workdays to weekend days, from exercise days to nonexercise days, and they may change over time. Therefore, ratios require periodic reevaluation.

To determine carbohydrate-to-insulin ratios, the grams of carbohydrate eaten at a meal are divided by the number of units of rapid- or short-acting insulin needed to meet blood glucose goals. For example, an individual who eats 75 g carbohydrate (5 carbohydrate choices) at a meal and requires 9 U of insulin has a ratio of 1 U insulin to every 8 g carbohydrate, or 2 U insulin for every 1 carbohydrate choice. Furthermore, individuals may discover they need food-specific insulin doses, i.e., a spaghetti dose, a pizza dose, a DQ Blizzard dose, etc. (26,27).

Individuals may also find that when they eat much larger amounts of meat and/or fat at a meal than usual, they need to make insulin adjustments (28,29). Large amounts of fat in a meal can delay the postprandial peak (29), and it has been suggested that for meals with a high fat content, administration of rapid-acting insulin after the meal may be preferable to administration of rapid-acting insulin before the meal (14). If a serving of food contains >5 g fiber, the grams of fiber may be subtracted from the total carbohydrate content because fiber is not considered an available source of glucose (30).

A yet-to-be-determined issue relates to a basic principle of intensive therapy, that is, whether it is better simply to adjust mealtime insulin doses based on whatever the individual decides to eat or better to be more consistent with meal carbohydrate choices and use carbohydrate-to-insulin ratios when deviating from the usual carbohydrate content of the meal. Clinically, some centers report better metabolic control with the second approach, but this concept has not been well studied.

Other Meal Planning Approaches

For many years, *Exchange Lists for Meal Planning* (31) has been a widely used method for planning food intake. It is the basis of carbohydrate counting. In the 1995 edition, the starch, fruit, milk, and other carbohydrate (dessert-type or snack foods that do not fit into the starch or starch plus 1 fat list) lists are in the Carbohydrate Group. It also expands the Meat and Meat Substitute Group into very lean, lean, medium-fat, and high-fat lists; and the Fat Group is divided into monounsaturated, polyunsaturated, and saturated fat lists.

Exchange lists still remain an excellent system for meal planning, especially for individuals who want or can benefit from detailed serving sizes and more precise food content. It is probably most useful for health professionals because exchange lists are usually the basis for assessing food and nutrient intake.

Total available glucose (TAG) is another meal planning system used at some centers (18). It is based on the assumption that 100% of the carbohydrate content, 58% of the protein content, and 10% of the fat content of foods become glucose. However, it has now been shown that although 50–60% of protein has the potential to be used for gluconeogenesis, protein has little effect on postmeal blood glucose levels (28,29). The system probably works because both protein and fat require insulin for metabolism even though they have minimal effects on postmeal glycemia (29).

Other systems of meal planning include more simplified approaches (18,32). For example, some DCCT centers used *Healthy Food Choices* (33) with excellent results. Other centers may use a point system or another approach (34). No one of the meal planning approaches has been scientifically validated or shown to result in better outcomes than any other. The individual with diabetes determines what meal planning approach should be selected. It should be one that an individual can understand and that helps the individual with diabetes select appropriate foods and plan meals that will facilitate the achievement of glycemic goals.

WEIGHT GAIN AND HYPOGLYCEMIA ASSOCIATED WITH IMPROVED METABOLIC CONTROL

Weight Gain

After the implementation of insulin therapy and improved glycemic control, individuals with diabetes may experience unwanted weight gain (35,36). Individuals with type 1 diabetes in the DCCT intensive therapy group experienced on average a gain of ~10 lb during the first year of the trial (35). Weight gain associated with improved control can be related to several factors: *1*) fewer calories being lost as glycosuria, *2*) euglycemia promoting rehydration, which can add 2–5 lb of weight, and *3*) need for frequent treatment, as well as overtreatment, of hypoglycemia. Carlson and Campbell (37) studied weight gain during intensified insulin therapy. A total of 70% of the weight gain can be accounted for by reduced glycosuria, and 30% of the reduction in energy expenditure can be accounted for by the reversal of catabolic changes in carbohydrate, protein, and lipid metabolism and by the decrease in futile metabolic cycling.

Patients on intensive therapy who count carbohydrates often ignore the calories from the meat and fat food groups. An increase in these foods can also contribute to weight gain. Furthermore, with increased flexibility from the use of intensive insulin therapy, individuals may experiment with the inclusion of higher-calorie foods, such as desserts or chocolates, on an ongoing basis. Therefore, it is essential that patients have a general concept of total daily calories needed as well as of carbohydrate counting. Self-management education about blood glucose goals, food choices, especially related to total caloric intake, insulin algorithms, and adjustments for exercise is essential for weight management.

Purnell et al. (38) have reported on the relationship of weight gain to changes in lipid levels in the subjects receiving intensive therapy in the DCCT. Subjects were divided into quartiles based on weight gain during the study, with all subjects achieving the same level of glycemic control. In the first quartile, in which weight did not change significantly, subjects experienced improvements in triglyceride, total cholesterol, and LDL cholesterol compared with baseline values. In the second and third quartiles, there was no change in these lipids; however, in the fourth quartile (average BMI 31 kg/m^2), besides becoming clinically obese, subjects experienced significantly higher levels of these lipids and apolipoprotein B compared with subjects in the first three quartiles. Therefore, the effect of weight gain on lipids does not become a concern until the gain is excessive (BMI >31). Because lipid changes with excessive weight gain may contribute to an increased risk of macrovascular disease, it is important that individuals receive appropriate nutrition counseling to prevent weight gain.

Hypoglycemia

All individuals on insulin therapy need to know how to treat hypoglycemia. In the DCCT feasibility phase, intensive therapy was accompanied by a threefold increase in severe hypoglycemia (39). Because of this risk, individuals on intensive insulin therapy and the people in their support system need a complete review of the causes, treatment, and prevention of hypoglycemia and the role and use of glucagon.

Hypoglycemia can result from administration of too much insulin, too little food intake, delayed or missed meals or snacks, exercise or other physical activity, or alcohol intake without food. Immediate treatment is essential and begins with testing blood glucose, consuming 15 g of carbohydrate, and waiting 15 min to test blood glucose levels again to determine whether additional carbohydrate is needed. When blood glucose levels are ~50–60 mg/dl (2.7–3.3 mmol/l), 15 g carbohydrate can be expected to raise blood glucose levels ~50 mg/dl (2.7 mmol/l) over ~40–45 min, with levels starting to fall after 60 min (40). If a meal or snack is not scheduled for this time, a snack is necessary to prevent recurrent hypoglycemia. A repeat blood glucose test is necessary to confirm the actual rise and possible need for additional treatment. In the previous study (40), injected glucagon raised glucose levels from 60 to 200 mg/dl.

This was a temporary measure because glucose levels fell at ~1.5 h and ingestion of food was also needed to prevent subsequent hypoglycemia. Slama et al. (41) treated hypoglycemia with 15 g each of seven forms of carbohydrate. Using glucose or sucrose in tablets or in solution or using a starch hydrolysate (corn syrup), the response was similar at 10 min and symptoms were alleviated in ~15 min. However, at 10 min there was no response to 15 g of glucose gel or orange juice. Brodows et al. (42) also treated hypoglycemia (55 mg/dl [3.0 mmol/l]) with either 20 g of carbohydrate as glucose tablets, orange juice, or milk or 40 g as orange juice. Twenty grams of carbohydrate as glucose tablets or 40 g orange juice raised blood glucose levels ~50–55 mg/dl (2.7–3.0 mmol/l), whereas there was minimal response to 20 g carbohydrate as milk or orange juice. Although commercially available glucose tablets have the advantage of being premeasured to help prevent overtreatment, all forms of carbohydrate eventually raise blood glucose levels. Frequently used terms such as quick, fast-acting, or simple sugar are difficult to define, and the treatment choice should be whatever is convenient, is readily available, is easily and quickly consumed, and does not spoil. Foods containing fat may have a delay in the peak effect.

In type 1 diabetes, the gastric emptying rate is twice as high during hypoglycemia and this response is similar for either liquids or solid foods. During euglycemia, 50% of liquid or solid food is emptied at ~48 min, compared with ~25 min during hypoglycemia (43). In contrast, hyperglycemia slows the gastric emptying rate (44).

Adding protein to the treatment of hypoglycemia is not helpful or necessary. Gray et al. (45) treated hypoglycemia (50 mg/dl [2.7 mmol/l]) in people with type 1 diabetes with 15 g of carbohydrate as either bread or bread plus meat (15 g carbohydrate plus 15 g protein and 5 g fat). Peak glucose levels after treatment with either snack were comparable, and time to subsequent hypoglycemia (~180 min) was similar for both snacks. Although it is frequently recommended that protein be added to treatment of hypoglycemia to prevent subsequent hypoglycemia, they concluded that treatment with a protein-enriched snack does not help in treatment and merely adds often unwanted calories.

OTHER NUTRITION-RELATED CONCERNS

Hyperglycemia/Sick Days

Hyperglycemia can lead to diabetic ketoacidosis (DKA). DKA is a life-threatening but reversible complication that is always caused by having inadequate insulin to utilize glucose. Acidosis results from increased production and decreased utilization of acetoacetic acid and 3-β-hydroxybutyric acid from fatty acids. Causes of DKA, other than undiagnosed diabetes, include infection, a commonly cited precipitating factor; acute illness, such as flu, cold, vomiting, or diarrhea; unrecognized subclinical illness; lack of diabetes education; psychological problems; and indeterminate causes. If untreated, DKA can lead to coma and death. Treatment includes supplemental insulin, replacement of fluids and electrolytes, and medical monitoring.

To prevent DKA, individuals with type 1 diabetes need to know how to handle acute illnesses appropriately. During acute illnesses with the accompanying increases in counterregulatory hormones, the need to take injected insulin continues or may increase. Testing blood glucose levels, testing urine for ketones, drinking adequate amounts of fluids, and ingesting carbohydrate, especially if blood glucose levels are <250 mg/dl (13.8 mmol/l), are also important during acute illnesses.

Although the production of glucose is increased in individuals with diabetes and is proportional to the fasting plasma concentration (46), providing the carbohydrate for normal physiological processes during the fasting and postabsorptive state should be sufficient to prevent starvation ketosis. In general, oral ingestion of ~200 g of carbohydrate per day in evenly divided doses (45–50 g, or three or four carbohydrate choices, every 3–4 h) should be sufficient, along with medication adjustment, to keep glucose in the goal range (47). If regular foods are not tolerated, liquid or soft carbohydrate-containing foods, such as regular soft drinks, soups, juices, and ice cream, should be eaten.

Liquids should also be increased to prevent dehydration. If nausea or vomiting occurs, small sips—1 or 2 Tbsp every 15–30 min—should be consumed. If vomiting continues or if the illness continues for more than 1 day, the health care team should be called for additional changes in the management plan.

Exercise

Both hypoglycemia and hyperglycemia are acute risks of exercise. Hypoglycemia can occur during prolonged exercise (usually >1 h) and for up to 24 h after unusually strenuous, prolonged, and/or sporadic exercise. However, hypoglycemia occurs most commonly 3–15 h after exercise (48,49). This hypoglycemia is not limited to people in good metabolic control and is more likely to occur in individuals who are untrained and who exercise on a sporadic basis, i.e., after periods of relative inactivity. Replenishment of muscle and liver glycogen stores, along with increased insulin sensitivity following exercise, causes insulin requirements to drop. Therefore, monitoring blood glucose levels as well as increasing carbohydrate and/or adjusting insulin after exercise is necessary. Before exercise it is important to consider not only absolute glycemic levels but also the rate at which any change in glycemia may be occurring. For example, a glucose level that is stable at 100 mg/dl (5.5 mmol/l) may be safe, but if the same level is indicative of a fall in blood glucose level from 150 mg/dl (8.3 mmol/l) an hour before, extra carbohydrate will be needed before exercise to prevent a further drop in blood glucose levels (50).

In contrast, in poorly controlled (underinsulinized) individuals, exercise can result in hyperglycemia. With a deficiency of insulin, the rise in counterregulatory hormones that occurs during exercise causes an increase in hepatic glucose production and in free fatty acids, whereas cellular uptake is minimal. This can result in both hyperglycemia and ketonemia (51). Exercise of a high intensity can also result in hyperglycemia. This also has been attributed to the effects of the counterregulatory hormones (52,53).

Blood glucose monitoring, both preexercise and postexercise, is the key to safety and to understanding how exercise affects diabetes control. It provides the needed feedback to help with insulin and carbohydrate adjustments. Moderate-intensity exercise increases whole-body glucose uptake by 2–3 mg/kg/min. For a 70-kg (150-lb) individual, an additional 8.4–12.6 g of carbohydrate is needed for every hour of exercise. During high-intensity exercise, the rate of whole-body glucose uptake may increase by 5–6 mg/kg/min. Despite this increased rate of glucose use, the demand on glucose stores and the risk of hypoglycemia are less, because exercise of this intensity cannot be sustained for long intervals (50). Rasmussen et al. (54) reported that if blood glucose levels are near-normal before eating 50 g of carbohydrate, 30 min of moderate exercise done postprandially reduces the blood glucose response by about one-third.

In general, an additional 15 g of carbohydrate should be sufficient for an hour of moderate activity. For more strenuous exercise, 30 g of carbohydrate per hour may be required (50). Depending on the time that exercise is undertaken, the extra carbohydrate can be eaten either before or after exercise. For exercise before breakfast or later in the afternoon, it is best to eat the carbohydrate before exercising. For exercise after meals, the carbohydrate, if needed, can be eaten after exercising. For exercise performed during the evening, it may be particularly important to add extra carbohydrate to the evening or bedtime snack. Moderate exercise of <30 min rarely requires any additional carbohydrate or insulin adjustment; however, a small snack is needed if the blood glucose levels are <80 mg/dl (4.4 mmol/l) before exercise.

It is often necessary also to adjust the insulin dosage before exercise to prevent hypoglycemia. This is especially important if exercise is undertaken for >45–60 min. For most people, a modest decrease (~20%) in the insulin component corresponding to the period of exercise is a good starting point. For more prolonged or vigorous exercise, a larger decrease in the total insulin dosage (by as much as one-third to one-half) may be necessary to prevent repeated hypoglycemic episodes. In contrast to these acute reductions in insulin dosages for sporadic exercise, individuals who participate in regular exercise sessions (at least every other day) often do not need to adjust insulin doses. In the process of training, they may have already decreased their total insulin doses as their bodies adjusted to the regular exercise (50).

Although increased physical activity has not been shown to improve glycemic control in individuals with type 1 diabetes, regular exercise can achieve the same health benefits in people with type 1 diabetes as in people without diabetes. Individuals with well-controlled type 1 diabetes who engaged in a regular exercise program (endurance sports) exercised safely and did not have more hypoglycemic episodes than they did before beginning the exercise program. Additional benefits were a loss of abdominal fat, a decrease in blood pressure and LDL cholesterol, and an increase in HDL cholesterol—all changes that contribute to improvement in cardiovascular risk factors (55).

NUTRITION PRACTICE GUIDELINES FOR TYPE 1 DIABETES

Nutrition practice guidelines (NPGs) for type 1 diabetes have been developed and field tested by the Diabetes Care and Education Practice Group of The American Dietetic Association (17,56). The purposes of the NPGs are to ensure the maximum effect of nutrition therapy in the management of type 1 diabetes and, through changes in nutrition behaviors, to empower individuals with diabetes to improve metabolic control (56). The practice guidelines describe responsibilities within the scope of practice for qualified dietetics professionals, guide practice decisions, promote self-management education for patients, and define state-of-the-art nutrition therapy based on available scientific evidence and experience of experts. In addition, the guidelines define levels of nutrition care (initial, continuing, and intensive) and state a minimum number of visits and amount of contact time. The guidelines define necessary and appropriate nutrition care for type 1 diabetes that should be provided by dietitians in all settings (17).

Using the approach of outcomes research, volunteer dietitians were randomly assigned to provide individuals with type 1 diabetes either usual care or practice guideline care and were followed for 3 months. Dietitians using practice guidelines paid greater attention to glycemic control goals at the first visit. They were more likely to do an assessment and discuss results at the first visit. In addition, dietitians using practice guidelines spent more time with patients (~1 h for the first visit) and were more likely to have a third or fourth visit in the 3-month period. Practice guideline patients achieved greater reductions in HbA$_{1c}$ levels than did usual care patients (–1.00% vs. –0.33%). This difference was statistically significant and clinically meaningful (56). When glycemic control goals became the focus of the nutrition visit, the emphasis of the interaction was shifted away from evaluation of the diet according to nutrition recommendations toward evaluation of the diet as one of many factors that affect blood glucose patterns (57).

SUMMARY

MNT is one of the main tools for improving metabolic control in people with type 1 diabetes. When the meal or food plan is developed first, both conventional and intensive insulin therapy can be integrated into the usual eating and exercise habits of the person with diabetes. Rapid-acting insulin before meals has proved helpful to many individuals with type 1 diabetes, and carbohydrate counting is a meal planning approach that can provide more flexibility and an increased number of food choices. However, with improved metabolic control, weight gain and increased frequency of hypoglycemia become more of a concern. Attention to total caloric intake and appropriate treatment of hypoglycemia can help alleviate these problems. Nutrition strategies for acute illnesses and changes in usual exercise patterns that require insulin and/or carbohydrate adjustments are other concerns. NPGs for type 1 diabetes define state-of-the-art nutrition care and can ensure consistent quality of care and positive clinical outcomes.

REFERENCES

1. Delahanty LM, Halford BN: The role of diet behaviors in achieving improved glycemic control in intensively treated patients in the Diabetes Control and Complications Trial. *Diabetes Care* 16:1453–1458, 1993

2. American Diabetes Association: Nutrition recommendations and principles for people with diabetes (Position Statement). *Diabetes Care* 21 (Suppl. 1):S32–S35, 1998

3. Franz MJ, Horton ES, Bantle JP, Beebe CA, Brunzell JD, Coulston AM, Henry RR, Hoogwerf BJ, Stacpoole PW: Nutrition principles for the management of diabetes and related complications (Technical Review). *Diabetes Care* 17:490–518, 1994

4. Zinman B, Chiasson JL, Tildesley H, Tsui E, Strack TR: Insulin lispro in CSII: results of a double-blind cross over study. *Diabetes* 46:400–443, 1997

5. American Diabetes Association: Standards of medical care for patients with diabetes mellitus (Position Statement). *Diabetes Care* 21 (Suppl. 1):S23–S31,1998

6. Diabetes Control and Complications Trial Research Group: The effect of intensive treatment of diabetes on the development and progression of long-term complications in insulin-dependent diabetes mellitus. *N Engl J Med* 329:977–986, 1993

7. Bantle JP, Neal L, Frankamp LM: Effects of the anatomical region used for insulin injections on glycemia in type 1 diabetes subjects. *Diabetes Care* 16:1592–1597, 1993

8. Ebeling P, Jansson, P-A, Smith U, Lalli C, Bolli GB, Koivisto VA: Strategies toward improved control during insulin lispro therapy in IDDM. *Diabetes Care* 20:1827–1832, 1997

9. Fineberg SE: Insulin analogs and human insulin lispro (Humalog). *Pract Diabetology* June 1997, pp. 16–23

10. Ter Braak EW, Woodwroth JR, Bianchi R, Cerimele B, Erkelens DW, Thisjssen JHH, Kurtz D: Injection site effects on the pharmacokinetics and glucodynamics of insulin lispro and regular insulin. *Diabetes Care* 19:1437–1440, 1996

11. Holcombe J, Zalani S, Arora V, Headlee S, Gill A: Insulin lispro (LP) results in less nocturnal hypoglycemia, compared with regular insulin in adolescents with type 1 diabetes (Abstract). *Diabetes* 46 (Suppl. 1):103A, 1997

12. Pfutzer A, Kustner E, Forst T, Schulze-Schleppinghoff B, Trautmann M, Haslbeck M, Schatz H, Beyer J, the German Insulin Lispro/IDDM Study Group: Intensive insulin therapy with insulin lispro in patients with type 1 diabetes reduces the frequency of hypoglycemic episodes. *Exp Clin Endocrinol* 104:25–30, 1996

13. Heinemann L, Heise T, Wahl LC, Trautmann ME, Ampudia J, Starke AAR, Berger M: Prandial glycaemia after a carbohydrate-rich meal in type 1 diabetic patients: using the rapid acting insulin analogue [Lys(B28), Pro(B29)] human insulin. *Diabetic Med* 13:625–629, 1995

14. Strachan MWJ, Frier BM: Optimal time of administration of insulin lispro. *Diabetes Care* 21:26–31, 1998

15. Tuominen JA, Karonen SL, Melamies L, Bolli G, Koivisto VA: Exercise-induced hypoglycaemia in IDDM patients treated with a short-acting insulin analogue. *Diabetologia* 38:106–111, 1995

16. Diabetes Control and Complications Trial Research Group: Implementation of treatment protocols in the Diabetes Control and Complications Trial. *Diabetes Care* 18:361–376, 1995

17. Diabetes Care and Education Practice Group of The American Dietetic Association, Kulkarni K, Castle G, Gregory R, Holmes A, Leontos C, Powers MA, Snetselaar L, Splett PL, Wylie-Rosett J: Nutrition practice guidelines for type 1 diabetes: an overview of the content and application. *Diabetes Spectrum* 10:248–256, 1997

18. The DCCT Research Group: Nutrition interventions for intensive therapy in the Diabetes Control and Complications Trial. *J Am Diet Assoc* 93:768–772, 1993

19. Nuttall FQ: Carbohydrate and dietary management of clients with insulin-requiring diabetes. *Diabetes Care* 16:1039–1042, 1993

20. Halfon P: Correlation between amount of CHO in mixed meals and insulin delivery by artificial pancreas in seven IDDM subjects. *Diabetes Care* 12:427–429, 1989

21. Gillespie S, Kulkarni K, Daly A: Using carbohydrate counting in diabetes clinical practice. *J Am Diet Assoc* 98:897–899, 1998

22. American Diabetes Association, The American Dietetic Association: *Carbohydrate Counting: Getting Started.* Alexandria, VA, and Chicago, IL, American Diabetes Association and The American Dietetic Association, 1995

23. American Diabetes Association, The American Dietetic Association: *Carbohydrate Counting: Moving On.* Alexandria, VA, and Chicago, IL, American Diabetes Association and The American Dietetic Association, 1995

24. American Diabetes Association, The American Dietetic Association: *Carbohydrate Counting: Carbohydrate/Insulin Ratios.* Alexandria, VA, and Chicago, IL, American Diabetes Association and The American Dietetic Association, 1995

25. Grinvalsky MA, Nathan DM: Diets for insulin pump and multiple daily injection therapy. *Diabetes Care* 6:241–244, 1983

26. Ahren JA, Gatcomb PM, Held NA, Pettit WA, Tamborlane WV: Exaggerated hyperglycemia after a pizza meal in well-controlled diabetes. *Diabetes Care* 16:578–580, 1993

27. Vlachokosta FV, Piper CM, Gleason R, Kinzel L, Kahn CR: Dietary carbohydrate, a Big Mac, and insulin requirements in type I diabetes. *Diabetes Care* 11:330–336, 1988

28. Franz MJ: Protein: metabolism and effect on blood glucose levels. *Diabetes Educ* 23:663–651, 1997

29. Peters AL, Davidson MB: Protein and fat effects on glucose responses and insulin requirements in subjects with insulin-dependent diabetes. *Am J Clin Nutr* 58:555–560, 1993

30. Wheeler ML, Franz MJ, Barrier P, Holler J, Cronmiller N, Delalanty LM: Macronutrient and energy database for the 1995 *Exchange Lists for Meal Planning*: a rationale for clinical practice decisions. *J Am Diet Assoc* 96:1165–1171, 1996

31. American Diabetes Association, The American Dietetic Association: *Exchange Lists for Meal Planning*. Alexandria, VA, and Chicago, IL, American Diabetes Association and The American Dietetic Association, 1995

32. International Diabetes Center: *My Food Plan*. Minneapolis, MN, IDC, 1996

33. American Diabetes Association, The American Dietetic Association: *Healthy Food Choices*. Alexandria, VA, and Chicago, IL, American Diabetes Association and The American Dietetic Association, 1985

34. Holler HJ, Pastors JG (Eds.): *Diabetes Medical Nutrition Therapy: A Guide to Management and Nutrition Education Resources*. Chicago, The American Dietetic Association, 1997

35. Diabetes Control and Complications Trial Research Group: Weight gain associated with intensive therapy in the Diabetes Control and Complications Trial. *Diabetes Care* 11:67–73, 1998

36. Wing RR, Klein R, Moss SE: Weight gain associated with improved glycemic control in population-based sample of subjects with type I diabetes. *Diabetes Care* 13:1106–1109, 1990

37. Carlson MG, Campbell PJ: Intensive insulin therapy and weight gain in IDDM. *Diabetes* 42:1700–1707, 1993

38. Purnell JQ, Hokanson JE, Marcovina SM, Steffes MW, Cleary PA, Brunzell JD: Effect of excessive weight gain with intensive therapy of type 1 diabetes on lipid levels and blood pressure. *JAMA* 280:140–146, 1998

39. The DCCT Research Group: Epidemiology of severe hypoglycemia in the Diabetes Control and Complications Trial. *Am J Med* 90:450–459, 1990

40. Cryer PE, Fisher JN, Shamoon H: Hypoglycemia (Technical Review). *Diabetes Care* 17:734–755, 1995

41. Slama G, Traynard P-Y, Desplanque N, Pudar H, Dhunputh I, Letanoux M, Bornet FRJ, Tchobroutsky G: The search for the optimized treatment of hypoglycemia: carbohydrates in tablets, solution, or gel in the correction of insulin reactions. *Arch Intern Med* 150:589–593, 1990

42. Brodows RG, Williams C, Amatruda JM: Treatment of insulin reactions in diabetics. *JAMA* 252:3378–3381, 1984

43. Schvarcz E, Palmer M, Aman J, Lindkvist B, Beckman K-W: Hypoglycemia increases the gastric emptying rate in patients with type 1 diabetes mellitus. *Diabetic Med* 10:660–663, 1993

44. Fraser RJ, Horowitz M, Maddox AF, Harding PE, Chatterton BE, Dent J: Hyperglycaemia slows gastric emptying rate in type 1 (insulin-dependent) diabetes mellitus. *Diabetologia* 33:675–668, 1990

45. Gray RO, Butler PC, Beers TR, Kryshak EJ, Rizza RA: Comparison of the ability of bread versus bread plus meat to treat and prevent subsequent hypoglycemia in patients with insulin-dependent diabetes mellitus. *J Clin Endocrinol Metab* 81:1508–1511, 1996

46. Dinneen S, Gerrich J, Rizza R: Carbohydrate metabolism in non-insulin-dependent diabetes mellitus. *N Engl J Med* 327:707–713, 1992

47. Schafer BG, Bohannon B, Franz M, Freeman J, Holmes A, McLaughlin S, Haas LB, Kruger DF, Lorenz RA, McMahon, MM: Translation of the diabetes nutrition recommendations for health care institutions (Technical Review). *Diabetes Care* 20:96–105, 1997

48. Campaigne BN, Wallberg-Henrikssen H, Gunnarsson R: 12-hour glycemic response following acute exercise in type 1 diabetes in relation to insulin dose and caloric intake. *Diabetes Care* 10:716–721, 1987

49. MacDonald MJ: Postexercise late-onset hypoglycemia in insulin-dependent diabetic patients. *Diabetes Care* 10:584–588, 1987

50. Wasserman DH, Zinman B: Exercise in individuals with IDDM (Technical Review). *Diabetes Care* 17:924–937, 1994

51. Berger MP, Berchtold HJ, Cuppers H, Drost H, Kley HK, Muller WA, Viegelman W, Zimmermann-Telschow H, Gries FA, Kruskemper HL, Zimmermann H: Metabolic and hormonal effects of exercise in juvenile type diabetes. *Diabetologia* 13:355–367, 1977

52. Mitchell TH, Abraham G, Schiffrin A, Leiter LA, Marliss EB: Hyperglycemia after intense exercise in IDDM subjects during continuous subcutaneous insulin infusion. *Diabetes Care* 11:311–317, 1988

53. Purdon C, Brousson M, Nyveen L, Miles PDG, Halter JB, Vranic M, Marliss EB: The roles of insulin and catecholamines in the glucoregulatory response to intense exercise and early recovery in insulin-dependent diabetic and control subjects. *J Clin Endocrinol Metab* 76:566–573, 1993

54. Rasmussen OW, Lauszus FF, Hermansen K: Effects of postprandial exercise on glycemic response in IDDM subjects. *Diabetes Care* 17:1203–1205, 1994

55. Lehman R, Kaplan V, Bingisser R, Bloch KE, Spinas GA: Impact of physical activity on cardiovascular risk factors for IDDM. *Diabetes Care* 20:1603–1611, 1997

56. Kulkarni K, Castle G, Gregory R, Holmes A, Leontos C, Powers M, Snetselaar L, Splett P, Wylie-Rosett J, the Diabetes Care and Education Dietetic Practice Group: Nutrition practice guidelines for type 1 diabetes mellitus positively affect dietitian practices and patient outcomes. *J Am Diet Assoc* 98:62–70, 1998

57. Delahanty LM: Clinical significance of medical nutrition therapy in achieving diabetes outcomes and the importance of the process. *J Am Diet Assoc* 98:28–30, 1998

Ms. Kulkarni is a diabetes clinician in Salt Lake City, UT, and Ms. Franz is Director of Nutrition and Professional Education at the International Diabetes Center, Institute for Research and Education, HealthSystem Minnesota, Minneapolis, MN.

4. Nutrition Therapy for Type 2 Diabetes

Christine A. Beebe, MS, RD, LD, CDE

Highlights

- Medical management of type 2 diabetes comprises nutrition therapy, increased physical activity, and medications when necessary. The goals of nutrition therapy are to achieve near-normal metabolic control—blood glucose, blood lipids, and blood pressure—and to prevent the acute and chronic complications of diabetes.
- Both moderate weight loss and reduced caloric intake improve blood glucose levels in type 2 diabetes. The primary benefit of weight loss is postulated to be the decrease in body fat, especially abdominal fat. Fat cells in the abdominal area have a higher turnover rate and greater release of free fatty acids (FFAs) and are most closely correlated with insulin resistance and type 2 diabetes.
- Glycemic improvement as a result of energy restriction is likely due to the combined effect of reduced calories and carbohydrate restriction. Carbohydrate restriction decreases hepatic glucose output, which lowers fasting glucose levels. Caloric restriction generally includes a reduction in dietary fat, which may reduce FFA levels.
- Individualizing the carbohydrate and fat content of the diet is crucial. Blood glucose monitoring responses are used to evaluate the impact of specific amounts of carbohydrate at meals and snacks.

INTRODUCTION

Current nutrition recommendations to achieve and maintain glucose, lipid, and blood pressure goals for individuals with type 2 diabetes are simple in their brevity: lose weight if overweight, restrict saturated fat, and spread nutrient intake throughout the day (1,2). At the same time, clinicians and patients alike find these recommendations to be extremely complex because of their vagueness. Two likely sources of this frustration are *1*) the heterogeneous nature of type 2 diabetes, which makes it impossible to provide one "ADA Diet," and *2*) the paucity of research available to substantiate more precise guidelines.

The primary goals of medical nutrition therapy in type 2 diabetes are, in their broadest sense, to prevent the acute (hyperglycemia and hypoglycemia) and chronic complications of diabetes and, more specifically, to achieve near-normal metabolic control, i.e., blood glucose, lipids (HDL, LDL, total cholesterol, and triglycerides), and blood pressure. An important additional goal is to promote overall health through good nutrition so as to enhance quality of life and reduce likelihood of other chronic diseases influenced by nutritional status. The *Dietary Guidelines for Americans* (3) and the U.S. Department of Agriculture (USDA) Food Guide Pyramid (4) serve as the basis for achieving and maintaining good health for most healthy Americans and for people with type 2 diabetes. Every person with diabetes should receive basic nutrition education in the primary components of the dietary guidelines, with particular emphasis on the benefits of fruits and vegetables and whole-grain carbohydrate sources and on the modest use of animal protein, animal fats, and sugars. Strategies to achieve optimal metabolic control in type 2 diabetes are much more specific and must be individualized using the principles of medical nutrition therapy (5).

METABOLIC PROBLEMS IN TYPE 2 DIABETES

Type 2 diabetes is the most common form of the disease, affecting 90% of individuals with diabetes. The hyperglycemia associated with the metabolic disorder of either type 1 or type 2 diabetes increases the risk of premature death and a variety of complications, including cardiovascular disease, stroke, visual impairment and blindness, nephropathy, and neuropathy. It is sometimes argued that type 2 diabetes is a milder form of diabetes or should be treated less aggressively because it occurs in individuals who are older. With the trend toward an increase in younger overweight individuals developing type 2 diabetes and the fact that at diagnosis most people with type 2 diabetes have had the disease for an average of 7 years, this argument has no scientific basis. The hyperglycemia in type 2 diabetes is no less deadly than that in type 1 diabetes; it is simply grounded in a different etiology.

Type 2 diabetes is due to a combination of a defect in insulin secretion from the pancreas and insulin resistance at the site of insulin action in the periphery (6). Either impairment may predominate, depending on the individual. Pancreatic defects include lack of first-phase insulin response (first

10 min after stimulation) and inadequate insulin secretion for a given glucose load. Insulin resistance occurs in the liver and manifests itself as a failure of insulin to shut off gluconeogenesis and subsequent excess glucose production. Indeed, fasting hyperglycemia is a hallmark of type 2 diabetes.

Peripheral insulin resistance occurs at the sites of insulin-mediated glucose uptake when fat and muscle cells fail to respond to insulin's anabolic action. Because muscle cells take up more glucose than do fat cells, they are the primary site of insulin resistance. Glucose transport for both oxidative (using glucose for energy) and nonoxidative (storing glucose as glycogen) processes is impaired by insulin resistance in muscle cells (7). Insulin's role in fat cells is to depress hormone-sensitive lipase (HSL), which is responsible for lipolysis and release of fatty acids from the adipocyte. In obesity and type 2 diabetes, HSL becomes resistant to insulin's action, resulting in elevated free fatty acid (FFA) concentrations. This elevated FFA flux to the liver drives gluconeogenesis and increases hepatic glucose output (HGO), which ultimately leads to fasting hyperglycemia (8). This combination of muscle cells that fail to utilize glucose and fat cells that release excess FFA for gluconeogenesis results in the hyperglycemia of type 2 diabetes when compensatory insulin secretion cannot occur because of a pancreatic defect.

Insulin resistance is thought to be a combination of genetic defects and metabolic changes brought about by environmental factors. Pancreatic defects are genetic in nature and must be present for diabetes to occur. Obesity, upper-body obesity in particular (9), aging, and sedentary lifestyle are independent environmental factors contributing to insulin resistance (10). Even visceral fatness (fat around the waist and abdomen) without overt obesity leads to insulin resistance and impaired glucose tolerance (11) and increases risk of type 2 diabetes.

Duration and degree of obesity affect insulin secretion rate; β-cell exhaustion is thought to occur over time. Once diabetes is diagnosed, time continues to be a factor as β-cell exhaustion progresses and eventually necessitates the use of insulin secretagogues or exogenous insulin therapy. Early detection followed by early intervention is hoped to slow this progression and reduce complications (6).

Ethnicity may influence metabolic defects. For example, African Americans with type 2 diabetes are more likely to lack first-phase insulin response than their age-, sex-, and weight-matched white counterparts (12) and are more insulin resistant as well (13). Future research will likely identify many different genetic defects responsible for type 2 diabetes.

MEDICAL MANAGEMENT OF TYPE 2 DIABETES

While defects in insulin secretion and insulin action are required for type 2 diabetes to present itself, day-to-day blood glucose regulation in type 2 diabetes is clearly affected by intestinal absorption of glucose from food. Thus, there are three things contributing to glucose control: hepatic glucose production, glucose uptake by the periphery, and absorption of glucose from food. The medical management of type 2 diabetes requires a three-pronged approach involving nutrition therapy, physical activity, and medication when necessary. Each is designed to compensate for metabolic abnormalities in the three modulators of glucose control (Table 4.1). Successful management involves understanding the potential of each therapy, the synergistic relationship between therapies, and the maximal utilization of each therapy.

The traditional general approach to medical management of type 2 diabetes consisting of monotherapy, a weight-loss or a "no sugar" diet, and advice to "get some exercise" will not yield desired medical outcomes for people with diabetes (Table 4.2). Targeted blood glucose control, whereby patients know and attempt to achieve their blood glucose goals for various times of the day, is the optimal way to achieve good blood glucose control. This kind of therapy is orchestrated by feedback from daily self-monitoring of blood glucose (SMBG) and routine laboratory evaluations.

SMBG is the most useful tool for evaluating medical therapy, including the nutrition plan, and should be beneficial to all people with type 2 diabetes. This is despite the fact that few studies have looked at the role of SMBG in the medical management of type 2 diabetes and that those that have found little improvement in terms of HbA_{1c} (14,15). All of these studies suffer from problems in methodology and from the complexity

Table 4.1 Components of Therapy in Type 2 Diabetes

Therapy	Expected Outcome
Medical nutrition therapy	Nutritional health; weight management; improve insulin sensitivity; optimize glucose load; minimize blood glucose swings; improve blood lipids; affect blood pressure and albuminuria
Physical activity	Improve insulin sensitivity; weight management; cardiovascular health
Oral medications	
Insulin secretagogues	Stimulate insulin production
Insulin sensitizers	Increase muscle glucose uptake; decrease hepatic glucose production
Glucose inhibitors	Retard carbohydrate absorption
Insulin therapy	Correct insulin deficiency

Table 4.2 Glycemic Control for Type 2 Diabetes

Biochemical Index	Normal	Goal	Additional Action Suggested
Fasting/preprandial glucose	<110 mg/l (<6.0 mmol/l)	80–120 mg/dl (<6.6 mmol/l)	<80 or >140 mg/dl (<4.4 or >7.8 mmol/l)
Bedtime glucose	<120 mg/dl (<6.7 mmol/l)	100–140 mg/dl (5.6–7.8 mmol/l)	<100 or >160 mg/dl (<5.6 or >8.9 mmol/l)
HbA$_{1c}$	<6%	<7%	>8%

From Zimmerman BR (Ed.): *Medical Management of Type 2 Diabetes.* 4th ed. Alexandria, VA, American Diabetes Association, 1998, p. 35.

of measuring short-term outcomes in diabetes. Checking daily pre- or postprandial blood glucose levels is probably not the key process quality indicator in diabetes. Use of the data to modify food, exercise, or medications through problem-solving techniques is more valuable. For example, weight-loss efforts in type 2 diabetes are often seriously undermined by medication-induced hypoglycemic episodes that require therapeutic action with food. Frequent blood glucose testing and education can identify when medication reductions are necessary and can prevent excess food consumption when treating reactions. Furthermore, individuals who use carbohydrate counting to achieve targeted postprandial blood glucose values could not do so without SMBG feedback to guide carbohydrate and medication adjustments.

More research is needed on the role of SMBG in the nutritional management of type 2 diabetes. What is the frequency of testing required to improve blood glucose control? When are the best times to test if testing is to be limited? Who benefits most from SMBG? Does SMBG enhance adherence to dietary modifications or ability to understand and manipulate the macronutrient content of the diet?

Nearly 80% of those with diagnosed type 2 diabetes are taking some form of diabetes medication, either oral agents or insulin (16). Advances in the types of medications available make their use more likely. Each has unique characteristics that make it valuable in improving blood glucose control (Table 4.3). The U.K. Prospective Diabetes Study (17) found that each of these medications can be safe and effective in achieving good blood glucose control in type 2 diabetes, yet current estimates suggest that only 12% of people with diabetes are achieving an HbA$_{1c}$ goal of ≤7% (18). Primary care physicians identify noncompliance and fear of hypoglycemia in their patients, especially elderly patients, as major deterrents to more aggressive therapy in type 2 diabetes. On the other hand, only 20–48% of people with type 2 diabetes say that they have seen a dietitian or a diabetes nurse educator for their diabetes (18,19). Thus, it appears that the small number of individuals controlling blood glucose without medication and the lack of tight blood glucose control in type 2 diabetes may be due in part to patients' failure to receive a crucial component of the medical management plan. This is despite the fact that medical nutrition therapy for type 2 diabetes has been shown to be both medically and financially effective (5,20).

NUTRITIONAL MANAGEMENT OF TYPE 2 DIABETES

The role of dietary modifications in the management of type 2 diabetes should not be underestimated (Table 4.4). Their impact on overall health, metabolic control, and treatment of acute and chronic complications can be substantial. Clinicians who have been involved with diabetes for many years recognize that individuals who managed to have good blood glucose control in times of few technological and medical advances were those who adhered to rigid dietary regimens.

Current nutrition guidelines are less restrictive than previous guidelines because of *1*) new oral medications that target specific metabolic

Table 4.3 Medications Commonly Used in Type 2 Diabetes

Class	Medication	Action
Sulfonylurea	Tolbutamide Chlorpropamide Tolazamide Glipizide Glipizide-XL Glyburide Glyburide-micronized Glimepiride	Stimulate insulin secretion
Meglitinide	Repaglinide	Stimulates insulin secretion in presence of glucose, short-acting (5 h)
Biguanide	Metformin	Decreases HGO, improves insulin sensitivity
Thiazolidinedione	Troglitazone	Decreases insulin resistance
α-glucosidase inhibitor	Acarbose Miglitol	Delay intestinal absorption of glucose
Human insulin	Rapid, short, intermediate, long	Replace missing endogenous insulin

Table 4.4 Nutrition Recommendations for Type 2 Diabetes

Recommendation	Expected Outcome
USDA Food Guide Pyramid	Leads to more healthful diet with more antioxidants, fiber, and minerals
Weight loss	Decreases insulin resistance/reduces insulin requirements
Calorie restriction	Decreases insulin resistance/reduces insulin requirements
Saturated fat restriction	Reduces LDL cholesterol
Low-fat, high-carbohydrate intake	Helps in weight loss; decreases LDL and total cholesterol
Modest carbohydrate and fat intake	Lowers triglycerides; raises HDL; minimizes glucose rise in response to carbohydrates
Spread-out food intake	Limits blood glucose rise and insulin need at any one time
Protein at meals/snacks*	Stimulates insulin
Low–glycemic index foods*	Reduce blood glucose rise

*Potential options but not included in 1994 American Diabetes Association recommendations.

defects and a variety of insulin preparations that make physiological insulin delivery possible, 2) blood glucose testing technology that yields on-the-spot evaluation of and reaction to nutrient intake, and 3) clinical research that dispels some of the myths and supports new philosophies regarding nutrition management in type 2 diabetes.

The complex, heterogeneous nature of type 2 diabetes and the different ages, lifestyles, and cultural backgrounds of people with type 2 diabetes provide the opportunity and the challenge to be creative in the nutritional management of the disease. In spite of the availability of more clinical diabetes research, research into the nutritional management of diabetes is truly in its infancy, and there are few rules without controversy. As a result, the nutritional plan must be driven by and evaluated on the basis of desired medical outcomes. Because the average person with type 2 diabetes is generally older and may have multiple comorbid conditions, dietary modifications should be implemented by prioritizing metabolic problems and instituting a plan based on those priorities. Having too many priorities can be confusing and frustrating to the person with diabetes and can lead to nonadherence. Priorities may include improving overall blood glucose control, minimizing blood glucose excursions, optimizing serum lipid levels, improving blood pressure, reducing albuminuria, and maintaining or reducing weight (which generally leads to improvements in the aforementioned problems).

Nutrition practice guidelines for medical nutrition therapy in type 2 diabetes define nutrition care and processes that should consistently lead to desired medical outcomes (21). They can be used for all people with type 2 diabetes, regardless of duration of the disease, form of therapy, or any other individualized characteristics. These guidelines outline responsibilities of the self-management team members, which include the dietitian, the physician, and the patient (Table 4.5). Individuals with type 2 diabetes should be referred for medical nutrition therapy at the time of diagnosis; whenever blood glucose targets are not being met, a change in therapy or lifestyle occurs, or weight, lipid level, or renal function fails to meet target goals; and for continuing education and support.

Table 4.5 Physician/Dietitian Responsibilities for Nutrition Care

Physician responsibilities
- Refer patient to dietitian for MNT.
- Provide referral data.
- Communicate medical treatment goals for patient care to dietitian.
- Provide medical clearance for exercise.
- Based on outcomes of nutrition intervention, adjust medical therapy for diabetes control as necessary.
- Reinforce nutrition self-management education.

Dietitian responsibilities
- Obtain referral data and treatment goals before initial nutrition intervention.
- Obtain and assess food, exercise, SMBG, psychosocial and economic issues.
- Evaluate patient's knowledge, skill level, and readiness to learn.
- Identify patient's goals.
- Determine and implement appropriate nutrition prescription.
- Provide education on food/meal planning and self-management using appropriate tools.
- Evaluate effectiveness of MNT on medical outcomes, and adjust MNT as needed.
- Make recommendations to physician based on outcomes of nutrition interventions.
- Communicate outcomes to all team members.
- Decide which patients will benefit from basic care and which patients require more frequent follow-up visits.
- Make recommendations for ongoing MNT and self-management education.

MNT, medical nutrition therapy. From Monk et al. (20).

OPTIMIZING BLOOD GLUCOSE LEVELS

A number of strategies have been identified to help individuals achieve an improvement in blood glucose control. The choice of strategy requires a thorough knowledge of the patient and the problem.

Moderate Weight Loss

Somewhere between 80 and 90% of people with type 2 diabetes are overweight. Evidence is unequivocal that weight loss improves blood glucose control by improving insulin action to enhance glucose uptake (i.e., decrease insulin resistance) and by reducing HGO (11). A practical and clinically relevant research question is, How much weight needs to be lost to improve blood glucose control? Studies that have evaluated blood glucose control during weight loss have demonstrated that metabolic changes responsible for improved control occur with a 10- to 20-kg weight loss (22–26). Blood glucose levels and insulin sensitivity continue to improve as weight loss progresses on a calorie-restricted constant diet (23). No studies have examined whether attaining desirable body weight, or BMI <25, is correlated with better or more sustained blood glucose control.

Unfortunately, improvement in metabolic control diminishes and returns to baseline levels when caloric intake resumes and weight is regained (22). Furthermore, not everyone who loses weight sees an improvement in glycemic control. Several studies have demonstrated what is often seen in clinical practice: that subjects with the highest fasting plasma glucose values who respond quickly, i.e., see a dramatic drop in fasting glucose levels within the first 2 weeks of restriction, are most likely to gain glucose control through weight-loss efforts (4,27,28). It is apparent that these individuals are secreting large amounts of insulin and are primarily insulin resistant. Losing weight reduces insulin resistance and allows them to maximize the use of their own endogenous insulin production. This suggests that early intervention, before β-cell exhaustion occurs, will provide the best possibility for improving blood glucose control with weight loss.

It is clear that peripheral insulin resistance improves as actual weight loss progresses. This may be attributed to a change in body composition, especially in the abdominal fat depot (24,29,30). Fat cells in the abdominal area have a higher turnover rate, release more FFAs, and are most closely correlated with insulin resistance and type 2 diabetes (31). Decreasing body fat, especially abdominal fat, may be the primary benefit of weight loss.

Caloric Restriction

Curiously, several research studies in type 2 diabetes have indicated that glycemic control improves within 24 h of calorie restriction, before any weight loss occurs (22–24). Only 10 days of a calorie-restricted diet are required to see 87% of the eventual drop in blood glucose. What is not clear is the role that caloric restriction plays in improved glycemic control independent of weight loss. When obese individuals with type 2 diabetes lost the same amount of weight (11%, or 11 kg) by consuming either a 400-kcal (1,674 kJ) or a 1,000-kcal (4,185 kJ) diet, those on the 400-kcal plan had greater improvements in insulin sensitivity and fasting plasma glucose (23). Of further interest is the finding that the effect of caloric restriction on improved blood glucose control closely corresponds to the reduction in carbohydrate intake (24,26). Indeed, high-carbohydrate diets have been implicated in worsening blood glucose control in type 2 diabetes (32,33); however, there are other studies in which high-carbohydrate, high-fiber diets have improved glycemic control in type 2 diabetes (34) This raises the question of whether it is truly caloric restriction (i.e., energy restriction) or rather carbohydrate restriction (i.e., a reduced glucose load) that improves blood glucose control in overweight individuals with type 2 diabetes.

Very-low-calorie diet (VLCD) therapy consisting of 400–800 kcal/day is a calorie-restriction technique that has enjoyed success in obese individuals with type 2 diabetes (35). In the short term, VLCD therapy appears to offer a slight additional benefit over traditional diet therapy in type 2 diabetes: greater improvement in glycemic control despite similar weight loss. This benefit may be due to the more severe carbohydrate restriction that is characteristic of VLCD therapy, since the improvement in blood glucose occurs early in the diet and is predominantly evident in fasting plasma glucose levels. This theory may be supported by studies using intermittent VLCD therapy in type 2 diabetes in which short periods of caloric restriction, ranging from 1 day/week to 1 week/month, improved glycemic control and enhanced weight-loss efforts (36,37).

The only currently available study to delineate the mechanism responsible for improved glycemic control with caloric restriction suggests that it is likely a combined effect of carbohydrate restriction and body fat reduction (24,26). Carbohydrate restriction is suspected of having an early impact by decreasing HGO. There appears to be no further reduction in HGO with continued weight loss. It is postulated that carbohydrate restriction depletes liver glycogen stores, thus resulting in a fall in HGO. Continued body fat reduction then reduces insulin resistance and insulin requirement.

On the other hand, high levels of circulating FFAs are present in central obesity and type 2 diabetes and are proposed as a primary cause of insulin resistance (8,29). Caloric restriction generally includes a reduction in dietary fat and a subsequent reduction in FFA levels. Perhaps caloric restriction functions through fat restriction, not carbohydrate restriction. More research is needed into the effect of substrate availability and its role in the improved glycemic control seen with weight loss.

The clinically relevant question a practitioner needs to ask is, Should an obese person with type 2 diabetes be placed on a hypocaloric diet with a goal of weight loss, a mildly calorie-restricted diet, or a carbohydrate-restricted diet? Once again, the principles of medical nutrition therapy guide the practitioner in basing decisions on desired medical outcomes, setting goals with the person with diabetes, and providing routine care and follow-up that include changing the course of action if goals are not being met. Any one of these techniques should produce a reduction in fasting blood glucose within 2–4 weeks (5). If a patient does not respond with a significant drop in fasting blood glucose levels, it is unlikely that he or she will respond to nutrition therapy in the form of weight loss or caloric restriction, and other methods of controlling blood glucose should be used.

One characteristic all current weight-loss methods have in common is that actual long-term weight loss is difficult and is not dramatically different between techniques. This illustrates the complexity of weight management. This has also led many clinicians to adopt the philosophy that weight maintenance, absence of weight gain, over a lifetime is in itself a reputable and lofty goal (38). Whether caloric restriction without weight loss or intermittent caloric restriction is beneficial to weight maintenance is yet another unanswered question.

Application of this philosophy is observed when instituting targeted, or tight, blood glucose control in type 2 diabetes with the introduction of any insulin secretagogue or insulin therapy. Improved substrate utilization and storage generally lead to weight gain or, at the very least, weight maintenance. The results can be discouraging to overweight patients, who are most likely struggling with a diet at the time. Caloric restriction without weight loss is beneficial in this situation as long as the patient and professional identify the marker of success as improved blood glucose and lipid control rather than weight loss.

Carbohydrate Modification

Calorie reduction and weight loss are extremely effective in the management of type 2 diabetes in obese individuals and should therefore be the first line of therapy. However, there are many individuals whose body weight is normal or who cannot, will not, or may not need to lose weight. For example, in the increasing number of individuals over the age of 70 with type 2 diabetes, aggressive weight loss efforts may be inappropriate and may not support the quality of life desired. How then do we best modify the macronutrient content of the diet to produce optimal blood glucose levels?

Studies conducted in type 2 diabetes in which carbohydrates have been reduced to 40–45% of calories and replaced with monounsaturated fat have yielded improved glycemia over diets containing 55–60% of calories from carbohydrate (32,33). Elevated triglyceride levels, commonly a problem in type 2 diabetes, generally improve on these diets of 40–45% carbohydrate. The hyperlipidemia associated with high-carbohydrate diets in type 2 diabetes is postulated to involve increased insulin-stimulated VLDL triglyceride production and increased lipoprotein lipase activity due to the hyperinsulinemia caused by a high carbohydrate intake (39).

The effect of carbohydrate on blood glucose and plasma lipids may depend on the severity of glucose intolerance. Type 2 individuals on hypoglycemic medication have greater postprandial blood glucose elevations in response to 60% carbohydrate diets than to 40% diets (40). Diet-controlled individuals also had higher glucose responses to the 60% diet, but the responses were less dramatic than those in their medication-taking counterparts. Clearly, individuals on diet alone are still capable of secreting a fair amount of insulin in response to a glucose load, whereas by the time one requires medication, the ability to secrete enough endogenous insulin in response to the same glucose load is diminished.

More and longer-term studies varying the amount of carbohydrate are needed. It appears that mild carbohydrate restriction may benefit some individuals with type 2 diabetes by minimizing blood glucose load and optimizing blood glucose responses. A major concern of clinicians is that the resulting increased fat intake will increase the likelihood of weight gain. Dietary fat seems to play a role in stimulating caloric consumption (41) and is strongly associated with obesity. An examination of energy-expenditure studies, both epidemiological and intervention, did not find this concern to be warranted (42). Careful attention to controlling the total calorie content of the diet can minimize concern over weight gain, and regular visits to a dietitian can assist in controlling calorie and fat intake while reducing carbohydrate intake.

What also remains unclear is what effect, if any, type of carbohydrate has in the day-to-day management of type 2 diabetes. Increasing research into the glycemic effects of various carbohydrates has shown that differences between carbohydrate foods do exist (43). High–glycemic index foods and low-fiber foods are postulated to affect blood glucose response and insulin secretion negatively in type 2 diabetes (44). The problem is how to make this information clinically relevant given the difficulty of predicting glycemic responses to mixed meals and in different individuals.

Individualization of the fat and carbohydrate content of the diet is crucial in people with type 2 diabetes because the heterogeneity of this disease makes it difficult to suggest anything otherwise. With the help of blood glucose monitoring, it is possible to evaluate the impact of specific amounts of carbohydrate at meals and snacks and to titrate carbohydrate intake appropriately.

Meal Spacing

Logic would suggest that if one of the primary metabolic problems of type 2 diabetes is a limited capacity to secrete insulin in response to a given glucose load, then partitioning food and particularly carbohydrate intake into small glucose loads would allow better utilization of endogenous insulin production. Controversy continues, however, because a limited number of studies have been conducted, each with its own limitations. Nondiabetic individuals who either sipped a glucose solution throughout the day or consumed six liquid meals every 4 h for 24 h (45) had lower blood glucose and insulin responses than when they consumed the calories as one or three meals a day. Another study in nondiabetic subjects (46) found no difference in blood glucose, but found flatter insulin responses in nibblers than in meal eaters. Cholesterol levels improved in the two studies in which they were measured.

Few studies have been performed in individuals with type 2 diabetes. One compared consumption of two versus six hypocaloric meals in an 8-h period and found blood glucose increases to be greater after two meals (47). However, overall blood glucose was the same for the 8-h period regardless of intake frequency. This was corroborated by comparing realistic, energy-balanced food intake patterns in type 2 individuals in a 24-h period (48). Individuals consumed three equal meals, each 30% of calories; three meals containing 10, 20, and 70% of calories for the morning, midday, and evening meals, respectively; or three equal meals plus three snacks. Only the snacking pattern showed a modest rise in overall 24-h blood glucose and insulin secretion. Interestingly, the late snack and large evening meal blunted the next day dawn phenomenon better than when the last meal was 30% of calories. A longer-term study (49) compared three- and nine-meal regimens in people with type 2 diabetes and found no difference in glucose, insulin, or HbA_{1c} responses.

Available data for type 2 diabetes suggest that more and longer-term studies are necessary before any conclusions can be drawn regarding blood glucose control and meal spacing. Because there appears to be no advantage or disadvantage to any one pattern, meal spacing should be determined by the patient and clinician and directed by the patient's lifestyle. Individual responses are likely to be different depending on insulin secretion capacity and degree of insulin resistance. SMBG is a valuable tool for evaluating daily meal-to-meal blood glucose fluctuations and the impact of snacks. Because carbohydrate foods have the greatest impact on blood glucose response, they can be distributed in a manner that yields an acceptable daily blood glucose pattern. The optimal distribution of carbohydrate is not yet known. The most realistic way to distribute carbohydrates is to evaluate a person's usual carbohydrate intake at meals and snacks, use carbohydrate counting to maintain consistency, and evaluate with pre- and postprandial blood glucose tests. The carbohydrate load at meals and snacks can be titrated up or down depending on the response. Medications such as short- and rapid-acting insulin, repaglinide, or α-glucosidase inhibitors can be added to reduce postprandial response.

Physical Activity

The benefit of physical activity for blood glucose control in type 2 diabetes is so well documented that exercise is generally prescribed for everyone with type 2 diabetes along with nutrition therapy. Indeed, dietitians often discuss physical activity when counseling people with type 2 diabetes because it is impossible to design a nutrition plan without knowing the level and timing of physical activity and coordinating it with the food and medication plan. Furthermore, dietitians are generally skilled in the nuances of behavior modification, which proves valuable when asking sedentary individuals with an average age of 55 to adopt an exercise regimen.

Physical activity improves blood glucose levels by enhancing muscle blood glucose uptake during or shortly after the activity and by improving insulin sensitivity. Exercise enhances weight-loss efforts, which in turn improve insulin sensitivity and blood glucose control. The training effect of decreasing insulin resistance with exercise is thought to improve both fasting and postprandial insulin levels, thus improving one of the major metabolic abnormalities in type 2 diabetes (50,51).

The association between physical activity and the prevention of type 2 diabetes is very strong. Numerous epidemiological studies show that increased participation in both vigorous and nonvigorous physical activity significantly improves insulin sensitivity and reduces risk of developing type 2 diabetes (52,53). This increase in insulin sensitivity in both normal and type 2 individuals is closely correlated with the improvement in maximum aerobic capacity that comes with training (54). It appears that exercise has its greatest impact early in the development of type 2 diabetes, when insulin resistance is the predominant abnormality (55,56); however, in later stages exercise can reduce medication requirements in people with type 2 diabetes taking oral agents or insulin.

If any controversy exists over the role of exercise in blood glucose control it is over when, how often, how much, and what type of exercise is most beneficial in type 2 diabetes. Intervention studies have identified that improved insulin sensitivity and the subsequent impact on blood glucose control are only as good as the last exercise bout. The enhanced insulin sensitivity effect is lost anywhere from 3 to 5 days after physical activity (57). Even with an improvement in insulin sensitivity, only one study has shown an improvement in fasting blood glucose or HbA_{1c} with regular physical activity in type 2 diabetes (50). The clinical interpretation is that exercise should be performed at least every 48 h and that it will likely improve average blood glucose values but may have little impact on either fasting or postprandial blood glucose responses. As with everything in diabetes, however, responses vary with individuals.

More research is needed to identify whether activity at specific times of the day, e.g., postprandially or before breakfast or bedtime, is more beneficial. Clinical experience suggests that any time a person can fit in an activity is the right time. There is no scientific basis for suggesting a specific time of day for people with type 2 diabetes. Even if they are on insulin or an oral hypoglycemic agent, they can exercise when they wish if they are taught how to recognize hypoglycemia and how properly to treat and prevent it.

Individuals most likely to develop hypoglycemia are those on a calorie-restricted diet or those on medication and very tightly controlled. An increase in the amount of exercise should be accompanied by a medication reduction to prevent hypoglycemia. This is especially true if weight loss is desired, because treatment of hypoglycemia with a minimum of 15 g of carbohydrate provides 60–100 extra calories, which, over time, can undermine even the best weight-loss efforts.

The type of physical activity recommended will vary with the individual and is influenced by personal preferences, age, and presence of complications that may contraindicate certain types of activity. According to a U.S. Surgeon General's Report, 60% of Americans do not engage in moderate physical activity and 30% do not engage in any activity at all (58). People with diabetes exercise even less frequently than the general population (59). As more epidemiological data suggest that even nonvigorous physical activity can enhance insulin sensitivity, it stands to reason that people with type 2 diabetes should be encouraged to increase their physical activity of daily living (home maintenance, gardening, cleaning, walking) as well as perform regular vigorous activities (lifting, digging, running, swimming, bicycling, weight lifting). This is where health professionals play a key role not only in encouraging activity but also in helping the individual figure out how to work a specific activity into his or her daily routine and which one to perform. A referral to an exercise professional is valuable. While exercise physiologists are skilled in the nuances of developing an aerobic plan, older individuals with type 2 diabetes generally benefit from a consultation with a physical therapist, who can help develop a plan that compensates for any physical problems, including exercise-induced incontinence. Behavior modification and motivation techniques are sorely needed in assisting patients to maintain an exercise regimen.

The frequency of physical activity necessary to improve blood glucose control is generally accepted to be a minimum of three times per week. Because the beneficial effect of physical activity is lost after 48 h, the three times should be spaced throughout the week. Studies on the benefit of exercise for weight loss suggest that the entire benefit is due to increased energy expenditure and that therefore physical activity must occur at least 5 days per week. Exercise has proven particularly beneficial in maintenance of weight loss, and a recent study indicated a threshold for weight maintenance of ~11 kcal/kg body wt/day (47 kJ/kg body wt/day) (60). This threshold corresponds to 80 min/day of moderate activity and 35 min/day of vigorous physical activity.

IMPROVING BLOOD LIPIDS

Hyperlipidemia is as much a hallmark of type 2 diabetes as is elevated fasting blood glucose. Increased triglyceride and decreased HDL cholesterol levels are the most common lipid abnormalities present in type 2 diabetes and appear more frequently in women than in men (61). Lipid levels can be related to glycemia, and glycemic control improves hypertriglyceridemia regardless of how the improved glycemic control is achieved (62). Other factors unrelated to glycemic control or insulin resistance, including renal disease, hypothyroidism, genetic disorders, and use of alcohol or estrogen, can affect lipid levels in type 2 diabetes.

In addition to improving glycemic control, the most valuable nutrition intervention for the dyslipidemia of type 2 diabetes is moderate weight loss, followed by restriction of saturated fat consumption. Considerable controversy exists over whether a low-fat diet actually worsens hypertriglyceridemia and lowers HDL, as many studies have shown in individuals with insulin-resistant type 2 diabetes (see chapter 8 on food fats and dyslipidemia for a thorough discussion). The negative effect of a fat-restricted diet cannot be attributed to sugar consumption, since it is found even with a complex-carbohydrate, high-fiber diet in healthy adults (63). More research is needed to identify whether or not total fat needs to be restricted and whether restricting the type of fat, i.e., saturated and *trans* fat, is more beneficial in both high-risk and type 2 diabetic individuals. This hypothesis is confounded by the concern that higher fat intakes increase insulin resistance and are associated with an increased recurrence rate of gestational diabetes (64).

The need for dietary cholesterol restriction in type 2 diabetes continues to be controversial, especially because many individuals have normal serum cholesterol levels. Age is a key factor to consider when deciding on the components of the nutrition plan, since increasing evidence supports that total serum cholesterol is not a strong predictor of cardiovascular disease after age 65.

Regular exercise has consistently been effective in decreasing triglycerides and increasing HDL in nondiabetic individuals. This has not been well documented in type 2 diabetes. However, experts speculate this is due to the modest intensity of exercise performed in the studies of people with type 2 diabetes. This is an area where much speculation and lack of data make firm recommendations difficult. This should not deter the clinician from recommending exercise for hyperlipidemic patients, since the therapeutic benefits are many and may have an additive effect.

Excess alcohol consumption will increase triglyceride levels in people with hypertriglyceridemia, but there is no evidence that a modest amount, i.e., one drink daily, will aggravate serum lipids. Careful and close monitoring of the patient's lipid levels at least annually allows evaluation and therapy changes that are based on clinical need, not speculation.

BLOOD PRESSURE CONTROL

Approximately 65% of those with type 2 diabetes have hypertension. There is good evidence that weight loss and exercise have a much greater effect on blood pressure than does salt restriction. Salt sensitivity is a controversial area in recommendations to the general public and probably fewer data are available in individuals with diabetes (see chapter 16 on hypertension). This should be considered when developing the nutrition plan for a person with type 2 diabetes. Excessive dietary restrictions lead to frustration and nonadherence. Calorie restriction almost always leads to sodium restriction, and the weight loss and increase in physical activity that accompanies a hypocaloric diet will positively improve both systolic and diastolic blood pressure.

SUMMARY

Data point to the fact that if a person with type 2 diabetes is overweight, every attempt should be made to encourage the person to lose a modest amount of weight and to reduce caloric intake by at least a modest amount while implementing an exercise regimen. There is no preferred way to do this. Focus should also be on the carbohydrate content of the diet. Partitioning carbohydrate intake between meals and snacks should be based on blood glucose response to a given glucose load not on an artificial pattern, since there is no current evidence to suggest otherwise. The macronutrient composition of the diet (carbohydrate, protein, and fat) is best individualized based on desired blood glucose and lipid levels, taking into consideration personal preferences, age, and level of glucose intolerance. The goal of therapy in type 2 diabetes is improved metabolic control. This needs to be communicated to individuals with type 2 diabetes, who traditionally view weight loss as their primary marker of success.

REFERENCES

1. American Diabetes Association: Nutrition recommendations and principles for people with diabetes mellitus (Position Statement). *Diabetes Care* 21:S32–S35, 1998

2. Franz MJ, Horton ES, Bantle JP, Beebe CA, Brunzell JD, Coulston AM, Henry RR, Hoogwerf BJ, Stacpoole PW: Nutrition principles for the management of diabetes and related complications (Technical Review). *Diabetes Care* 17:490–518, 1994

3. U.S. Department of Agriculture, U.S. Department of Health and Human Services: *Nutrition and Your Health: Dietary Guidelines for Americans.* 4th ed. Hyattsville, MD, USDA's Human Nutrition Information Service, 1995

4. U.S. Department of Agriculture: *The Food Guide Pyramid.* Hyattsville, MD, USDA's Human Nutrition Information Service, 1992

5. Franz MJ, Monk A, Barry B, McLain K, Weaver T, Cooper N, Upham P, Bergenstal R, Mazze R: Effectiveness of medical nutrition therapy provided by dietitians in the management of non-insulin-dependent diabetes mellitus: a randomized, controlled clinical trial. *J Am Diet Assoc* 95:1009–1017, 1995

6. American Diabetes Association: Report of the Expert Committee on the Diagnosis and Classification of Diabetes Mellitus. *Diabetes Care* 21 (Suppl. 1):S5–S19, 1998

7. Chung JW, Suh K, Joyce M, Ditzler T, Henry R: Contribution of obesity to defects of intracellular glucose metabolism in NIDDM. *Diabetes Care* 18:666–673, 1995

8. Foley JE, Anderson R: Fatty acid oxidation inhibitors. In *Diabetes Mellitus: A Fundamental and Clinical Text.* LeRoith D, Taylor S, Olefsky JM, Eds. Philadelphia, Lippincott-Raven, 1996, pp. 668–674

9. Kissebah AH, Vydelingum N, Murray R, Evans DF, Hartz AJ, Kalkhoff RK, Adams PW: Relationship of body fat distribution to metabolic complications of obesity. *J Clin Endocrinol Metab* 54:254–260, 1982

10. Eriksson KF, Lindgarde F: Poor physical fitness, and impaired early insulin response but late hyperinsulinaemia, as predictors of NIDDM in middle-aged Swedish men. *Diabetologia* 39:573–579, 1996

11. Ruderman N, Chisholm D, Pi-Sunyer X, Schneider S: The metabolically obese, normal-weight individual revisited. *Diabetes* 47:699–713, 1998

12. Osei K, Gailllard T, Schuster D: Pathogenetic mechanisms of impaired glucose tolerance and type 2 diabetes in African-Americans. *Diabetes Care* 20:396–404, 1997

13. Haffner S, D'Agostino R, Saad MF, Rewers M, Mykinen L, Selby J, Howard G, Savage PJ, Hamman RF, Wagenknecht LE, Bergman RN: Increased insulin resistance and insulin secretion in nondiabetic African-Americans and Hispanics compared with non-Hispanic whites: the Insulin Resistance Atherosclerosis Study. *Diabetes* 45:742–748, 1996

14. Faas A, Schellevis FG, Van Eijk JTM: The efficacy of self-monitoring of blood glucose in NIDDM subjects, a criteria-based literature review. *Diabetes Care* 20:1482–1486, 1997

15. Oki J, Flora DP, Isley WL: Frequency and impact of SMBG on glycemic control in patients with NIDDM in an urban teaching hospital clinic. *Diabetes Educ* 23:419–424, 1997

16. American Diabetes Association: *Diabetes 1996: Vital Statistics*. Alexandria, VA, American Diabetes Association, 1996

17. U.K. Prospective Diabetes Study Group: Intensive blood glucose control with sulfonylureas or insulin compared with conventional treatment and risk of complications in patients with type 2 diabetes (UKPDS 33). *Lancet* 352:837–853, 1998

18. Fertig BJ, Simmons DA, Martin DB: Therapy for diabetes. In *Diabetes in America*. 2nd ed. Harris MI, Cowie CC, Stern MP, Boyko EJ, Reiber GE, Bennett PH, Eds. Bethesda, MD, National Institutes of Health, National Institute of Diabetes and Digestive and Kidney Diseases, 1995 (NIH publ. no. 95-1468), pp. 519–540

19. Stolar M, Endocrine Fellows Foundation Study Group: Clinical management of the NIDDM patient. *Diabetes Care* 18:701–707, 1995

20. Franz MJ, Splett PL, Monk A, Berry B, McClain K, Weaver T, Upham P, Bergenstal R, Mazze RS: Cost-effectiveness of medical nutrition therapy provided by dietitians for persons with non-insulin-dependent diabetes mellitus. *J Am Diet Assoc* 95:1018–1024, 1995

21. Monk A, Barry B, McClain K, Weaver T, Cooper N, Franz MJ: Practice guidelines for medical nutrition therapy provided by dieti-

tians for persons with non-insulin-dependent diabetes mellitus. *J Am Diet Assoc* 95:999–1006, 1995

22. Henry RR, Schaefer L, Olefsky JM: Glycemic effects of intensive caloric restriction and isocaloric refeeding in noninsulin dependent diabetes mellitus. *J Clin Endocrinol Metab* 61:917–925, 1985

23. Wing RR, Blair EH, Bononi P, Marcus MD, Watanabe R, Bergman RN: Caloric restriction per se is a significant factor in improvements in glycemic control and insulin sensitivity during weight loss in obese NIDDM patients. *Diabetes Care* 17:30–36, 1994

24. Markovic TP, Jenkins AB, Campbell LV, Furlher SM, Kraegen EW, Chisholm DJ: The determinants of glycemic responses to diet restriction and weight loss in obesity and NIDDM. *Diabetes Care* 21:687–694, 1998

25. Lasko M, Usitupa M, Takala J, Majander H, Reijonen T, Penttila I: Effects of hypocaloric diet and insulin therapy on metabolic control and mechanisms of hyperglycemia in obese noninsulin dependent diabetic patients. *Metabolism* 37:1092–1100, 1988

26. Wing RR, Koeske R, Epstein LH, Nowalk MP, Gooding W, Becker D: Long-term effects of modest weight loss in type II diabetic patients. *Arch Intern Med* 147:1749–1753, 1987

27. Henry RR, Wallace P, Olefsky JM: Effects of weight loss on mechanisms of hyperglycemia in obese non-insulin-dependent diabetes mellitus. *Diabetes* 35:990–998, 1986

28. Nagulesparan M, Savage PJ, Bennion LJ, Unger RH, Bennett PH: Diminished effect of caloric restriction on control of hyperglycemia with increasing duration of type II diabetes mellitus. *J Clin Endocrinol Metab* 53:560–568, 1981

29. Carey DG, Jenkins AB, Campbell LV, Freund J, Chisholm DJ: Abdominal fat and insulin resistance in normal and overweight women: direct measurements reveal a strong relationship in subjects at both low and high risk of NIDDM. *Diabetes* 45:633–638, 1996

30. Watts NB, Spanheimer RG: Prediction of glucose response to weight loss in patients with non-insulin-dependent diabetes mellitus. *Arch Intern Med* 150:803–806, 1990

31. Marin P, Anderson B, Ottosson M, Olbe L, Chowdhury B, Kvist H, Holm G, Sjostrom L, Bjorntorp P: The morphology and metabolism of intraabdominal adipose tissue in men. *Metabolism* 41:1242–1248, 1992

32. Garg A, Bantle JP, Henry RR, Coulston AM, Griver KA, Raatz SK, Brinkley L, Chen Y-DI, Grundy SM, Huet BA, Reaven GM: Effects of varying carbohydrate content of the diet in patients with non-insulin-dependent diabetes mellitus. *JAMA* 271:1421–1428, 1994

33. Hollenbeck CB, Coulston AM: Effects of dietary carbohydrate and fat intake on glucose and lipoprotein metabolism in individuals with diabetes mellitus. *Diabetes Care* 14:774–785, 1991

34. Anderson JW, Gustafson NJ, Bryant CA, Tietyen-Clark J: Dietary fiber and diabetes: a comprehensive review and practical application. *J Am Diet Assoc* 87:1189–1197, 1987

35. Wadden TA, Stunkard AJ: Controlled trial of very low calorie diet, behavior therapy, and their combination in the treatment of obesity. *J Consult Clin Psychol* 54:482–488, 1986

36. Wing RR, Blair E, Marcus M: Year-long weight loss treatment for obese patients with type 2 diabetes: does inclusion of an intermittent very low calorie diet improve outcome? *Am J Med* 97:354–362, 1994

37. Williams K, Mullen M, Kelley D, Wing R: The effect of short periods of caloric restriction on weight loss and glycemic control in type 2 diabetes. *Diabetes Care* 21:2–8, 1998

38. St. Jeor ST: New trends in weight management. *J Am Diet Assoc* 97:1096–1098, 1997

39. Chen Y-D, Coulston AM, Zhou M-Y, Hollenbeck CB, Reaven GM: Why do low-fat high-carbohydrate diets accentuate postprandial lipemia in patients with NIDDM? *Diabetes Care* 18:10–16, 1995

40. Parillo M, Giacco R, Ciardullo AV, Rivellese AA, Riccardi G: Does a high-carbohydrate diet have different effects in NIDDM patients treated with diet alone or hypoglycemic drugs? *Diabetes Care* 19:498–500, 1996

41. Lissner L, Levitsky DA, Strupp BJ: Dietary fat and the regulation of energy intake in human subjects. *Am J Clin Nutr* 46:886–892, 1987

42. Shah M, Garg A: High-fat and high-carbohydrate diets and energy balance. *Diabetes Care* 19:1142–1152, 1996

43. Wolever T, Jenkins D, Vuskan V, Jenkins A, Wong G, Josse R: Beneficial effect of low-glycemic index diet in overweight NIDDM subjects. *Diabetes Care* 15:562–564, 1992

44. Cummings J, Englyst H: Gastrointestinal effects of food carbohydrate. *Am J Clin Nutr* 61:938S–945S, 1995

45. Jones PJH, Leitch CA, Pederson RA: Meal-frequency effects on plasma hormone concentrations and cholesterol synthesis in humans. *Am J Clin Nutr* 57:868–874, 1993

46. Jenkins DJ, Wolever TMS, Vuksan V: Nibbling versus gorging: metabolic advantages of increased meal frequency. *N Engl J Med* 321:929–934, 1989

47. Bertelsen J, Christiansen C, Thomsen C, Poulsen P, Vestergaard S, Steinov A, Rasmussen L, Rasmussen O, Hermansen K: Effect of meal frequency on blood glucose, insulin, and free fatty acids in NIDDM subjects. *Diabetes Care* 16:4–7, 1993

48. Beebe CA, Van Cauter E, Shapiro T, Tillel H, Lyons R, Rubenstein A, Polonsky K: Effect of temporal distribution of calories on diurnal patterns of glucose levels and insulin secretion in NIDDM. *Diabetes Care* 13:748–755, 1990

49. Arnold L, Mann J, Ball MJ: Metabolic effects of alterations in meal frequency in type 2 diabetes. *Diabetes Care* 20:1651–1654, 1997

50. Schneider SH, Amoroso LF, Khasdurian AK, Ruderman NB: Studies on the mechanism of improved glucose control during exercise in type 2 (noninsulin dependent) diabetes. *Diabetologia* 26:355–360, 1984

51. Bjorntorp P, DeJonge K, Sjostrom L, Sullivan L: The effect of physical training on insulin production in obesity. *Metabolism* 19:631–638, 1970

52. James SA, Jamjoum L, Raghunathan TE, Strogatz DS, Furth E, Khazanie PG: Physical activity and NIDDM in African-Americans. *Diabetes Care* 21:555–564, 1998

53. Mayer-Davis E, D'Agostino R, Karter A, Haffner S, Rewers M, Saad M, Bergman R: Intensity and amount of physical activity in relation to insulin sensitivity: the Insulin Resistance Atherosclerosis Study. *JAMA* 279:669–674, 1998

54. Yki-Jarvinen H, Kovisto VA: Effects of body composition on insulin sensitivity. *Diabetes* 32:965–969, 1983

55. Barnard RJ, Jung T, Inkeles SB: Diet and exercise in the treatment of NIDDM. *Diabetes Care* 17:1469–1472, 1994

56. American Diabetes Association: Diabetes mellitus and exercise (Position Statement). *Diabetes Care* 21:S40–S44, 1998

57. Bogardus C, Ravussin E, Robbins D: Effects of physical training and diet therapy on carbohydrate metabolism in patients with glu-

cose intolerance and non-insulin-dependent diabetes. *Diabetes* 33:311–317, 1984

58. U.S. Department of Health and Human Services, Centers for Disease Control and Prevention: *Physical Activity and Health: A Report of the Surgeon General.* Washington DC, U.S. Govt. Printing Office, 1996

59. National Diabetes Data Group: *Diabetes in America.* 2nd ed. Harris MI, Cowie CC, Stern MP, Boyko EJ, Reiber GE, Bennett PH, Eds. Bethesda, MD, National Institutes of Health, National Institute of Diabetes and Digestive and Kidney Diseases, 1995 (NIH publ. no. 95-1468)

60. Schoeller D, Shay K, Kushner R: How much physical activity is needed to minimize weight gain in previously obese women? *Am J Clin Nutr* 66:551–556, 1997

61. Barrett-Connor E, Grundy SM, Holdbrook JJ: Plasma lipids and diabetes mellitus in an adult community. *Am J Epidemiol* 115:657–663, 1982

62. Haffner SM: Management of dyslipidemia in adults with diabetes (Technical Review). *Diabetes Care* 21:160–178, 1998

63. Mensink RP, Katan MB: Effect of monounsaturated fatty acids versus complex carbohydrates on high-density lipoproteins in healthy men and women. *Lancet* i:122–125, 1987

64. Moses R, Shand J, Tapsell L: The recurrence of gestational diabetes: could dietary differences in fat intake be an explanation? *Diabetes Care* 20:1647–1650, 1997

Ms. Beebe is Director of the Center for Diabetes at St. James Hospital and Health Centers, Chicago Heights, IL.

5. Weight-Loss Treatments for Overweight Individuals with Type 2 Diabetes

JOHN P. BANTLE, MD

Highlights

- Most individuals with type 2 diabetes are overweight. Their increased adiposity aggravates insulin resistance and impairs glucose disposal. Because energy intake, energy balance, and thereby body weight are probably controlled by the central nervous system, when patients are asked to diet and lose weight, they are probably being asked to override a powerful biological control system.
- Standard weight-reduction diets are usually not effective. However, some people may achieve long-term weight loss with them. For these people, there is often a triggering event, such as a new medical diagnosis.
- Very-low-calorie diets can produce substantial weight loss. However, the weight loss usually is not maintained.
- Gastric-reduction surgery is the most effective weight-loss treatment for obese type 2 diabetic patients and should be considered in those with a BMI ≥ 35 kg/m^2. However, the efficacy and the safety of gastric-reduction surgery for type 2 diabetes have not been defined.
- Weight-loss drugs appear to be an important new avenue of treatment for obese patients with type 2 diabetes. However, the available drugs have limited efficacy. Moreover, long-term safety remains a concern. Additional weight-loss drugs should soon become available.

INTRODUCTION

Most individuals with type 2 diabetes are overweight. Approximately 36% have a BMI ≥30 kg/m^2 and can thus be classified as frankly obese (1). The prevalence of obesity is even higher in women and minorities with type 2 diabetes (1). As body adiposity increases in diabetic or nondiabetic subjects, so does insulin resistance (2–4). Body weight of 120% of ideal (BMI ~27 kg/m^2) appears to be the threshold at which insulin resistance begins to impair glucose disposal and thereby aggravate hyperglycemia (2). Obesity may also aggravate hyperlipidemia and hypertension in people with type 2 diabetes (5).

Because of the effects of obesity on insulin resistance, weight loss may be the single most important therapeutic objective for individuals with type 2 diabetes (6). Consistent with this, short-term studies lasting 6 months or less have demonstrated that weight loss in type 2 diabetic subjects is associated with decreased insulin resistance, improved glycemia, reduced serum lipids, and reduced blood pressure (7–9). However, long-term data assessing the extent to which these improvements can be maintained are not available. This is because no study has yet accomplished long-term weight loss in a group of carefully studied subjects with diabetes. Thus, weight-loss treatments available at present fall into one of two categories: the ineffective and the unproven.

The reason that long-term weight loss is difficult for most people to accomplish is probably because energy intake, energy balance, and thereby body weight are controlled by the central nervous system (10,11). When we ask overweight type 2 diabetic patients to diet and lose weight, we may be asking them to override by force of will a powerful biological control system. This is something most people simply cannot do.

Although understanding of central nervous system regulation of energy balance is incomplete, the hypothalamus appears to be the center of control. Neuropeptide Y is a peptide abundantly expressed in the hypothalamus that is a potent stimulator of food intake (12). Neuropeptide Y may also inhibit sympathetic nervous system activity and thereby lower energy expenditure. Leptin, a peptide produced in adipose tissue, inhibits hypothalamic neuropeptide Y (13). Serum leptin is increased in obese human subjects and is strongly correlated with body fat stores (14). Leptin may help define the extent of body fat stores for the brain and appears to exert negative feedback on neuropeptide Y and feeding behavior when body fat stores are high. Fasting serum insulin levels in nondiabetic subjects vary in proportion to body adiposity, suggesting that circulating insulin may also help define body fat stores. Thus, both leptin and insulin appear to be afferent signals that describe adipose stores for the brain.

Our preliminary understanding of the regulation of energy balance points out how much remains to be learned. Clearly there is a complicated and redundant control system. In addition to neuropeptide Y, leptin, and insulin, a variety of other neural, endocrine, and gastrointestinal signals are involved. A partial list of such signals includes corticotropin-releasing hormone, glucocorticoids, serotonin, triiodothyronine, and cholecystokinin. Effector systems such as uncoupling proteins and brown adipose tissue may also be important in energy dissipation.

General support for the concept of central nervous system regulation of energy metabolism, as described above, is provided by two distinct lines of evidence. First, in parabiosis experiments in rodents, the feeding behavior of one rodent inhibited feeding in the other member of the pair (15,16). This suggests that a circulating factor or factors crossed from the feeding rodent to the other rodent to inhibit feeding. Second, body weight and adipose stores tend to remain constant over long periods of time in virtually all adult mammalian species (10). This latter point might be underscored for each of us by comparing our weight today to our weight 1 year ago. Most of us will have experienced little change in body weight in spite of the fact that ~1 million calories passed our lips during that time. The idea that constant weight was maintained because of conscious decisions we made about what we ate is probably naive.

Individual characteristics of central nervous system control of energy metabolism appear to be genetically determined. For instance, in a remarkable study of Danish adoptees, there was a strong relationship between the BMIs of the adoptees and those of their biological parents and no relationship whatsoever between the BMIs of the adoptees and those of their adoptive parents (the people with whom they ate) (17). This study suggests in a powerful way that genetic factors have an important role in determining body fatness. Other data support this conclusion (18,19).

A hypothetical example of how energy balance might work in a given individual is provided in Table 5.1. A 50-year-old man with height 1.78 m, weight 98 kg, and BMI 30.9 kg/m² might have an average energy

---

Table 5.1 Hypothetical Example of How Energy Balance Might Work

50-year-old man
Height 1.78 m (70 inches)
Weight 98 kg (216 lb)
BMI 30.9 kg/m²
Average daily energy intake 2,800 calories

Compensatory mechanisms may allow weight maintenance as long as average daily energy intake falls between 2,400 and 3,200 calories.

intake of 2,800 calories daily. Compensatory mechanisms may allow him to maintain that weight as long as average daily energy intake falls between 2,400 and 3,200 calories. If he should develop type 2 diabetes and reduce average daily energy intake to 2,500 calories in an effort to lose weight, compensatory mechanisms, such as reduction in metabolic rate, decrease in spontaneous physical activity, and others not yet understood, would defeat weight loss. If he decreased average daily energy intake to 2,200 calories, compensatory mechanisms would no longer be able to sustain a weight of 98 kg and he would begin to lose weight. If, however, after several weeks his resolve lessened and he allowed average daily energy intake to increase to 2,500 calories, he would begin to regain weight and would return to his starting weight. Should he decide to increase his level of exercise and, for instance, walk 20 miles a week, the range of average daily energy intake that would allow him to maintain his weight might increase to 2,800–3,600 calories. This would facilitate weight loss with even a modest reduction in average daily energy intake. Moreover, with this level of habitual exercise, his hypothalamic control center might find it necessary to defend a lower body weight.

The available information thus suggests that obesity is caused by *1)* a defect in the hypothalamic control center or its biochemical signals (genetic obesity), *2)* caloric intake in excess of that for which the control center can compensate (environmental obesity), or *3)* some combination of these two factors. With this in mind, what should we recommend to our overweight type 2 diabetic patients? A list of treatment options is provided in Table 5.2.

Standard Weight-Reduction Diets

Standard weight-reduction diets provide 500–1,000 fewer calories than are estimated to be necessary for weight maintenance. Although many people can lose some weight (as much as 10% of initial weight) with such diets, the medical literature documents that long-term outcomes are usually poor (20–22). Most people regain most of the weight

---

Table 5.2 Weight-Loss Treatment Options

1. Standard weight-reduction diet
2. Very-low-calorie diet
3. Gastric-reduction surgery
4. Pharmacolgical therapy

they lose. However, standard weight-reduction diets might still be recommended for overweight patients with type 2 diabetes, since some people can lose weight with them and maintain the weight loss. Klem et al. (23) described a group of nearly 800 people who lost an average of 30 kg and maintained a minimum weight loss of 13.6 kg (30 lb) for 5 years. Slightly more than half lost weight through formal programs, whereas the remainder lost weight with a program of their own. Most of the people used both diet and exercise. Importantly, nearly 77% of this sample of people who were successful in achieving and maintaining weight loss reported a triggering event that preceded weight loss. The most common triggering events were medical conditions and emotional problems. Thus, a new diagnosis of type 2 diabetes could trigger lifestyle changes that would cause a patient to reduce energy intake, increase physical activity, or both and thereby lose weight.

When a person is dieting to lose weight, fat is probably the most important nutrient to restrict. Spontaneous food consumption and total energy intake are increased when the diet is high in fat and decreased when the diet is low in fat (24,25). Moreover, epidemiological studies have demonstrated that dietary fat intake is positively associated with adiposity and BMI (26,27). Simply reducing the fat content of the diet can result in reduced energy intake and therefore weight loss (25). For those people who have difficulty reducing the fat content of their diets, use of foods made with the nondigestible fat olestra can reduce available energy intake (28).

VERY-LOW-CALORIE DIETS

Very-low-calorie diets (VLCDs) provide 800 or fewer calories daily, primarily from high-quality protein and carbohydrate with mineral and vitamin supplementation. VLCDs can produce substantial weight loss and rapid improvements in glycemia and lipemia in patients with type 2 diabetes (29,30). Of note, reductions in glycemia occur before significant weight loss, suggesting that caloric restriction plays an important role in correcting hyperglycemia. Unfortunately, when VLCDs are stopped and food eaten in the usual way is reintroduced into the diet, recidivism is common (31,32). Most people treated with VLCDs are not able to maintain weight loss long term. Thus, VLCDs appear to have limited utility in the treatment of type 2 diabetes.

An interesting possibility is that VLCDs could be used repetitively to treat overweight type 2 diabetic patients. However, only limited data about this treatment approach are available. A study by Smith and Wing (33) found that a second application of VLCD was not as effective as the first application because of reduced subject compliance. Intermittent use of VLCD therapy has been proposed by Williams et al. (34). In a 20-week study, they reported a 9.6-kg weight loss using a VLCD 1 day/week and a 10.4-kg weight loss using a VLCD 5 days/week once every 5 weeks. The drops in fasting plasma glucose and HbA_{1c} were comparable between the two groups and were greater than those in the standard behavior therapy group, in which subjects lost 5.4 kg.

GASTRIC-REDUCTION SURGERY

At present, the most effective weight-loss treatment for obese type 2 diabetic patients is gastric-reduction surgery. However, a National Institutes of Health Consensus Development Panel recommended that such surgery be considered only in type 2 diabetic patients with BMIs ≥35 kg/m² (35). Most patients who meet this criterion will be at least 40 kg overweight. The two surgical procedures most widely used are vertical banded gastroplasty and gastric bypass (Figure 5.1) (36). Both procedures involve creation of a small (25- to 50-ml) gastric pouch to receive food. This small pouch permits consumption of small meals without epigastric pain or vomiting. Larger meals cause pain and vomiting. Although

Vertical Banded Gastroplasty   **Gastric Bypass**

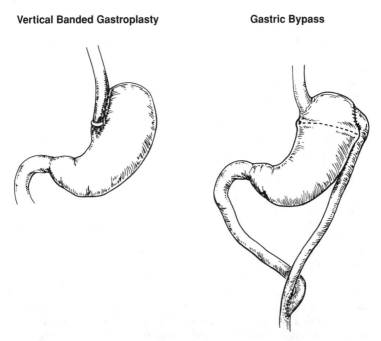

Figure 5.1 Surgical procedures used for weight loss.

weight loss may be greater with gastric bypass, the proximal small intestine is bypassed and malabsorption of certain nutrients such as iron and vitamin B_{12} can be expected. Vertical banded gastroplasty does not bypass any portion of the gastrointestinal tract and is thus less likely to produce malabsorption. For this reason, vertical banded gastroplasty may be preferable to gastric bypass.

In a series of 70 obese patients treated with vertical banded gastroplasty, median weight losses 1 and 3 years after surgery were 37 and 32 kg, respectively (37). In a large series of 515 obese patients treated with gastric bypass, mean weight losses at 1 and 3 years were 50 and 45 kg, respectively (38). Moreover, weight loss was well maintained in 44 patients who achieved 10 years of follow-up. A subgroup of 137 patients in this study had type 2 diabetes. Of these 137 diabetic patients, 107 (78%) experienced "clinical remission" of their diabetes. How long the remissions were maintained, however, was not reported.

Potential adverse effects of gastric-reduction surgery include perioperative mortality in 1–2% of patients, vitamin and mineral deficiencies, cholelithiasis, inability to eat certain foods (particularly meats, untoasted breads, and raw fruits), and persistent vomiting (36–38). Prophylactic treatment with ursodiol may prevent gallstone formation (39). Unfortunately, there are no data comparing medical and surgical treatments of obese type 2 diabetic patients. In the absence of data defining benefits and risks, gastric-reduction surgery probably should be considered unproven and experimental. Nevertheless, gastric-reduction surgery may be an attractive treatment option for some type 2 diabetic patients. It can produce substantial weight loss and thereby normalize glycemia without medication. Lipemia and blood pressure are also favorably influenced.

PHARMACOLOGICAL THERAPY

If energy balance is regulated by a hypothalamic control center that produces and responds to biochemical signals, it might be possible to influence the control center pharmacologically. This possibility first received widespread attention with the publication of a landmark study by Weintraub (40). In this study, a complex 4-year protocol was used to evaluate the ability of the drugs fenfluramine and phentermine to produce weight loss. The most important part of the study was a 34-week randomized, double-blind clinical trial comparing fenfluramine (60 mg daily) and phentermine (15 mg daily) to placebos in 112 participants ranging from 130 to 180% of ideal body weight. In addition to fenfluramine and phentermine or placebos, all subjects were asked to follow reduced-calorie diets and to exercise regularly. Mean weight loss at 34 weeks in the drug-treatment group was 14.3 kg and in the placebo group was 4.6 kg

($P < 0.001$). When fenfluramine and phentermine were discontinued, most subjects in the drug-treatment group rapidly regained weight.

Fenfluramine is a serotonergic sympathomimetic amine. Its mechanism of action appears to be appetite suppression. Phentermine is a noradrenergic sympathomimetic amine. Its mechanism of action may be appetite suppression or, perhaps, stimulation of metabolic rate. When the Weintraub study was published in 1992, it initiated a stampede in the U.S. to use fenfluramine and phentermine (fen-phen) for weight loss. It was estimated that in 1996 the total number of prescriptions written in the U.S. for fenfluramine and phentermine exceeded 18 million (41). The stampede came to an abrupt halt in 1997, when an association between fenfluramine usage and valvular heart disease was demonstrated (41). In September 1997, fenfluramine was voluntarily withdrawn from the U.S. market by its manufacturer. Dexfenfluramine, the dextroenantiomar of fenfluramine, was also withdrawn from the U.S. market.

Although fenfluramine and phentermine produced significant weight loss and were widely used in the U.S., only limited information about their effects on patients with type 2 diabetes is available. Treatment of type 2 diabetic patients with dexfenfluramine or placebo has been compared in four clinical trials, each lasting for 3 months (42–45). All four trials showed that dexfenfluramine produced greater weight loss than did placebo and led to significant reductions in HbA_{1c}. A clinical trial comparing phentermine to placebo in type 2 diabetic patients demonstrated significantly more weight loss with phentermine, but no significant reduction in glycemia or glycosuria (46).

In 1996, we at the University of Minnesota initiated a randomized, double-blind, placebo-controlled trial of fenfluramine and phentermine as treatment for overweight patients with type 2 diabetes. Forty-four type 2 diabetic patients were enrolled and randomly assigned to fenfluramine and phentermine or dual placebos. All participants received instruction in a hypocaloric diet, behavior modification techniques, and an exercise program. When fenfluramine was withdrawn from the U.S. market in September 1997, all subjects were unmasked and those taking fenfluramine discontinued it. Data from the last study visit before subjects were unmasked are presented in Table 5.3. At 2, 4, and 6 months of treatment, fenfluramine and phentermine produced significantly greater reductions than did placebo in body weight, BMI, and HbA_{1c}. Whether these beneficial effects could be maintained was not clear because few subjects reached 8 months or more of treatment and the study had little power to detect treatment differences at these later time points. Nevertheless, the study suggested that weight-loss drugs could be a powerful treatment for type 2 diabetes.

With the withdrawal of fenfluramine and dexfenfluramine, only a limited number of weight-loss drugs remain available in the U.S. These are listed in Table 5.4. Phentermine continues to be available, but appears

Table 5.3 Change from Baseline in Placebo and Fenfluramine-Phentermine–Treated Type 2 Diabetic Patients

	2 months	4 months	6 months
Number of subjects			
Placebo group	18	17	13
Drug group	21	17	13
Body weight (kg)			
Placebo group	−1.6 ± 0.5	−1.9 ± 0.9	−2.7 ± 1.4
Drug group	−7.9 ± 1.2	−10.3 ± 1.7	−9.6 ± 1.5
P value	<0.001	<0.001	0.003
BMI (kg/m²)			
Placebo group	−0.5 ± 0.2	−0.7 ± 0.3	−0.8 ± 0.5
Drug group	−2.5 ± 0.4	−3.2 ± 0.5	−3.2 ± 0.5
P value	<0.001	<0.001	0.003
Fasting plasma glucose (mg/dl)			
Placebo group	−12 ± 6	3 ± 15	−11 ± 14
Drug group	−71 ± 9	−54 ± 12	−47 ± 13
P value	<0.001	0.005	0.074
HbA$_{1c}$ (%)			
Placebo group	−0.4 ± 0.1	−0.5 ± 0.3	−0.3 ± 0.2
Drug group	−1.7 ± 0.2	−1.9 ± 0.3	−1.6 ± 0.3
P value	<0.001	<0.001	0.002

Data are means ± SE.

to have limited efficacy when used as a single agent. Sibutramine suppresses appetite by inhibiting reuptake of serotonin and norepinephrine in the central nervous system. In a double-blind, placebo-controlled study of obese patients treated with sibutramine, mean weight loss at 1 year for study completers was a somewhat disappointing 6.9 kg. No published data are yet available about the use of sibutramine in patients with type 2 diabetes. Orlistat is a drug that inhibits pancreatic lipase and thus has a different mechanism of action from the other drugs presently available. In a 1-year randomized, double-blind, placebo-controlled study comparing orlistat to placebo in type 2 diabetic patients, the orlistat group lost 6.2% of initial body weight, as compared with a 4.3% loss with placebo (*P* < 0.001) (47). In the orlistat group, HbA$_{1c}$ decreased by 0.28%, whereas there was a 0.18% increase in the placebo group (*P* < 0.001). Although the difference in HbA$_{1c}$ between the two groups was modest, more patients in the orlistat group required a reduction in hypoglycemic medications. Thus, orlistat may have a more potent effect on HbA$_{1c}$ than these data suggest. At the time this chapter was written, orlistat had not yet been approved by the U.S. Food and Drug Administration.

Table 5.4 Weight-Loss Drugs

Drug	Mechanism of Action	FDA Labeling
Phentermine	Nonadrenergic; appetite suppression and/or stimulation of metabolic rate	Short-term usage
Sibutramine	Serotonin and norepinephrine reuptake inhibitor; appetite suppression	Safety and effectiveness beyond 1 year not determined
Orlistat (approval pending)	Inhibition of pancreatic lipase; partial malabsorption of fat	Not yet determined

The available data suggest that weight-loss drugs are an important new approach to the treatment of overweight patients with type 2 diabetes. The data also suggest that these drugs work only as long as they are taken; that is, like antihypertensive and antihyperlipidemic medications, these drugs must be continued to maintain any beneficial effect. Fenfluramine is probably the most potent of the present weight-loss drugs, but it is no longer available in the U.S. because of its association with valvular heart disease. Only limited data are available about the efficacy and safety of phentermine, sibutramine, and orlistat. Thus, the use of these drugs to treat type 2 diabetes is unproven and should be considered experimental. However, for those type 2 diabetic patients who understand the issues, use of these drugs is probably acceptable. As we learn more about the regulation of energy balance, new and potentially more potent drugs should become available.

REFERENCES

1. Cowie CC, Harris MI: Physical and metabolic characteristics of persons with diabetes. In *Diabetes in America*. 2nd ed. Harris MI, Cowie CC, Stern MP, Boyko EJ, Reiber GE, Bennett PH, Eds. Bethesda, MD, National Institutes of Health, National Institute of Diabetes and Digestive and Kidney Diseases, 1995 (NIH publ. no. 95-1468), pp. 117–164

2. Campbell PJ, Gerich JE: Impact of obesity on insulin action in volunteers with normal glucose tolerance: demonstration of a threshold for adverse effect of obesity. *J Clin Endocrinol Metab* 70:1114–1118, 1990

3. Olefsky JM, Kalterman OG, Scarlett JA: Insulin action and resistance in obesity and non insulin-dependent diabetes mellitus. *Am J Physiol* 243:E15–E30, 1982

4. Campbell PJ, Carlson MG: Impact of obesity on insulin action in NIDDM. *Diabetes* 42:405–410, 1993

5. Maggio CA, Pi-Sunyer FX: The prevention and treatment of obesity: application to type 2 diabetes. *Diabetes Care* 20:1744–1766, 1997

6. Consensus Development Panel: Consensus development conference on diet and exercise in non-insulin-dependent diabetes mellitus. *Diabetes Care* 10:639–644, 1987

7. Hughes TA, Gwynne JT, Switzer BR, Herbst C, White G: Effects of caloric restriction and weight loss on glycemic control, insulin release and resistance, and atherosclerotic risk in obese patients with type II diabetes mellitus. *Am J Med* 77:7–17, 1984

8. Henry RR, Wiest-Kent A, Scheaffer L, Kolterman OG, Olefsky JM: Metabolic consequences of very-low-calorie diet therapy in obese non-insulin-dependent diabetic and nondiabetic subjects. *Diabetes* 35:155–164, 1986

9. Amatruda JM, Richeson JF, Welle SL, Brodows RG, Lockwood DH: The safety and efficacy of a controlled low energy (very-low-calorie) diet in the treatment of non-insulin dependent diabetes and obesity. *Arch Intern Med* 148:873–877, 1988

10. Schwartz MW, Seeley RJ: The new biology of body weight regulation. *J Am Diet Assoc* 97:54–58, 1997

11. Rosenbaum M, Leibel RL, Hirsch J: Obesity. *N Engl J Med* 337:396–407, 1997

12. Schwart MW, Seely RJ: Neuroendocrine responses to starvation and weight loss. *N Engl J Med* 336:1802–1811, 1997

13. Caro JF, Sinha MK, Kolaczynski JW, Zhang PL, Considine RV: Leptin: the tale of an obesity gene. *Diabetes* 45:1455–1462, 1996

14. Considine RV, Sinha MK, Heiman ML, Kriauciunas A, Stephens TW, Nyce MR, Ohannesian JP, Marco CC, McKee LJ, Bauer TL, Caro JF: Serum immunoreactive-leptin concentrations in normal-weight and obese humans. *N Engl J Med* 334:292–295, 1996

15. Coleman DL: Effects of parabiosis of obese with diabetes and normal mice. *Diabetologia* 9:294–298, 1973

16. Koopman HS: Internal signals cause large changes in food intake in one-way crossed intestine rats. *Brain Res Bull* 14:595–603, 1985

17. Stunkard AJ, Sorensen TIA, Hanis C, Teasdale TW, Chakraborty R, Schull WJ, Schulsinger F: An adoption study of human obesity. *N Engl J Med* 314:193–198, 1986

18. Bouchard C, Tremblay A, Despres, JP, Nadeau, Lupien PJ, Theriault G, Dussault J, Moorjani S, Pinault S, Fournier G: The response to long-term overfeeding in identical twins. *N Engl J Med* 322:1477–1482, 1990

19. Stunkard AJ, Harris JR, Pedersen NL, McClearn GE: The body mass index of twins who have been reared apart. *N Engl J Med* 322:1483–1487, 1990

20. Stunkard A, McLaren-Hume M: The results of treatment for obesity. *Arch Intern Med* 103:79–85, 1959

21. Fitzgerald FT: The problem of obesity. *Ann Rev Med* 32:221–231, 1981

22. NIH Technology Assessment Conference Panel: Methods for voluntary weight loss and control. *Ann Intern Med* 116:942–949, 1992

23. Klem ML, Wing RR, McGuire MT, Seagle HM, Hill JO: A descriptive study of individuals successful at long-term maintenance of substantial weight loss. *Am J Clin Nutr* 66:239–246, 1997

24. Lissner L, Levitsky DA, Strupp BJ, Kalkwarf HJ, Roe DA: Dietary fat and the regulation of energy intake in human subjects. *Am J Clin Nutr* 46:886–892, 1987

25. Kendall A, Levitsky DA, Strupp BJ, Lissner L: Weight loss on a low-fat diet: consequence of the imprecision of the control of food intake in humans. *Am J Clin Nutr* 53:1124–1129, 1991

26. Tucker LA, Kano MJ: Dietary fat and body fat: a multivariate study of 205 adult females. *Am J Clin Nutr* 56:612–622, 1992

27. Westsrate JA: Fat and obesity. *Int J Obesity* 19 (Suppl.):S38–S43, 1995

28. Hill JO, Seagle HM, Johnson SL, Smith S, Reed GW, Tran ZV, Cooper D, Stone M, Peters JC: Effects of 14 d covert substitution of olestra for conventional fat on spontaneous food intake. *Am J Clin Nutr* 67:1178–1185, 1998

29. Henry RR, Weist-Kent TA, Scheaffer L, Kolterman OG, Olefsky JM: Metabolic consequences of very-low-calorie diet therapy in obese non-insulin-dependent diabetic and nondiabetic subjects. *Diabetes* 35:155–164, 1986

30. Wing RR, Marcus MD, Salata R, Epstein LH, Miaskiewicz S, Blair EE: Effects of a very low calorie diet on long-term glycemic control

in obese type 2 diabetic subjects. *Arch Intern Med* 151:1334–1340, 1991

31. Henry RR, Gumbiner B: Benefits and limitations of very-low-calorie diet therapy in obese NIDDM. *Diabetes Care* 14:802–823, 1991

32. Wing RR: Use of very-low-calorie diets in the treatment of obese persons with non-insulin dependent diabetes mellitus. *J Am Diet Assoc* 95:569–572, 1995

33. Smith DE, Wing RR: Diminished weight loss and behavioral compliance during repeated diets in obese patients with type II diabetes. *Health Psychol* 10:378–383, 1991

34. Williams KV, Mullen ML, Kelley DE, Wing RR: The effect of short periods of caloric restriction on weight loss and glycemic control in type 2 diabetes. *Diabetes Care* 21:2–15, 1998

35. Consensus Development Conference Panel: Gastrointestinal surgery for severe obesity. *Ann Intern Med* 115:956–961, 1991

36. Gastric operations for obesity. *Med Lett Drugs Ther* 26:113–115, 1984

37. Nightengale ML, Sarr, MG, Kelly KA, Jensen MD, Zinsmeister AR, Palumbo PJ: Prospective evaluation of vertical banded gastroplasty as the primary operation for morbid obesity. *Mayo Clin Proc* 66:773–782, 1991

38. Pories WJ, MacDonald KG, Flickinger EG, Dohm GL, Sinha MK, Barakat HA, May HJ, Khazanie P, Swanson MS, Morgan E, Leggett-Frazier N, Long SD, Brown BM, O'Brien K, Caro JF: Is type II diabetes mellitus (NIDDM) a surgical disease? *Ann Surg* 633–643, 1992

39. Sugerman HJ, Brewer WH, Shiffman ML, Brolin RE, Fobi MAL, Linner JH, MaDonald KG, MacGregor AM, Martin LF, Oram-Smith JC, Popoola D, Schirmer BD, Vickers FF: A multicenter, placebo-controlled, randomized, double-blind, prospective trial of prophylactic ursodiol for the prevention of gallstone formation following gastric-bypass-induced rapid weight loss. *Am J Surg* 169:91–97, 1995

40. Weintraub M: Long-term weight control: the National Heart, Lung, and Blood Institute multimodal intervention study. *Clin Parmacol Ther* 51:586–646, 1992

41. Connolly HM, Crary JL, McGoon MD, Hensrud DD, Edwards BS, Edwards WD, Schaff HV: Valvular heart disease associated with fenfluramine-phentermine. *N Engl J Med* 337:581–588, 1997

42. Willey KA, Molyneaux LM, Overland JE, Yue DK: The effects of dexfenfluramine on blood glucose control in patients with type 2 diabetes. *Diabetic Med* 9:341–343, 1992

43. Stewart GO, Stein GR, Davis TME, Findlater P: Dexfenfluramine in type II diabetes: effect on weight and diabetes control. *Med J Aust* 158:167–169, 1993

44. Willey KA, Molyneaux LM, Yue DK: Obese patients with type 2 diabetes poorly controlled by insulin and metformin: effects of adjunctive dexfenfluramine therapy on glycaemic control. *Diabetic Med* 11:701–704, 1994

45. Chow C-C, Ko GTC, Tsang LWW, Yeung VTF, Chan JCN, Cockram CS: Dexfenfluramine in obese Chinese NIDDM patients. *Diabetes Care* 20:1122–1127, 1997

46. Campbell CJ, Bhalla IP, Steel JM, Duncan LJP: A controlled trial of phentermine in obese diabetic patients. *The Practitioner* 218:851–855, 1977

47. Hollander PA, Elbein SC, Hirsch IB, Kelley D, McGill J, Taylor T, Weiss SR, Crockett SE, Kaplan RA, Comstock J, Lucas CP, Lodewick PA, Canovatchel W, Chung J, Hauptman J: Role of orlistat in the treatment of obese patients with type 2 diabetes: a 1-year randomized double-blind study. *Diabetes Care* 21:1288–1294, 1998

Dr. Bantle is Professor of Medicine, Division of Endocrinology and Diabetes, at the University of Minnesota Medical School, Minneapolis, MN.

Nutrition Issues Related to Glucose and Lipid Goals/Outcomes

6. Carbohydrates and Diabetes

FRANK Q. NUTTALL, MD, PhD, AND MARY C. GANNON, PhD

Highlights

- The amount of glucose absorbed from a meal largely determines the blood glucose response. However, the response will be modified by gastric emptying rate, intestinal motility, and factors that affect glucose removal from the circulation, such as the insulin response, insulin resistance, etc.
- The starch in foods is composed exclusively of glucose molecules. Thus, starchy foods will raise the blood glucose concentration. Generally, the rise will be greater than when sucrose, fruits, or milk is ingested. Nevertheless, the increase in blood glucose will depend on the rate and completeness of digestion of the starch in a food, which is influenced by many factors.
- Fructose and galactose (e.g., from sucrose, fruits, and milk) have only a minimal effect on blood glucose in normal people or people with type 2 diabetes. With severe insulin deficiency, the response may be greater.
- From a clinical perspective, helping people with diabetes understand the total carbohydrate content of foods and the likely effects of specific carbohydrates on blood glucose and insulin levels should prove useful.
- Currently, there is no evidence to suggest that the percentage of calories from carbohydrate in the diet of people with diabetes should be any different from that in the diet of other family members or their cultural group.

INTRODUCTION

In England in 1776, Dodson reported that the sweet taste of urine from people with diabetes was due to the presence of glucose. This observation indicated an abnormality in carbohydrate metabolism in diabetes mellitus. Dodson also clearly demonstrated an excessive production of glucose in people with diabetes. Subsequently, a high-carbohydrate diet was noted to increase glucosuria, whereas glucosuria was diminished or even eliminated by a low-carbohydrate diet (methods for measuring blood glucose did not become available until about 1917). This observation suggested that another abnormality in diabetes was the inability to store or utilize ingested carbohydrates rapidly.

Whether the major abnormality in people with diabetes was an overproduction of glucose from endogenous noncarbohydrate sources, such as protein or glycerol, or an impaired utilization of ingested carbohydrates was vigorously debated by diabetologists until the early part of this century. It now is known that both abnormalities are present. With increasing degrees of insulin insufficiency, both become more severe (1).

Overproduction of glucose is the predominant and life-threatening problem in people with poorly controlled diabetes. However, an inability to rapidly clear ingested glucose from the circulation is considered to be the earliest diagnostic manifestation of the various syndromes lumped together and phenotypically referred to as "diabetes."

Before the availability of insulin and other pharmaceutical agents, both glucose overproduction and the impaired ability to metabolize absorbed glucose were shown to be treatable by dietary manipulations. Early physicians clearly demonstrated that glucose overproduction could be controlled by starvation or by a semi-starvation (low-calorie) diet. They also observed that the amount of glucose derived from the diet that could be metabolized, i.e., did not cause glucose to appear in the urine, depended on the severity of the diabetes. Thus, they would tailor the amount of carbohydrate (primarily starch-containing foods) to the individual's ability to utilize it. This was done by substitution of fats and, less commonly, foods high in protein (meats) for carbohydrate-containing foods. These dietary manipulations were quite effective. However, as expected, compliance was a serious problem, and people could not live indefinitely on a semi-starvation diet. Of some interest, we have more recently shown that the plasma glucose concentration can be normalized with starvation lasting less than 24 h in people with moderately severe, untreated type 2 diabetes (2). A review of published data on very-short-term starvation indicates that a decrease in glucose concentration of ~20–40% can be expected in people with type 2 diabetes, regardless of the initial blood glucose concentration and without significant weight loss

(2). This indicates the extreme sensitivity of glucose overproduction by the liver to an adequate dietary fuel supply.

Since the availability of insulin and oral agents for the treatment of diabetes, food energy restriction and limitation in carbohydrate content of the diet have generally been considered not to be necessary. In fact, there has been a trend toward advocating a higher and higher carbohydrate content in the diet, not only for people with diabetes, but also for the population at large. Foods containing complex carbohydrates (presumably starch) are being emphasized (cereal grains, etc.) (3–5). An increase in carbohydrate intake would result in a decrease in fat intake, since the protein content of the diet is relatively constant. Thus, the high-carbohydrate recommendation is being driven by the concern that dietary fat is pathogenetically important in the development of atherosclerosis and in turn the development of coronary heart disease in most people. The amount of saturated fatty acids is of particular concern. In the nondiabetic population there are epidemiological data to support this hypothesis, but it has been difficult to demonstrate in prospective studies (6).

Whether the general population actually benefits from a high-carbohydrate, low-fat diet is uncertain and is currently being debated (7,8). Whether such a diet benefits a diabetic population is also uncertain (9). A case for a relatively high-fat (40–45% of food energy) diet in which monounsaturated and polyunsaturated fatty acids are emphasized can be made. The lipid profile is improved and the increase in mono- and polyunsaturated fatty acids does not appear to affect disposal of a glucose load (insulin resistance is unchanged) (10). In addition, the amount of ingested glucose requiring disposition is reduced. As indicated above, a cardinal manifestation of diabetes is an impaired ability to clear absorbed glucose from the blood rapidly. As a consequence, the post-meal rise in glucose concentration is greater and, perhaps more importantly, is more sustained. Thus, the load of glucose derived from a meal and requiring disposition will have a major effect on the 24-h integrated glucose concentration.

That an elevated glucose concentration integrated over several years is pathogenetically important in the development of the microvascular and neuropathic complications of diabetes in people with type 1 diabetes and in people with type 2 diabetes is now generally accepted (11,12).

There is concern that a higher-fat diet will promote obesity (13). However, this is also a contentious issue (10) and requires further research.

Cardiovascular disease is more common in people with diabetes. The reason for this is uncertain. In people with type 2 diabetes, current evidence based on epidemiological data and prospective studies in which the triglyceride-lowering agent gemfibrozil (14) or HMG-CoA reductase inhibition by so-called statin drugs was used to lower cholesterol synthesis (15,16) suggests that an associated dyslipidemia is playing a significant role in the development of coronary heart disease. However, it is becoming increasingly clear that coronary heart disease is a multifactorial disease with a significant genetic component (17).

Whether a chronically elevated glucose concentration contributes to cardiovascular disease, particularly coronary heart disease, is at present uncertain (18,19). Nevertheless, it is a reasonable expectation. In any case, because a high glucose concentration results in the development of the microvascular complications of diabetes (11,12), a diet that both improves glucose concentration and results in an improved lipid profile would be ideal, at least theoretically. This may be accomplished by increasing the fat content of the diet without a corresponding increase in saturated fatty acids and by selecting carbohydrate-containing foods that reduce the rate and amount of absorbed glucose requiring metabolic disposition. This goal also may be accomplished by increasing the protein content of the diet (see chapter 7 on protein and diabetes) or by combining all three approaches.

Because carbohydrates have been emphasized in the diet for people with diabetes and not all carbohydrate-containing foods affect the blood glucose concentration to a similar degree, it is important to understand the structure of the various dietary carbohydrates, how they are affected by food preparation, their metabolism, and their possible interaction with other food substances.

DIETARY CARBOHYDRATES

In this chapter, we discuss briefly the structure, digestion, metabolism, and blood glucose response to the ingestion of digestible and nondigestible carbohydrates in people eating a weight-maintenance, typical Western European or American diet.

Through better understanding of the structure, digestion, and metabolism of the various dietary carbohydrates, one can largely predict their effects on blood glucose concentration, at least when ingested independently. We will focus primarily on data obtained in nondiabetic people and in people with type 2 diabetes. There is little scientific data available on the effects of various carbohydrate-containing foods in people with type 1 diabetes. They are difficult to study because of the variability in adequacy of insulin replacement. The latter will affect the metabolic response to foods. In well-insulinized individuals, the response may approach normal. However, in individuals treated with insulin, it should be understood that the insulin enters the circulation from under the skin rather than being secreted from the pancreas into the portal vein. Thus, even under the best of circumstances, cells in peripheral organs will be relatively overinsulinized. The most important peripheral organs in regard to fuel metabolism are skeletal muscle and adipose tissue. The liver, through which all of the portal blood must pass, will be under-insulinized.

Normally the insulin concentration entering the liver is twofold or greater than that in the peripheral circulation. Thus, the balance between an insulin-stimulated decrease in glucose production by the liver and an insulin stimulation of glucose uptake by skeletal muscle is disrupted when insulin is injected under the skin.

The circulating fatty acid concentration depends principally on the rate at which the fatty acids are released from the adipose cells. This is regulated by the insulin concentration. An increase in insulin inhibits fatty acid release, which results in a lower circulating fatty acid concentration. With a low fatty acid concentration, some organs will switch from a fatty acid–based fuel to glucose. The output of glucose by the liver is also determined in part by the fatty acid concentration (20). Thus, the normal functioning of this regulatory system will be disrupted when insulin is injected under the skin.

In this discussion, we specifically avoid the terms "complex" and "simple" carbohydrates. As indicated previously, these terms have never been defined (21). They are imprecise and confusing. To improve communication and understanding of the metabolic consequences of carbohydrate ingestion, they should be abandoned. Instead, dietary carbohydrates should be referred to by the names indicated below.

At a minimum, the mono- and disaccharides should be referred to as "sugars." The polysaccharides should be referred to as "starch" or "fiber," respectively. Nondigestible carbohydrate components of plants are commonly referred to as food fiber; more properly, they should be referred to as nonstarch polysaccharides. Of the major nondigestible structural components of plants, only lignin is not a polysaccharide, i.e., is not a carbohydrate.

Classification and Structure of Carbohydrates

The carbohydrates quantitatively most important in human nutrition are the monosaccharides, glucose and fructose; the disaccharides, sucrose and lactose; and the polysaccharides, starch and the nonstarch polysaccharides (fiber) (Table 6.1).

Sucrose (table sugar) is composed of a molecule of glucose attached to a molecule of fructose through the anomeric carbon atom of each. Lactose is composed of a molecule of glucose attached to a molecule of galactose through a β-1,4 bond. Starch is a long-chain polymer of glucose molecules in α-1,4 linkages. It is composed of a mixture of two polymers, a highly branched polymer referred to as amylopectin and a helical polymer referred to as amylose. The ratio of amylopectin to amylose is most commonly ~70:30, but it varies considerably in starch from different plant

Table 6.1 Classification and Structure of Carbohydrates

Monosaccharides	Disaccharides	Polysaccharides
Glucose	Sucrose (glucose + fructose)	Starch (amylopectin + amylose)
Fructose	Lactose (glucose + galactose)	Nonstarch polysaccharides (fiber)

sources. Amylose is poorly soluble in water and is difficult to digest. Amylopectin is readily digestible. The starch molecules also may be derivatized with phosphate or other compounds.

Free glucose and fructose as well as sucrose are common natural constituents of fruits and some vegetables. In fruits and fruit juices (and soft drinks), the total sugar content is generally about 10% by weight. However, in some grapes it is considerably higher (up to 22%). In dried fruits such as raisins, figs, and dates, the total sugar content is often as high as 50–70% by weight. Most commonly, the sugar present in fruits is sucrose or its equivalent, i.e., an approximately equal molar ratio of glucose and fructose. In vegetables, the sugar content varies but rarely exceeds 5–8%.

Traditionally it was taught that refined sucrose (table sugar) should be eliminated from the diets of people with diabetes. The scientific rationale for this was never defined (1). More recently, evidence has been developed indicating that amounts of sucrose typically found in the American diet are not likely to be harmful (22,23) or to affect blood glucose control adversely (1).

The so-called high-fructose corn syrups that are being widely used in the food industry are not extraordinarily high in fructose. Generally they are composed of 42% fructose and 53% glucose, or 55% fructose and 42% glucose. The remainder is composed of higher starch-derived saccharides (24). That is, the ratio of glucose to fructose resembles that of sucrose. Indeed, these syrups are used as sweetening agents in replacement of sucrose because they are less expensive in the U.S. because of tariffs on imported sugar (sucrose). Regular corn syrup is composed of hydrolyzed starch. It is composed mostly of glucose and glucose polymers (dextrins) and is excellent for treating hypoglycemic reactions (25).

Lactose is present only in milk and milk products. It often is referred to as "milk sugar." In cow's milk, the lactose content is ~5% by weight.

Starch is present in cereal grains, tubers (potato, cassava, etc.), legumes (peas, beans, and lentils), and some fruits, such as bananas. In cereal grains and cereal grain products, the starch content varies but is usually in the range of 70–100% by weight. In potatoes and legumes, the starch content is ~20–25%. In bananas, the starch content varies with ripeness. When the banana is green, starch makes up 25% by weight of the edible portion (minus the skin). As the banana ripens, this is converted into sugars. Starch is quantitatively the single most important nutrient throughout the world.

In a typical Western diet, it can be calculated that after digestion the proportion of absorbed monosaccharides would be ~75% glucose, ~22% fructose, and ~3% galactose. Thus, the major (70–80%) absorbed carbohydrate that will require metabolic disposition is glucose, either as such or as that derived from sucrose, lactose, or starch (26).

Carbohydrate Digestion

Sucrose is hydrolyzed by a sucrase enzyme present in the brush border of the mucosa of the duodenum and jejunum. Normally, this enzyme is present in excess. As a consequence, the rate-limiting step is not the hydrolysis of the sucrose but rather the rate at which the resulting glucose and fructose can be absorbed.

Lactose is hydrolyzed by a lactase enzyme also present in the brush border of the upper intestinal mucosa. In infants, the enzyme is present in large amounts. However, at the end of infancy, this diminishes. In adults, there is considerable uncertainty regarding the amount of enzyme present. In Northern Europeans and Northern European immigrants to North America, an amount of enzyme sufficient to prevent lactose malabsorption is usually present. Whether hydrolysis of lactose or absorption of glucose and galactose products is rate limiting probably depends on the amount of lactose ingested. With the usual amounts of milk consumed, hydrolysis does not appear to be limiting. In other ethnic groups, this may not be the case (27,28).

Ingested starch is hydrolyzed into its constituent glucose molecules by a combination of pancreatic amylase and intestinal mucosal glucosidase and maltase enzymes. These enzymes are present in excess. Thus, theoretically, the rate-limiting process should not be the rate at which starch is hydrolyzed but rather the rate at which the resulting glucose is absorbed. However, it was shown many years ago that uncooked corn starch is poorly digestible and results in only a small increase in blood glucose, whereas cooked starch is very readily hydrolyzed and as a consequence results in a very rapid and large rise in the circulating glucose concentration (29). Subsequently, it was reported that uncooked potato and banana starches are also poorly digestible, but that when cooked, they are readily digestible (30). These results clearly indicate that the physical state of the starch has a large effect on its digestibility.

Starch is present in plants in the form of large granules. There are major differences in size and structure, but they are unique for each plant species. Before the starch can be hydrolyzed by intestinal enzymes, the granule must be disrupted. When heated in water, starch granules imbibe water, swell, and eventually burst. This process is referred to in the food industry as gelatinization. How readily the granules swell and the temperature at which gelatinization occurs are characteristic for each plant species. The reasons for the differences in resistance to gelatinization are not well understood and are probably multifactorial. It is known that starches with a high amylose-to-amylopectin ratio are more rigid and resistant to swelling and disruption (31). It also has been known for many years that starch granules in legumes are difficult to disrupt by heating in water and thus are not readily digestible (32). Bean starch is not extraordinarily high in amylose (~30% of total starch), and highly purified bean starch is readily hydrolyzed by enzymes (33). These data, then, suggest that it is the organization of the starch granules in the leguminous seed that limits its gelatinization and digestibility. Grinding may be used to disrupt starch granules. In addition, they may be disrupted by extensive chewing (34).

The digestibility of starches is affected by other factors as well. Cooking may cause starch molecules to form insoluble complexes. Starch also may form insoluble complexes with proteins when cooked at high temperatures. This is the so-called browning reaction (Maillard reaction) and is the reason that bread crust, for example, turns brown when baked.

Cooling of a gelatinized starch followed by reheating results in formation of insoluble starch complexes, referred to as retrogradation of the starch. This form of the starch is not hydrolyzable by enzymes in the small intestine.

Because of the above factors, it is becoming increasingly clear that the starch in many foods, including bread, is not completely digestible. In addition, the rate at which starch is hydrolyzed by intestinal enzymes may differ. It will depend on the food source, the structure of the starch, and the preparation method used. Indeed, it has been proposed that the starch in a food be subdivided into readily digestible starch (RDS), slowly digestible starch (SDS), and resistant starch (RS) fractions, depending on the rate and the extent of digestion of the starch in a food by a mixture of enzymes in an in vitro system of analysis. For example, nearly all of the starch present in Rice Krispies cereal is RDS (~94%); whereas, in beans, chickpeas, or peas, RDS is only ~27–60% of the total starch present. The glucose that may be readily available for absorption can also be estimated using this system (35).

Inclusion of poorly digestible starches, such as those in beans and peas, has been advocated in the diet of people with diabetes because their ingestion results in only a small rise in blood glucose concentration (36). Inhibitors of amylase and sucrase enzyme activity as a means of reducing the postmeal glucose concentration are also currently being used to treat people with diabetes (acarbose). They generally reduce glycated hemoglobin levels by ~0.5–0.8% (37). In theory, similar results should be obtainable with a proper selection of dietary carbohydrates (38).

Carbohydrate Absorption

Glucose and galactose are absorbed from the duodenum and upper jejunum by a common carrier-mediated, active-transport mechanism. This is a rapid process. They appear in significant quantities in peripheral blood within 2–5 min after ingestion of either monosaccharide. Fructose is also absorbed by a carrier-mediated process. The transporter involved may be different (39), however; and the rate of absorption generally is only ~40–60% as rapid as with glucose or galactose (40) and may be even less (41).

Carbohydrate Metabolism

Glucose derived from the different food sources is absorbed by the intestinal mucosa and transferred to the portal venous circulation. Because all of the portal blood passes through the liver, the liver is exposed to a higher concentration of monosaccharides, including glucose, than any other organ in the body, with the exception of the gastrointestinal tract. However, the liver removes only a small amount of the glucose in normal people (42,43) and even less, if any, in people with poorly controlled diabetes. As a consequence, the absorbed glucose causes a prompt rise in glucose concentration in the general circulation. The liver does store a large amount of glucose as glycogen, but in part this occurs indirectly. The glucose is first converted to lactate and pyruvate in other organs, and these then are used by the liver to form glycogen (41,44,45).

Absorbed fructose entering the portal venous system is largely removed by the liver and converted into glycogen or possibly triglyceride. A small amount is converted to glucose and returned to the circulation. The relative amounts of fructose converted to glucose or to glycogen depend on the degree of insulin insufficiency (40,46). With increasing insulin deficiency and severity of diabetes, more fructose will be converted to glucose.

Interestingly, the slow rate of fructose absorption normally allows the liver to remove nearly completely all of the absorbed fructose on its first pass through the liver; very little gets into the peripheral circulation. As a result, the concentration rarely exceeds 0.5–1.0 mmol/l (9–18 mg/dl) (41,47). Overall, there is a beautiful balance between the rate at which fructose is absorbed and the rate at which the liver can remove it from the portal circulation (48).

Absorbed galactose is also rapidly removed by the liver, particularly when absorbed with glucose, as is the case when lactose is ingested. After lactose ingestion, the concentration of galactose in the peripheral circulation remains nearly unmeasurable (49). In the liver, a small amount of galactose is converted to glucose, but the majority is ultimately stored as glycogen (50). In normal people and in people with type 2 diabetes

(49,51), galactose ingestion results in only a slight rise in the peripheral glucose concentration. Data in people with severe, poorly treated diabetes are not available, but the rise in glucose is likely to be greater (52).

In summary, the absorption of the glucose and fructose resulting from the hydrolysis of sucrose in the intestine is rate limiting, as is the absorption of the glucose and galactose resulting from the hydrolysis of lactose, unless severe lactase deficiency is present. For starches, the rate and completeness of digestion will depend on the structure of the starch, how it is packaged in the plant source, and how the starch-containing food is processed and cooked. Food-derived fructose and galactose are rapidly removed by the liver and are largely stored as glycogen in people in whom an adequate effect of insulin in the liver is present; therefore, the rise in glucose concentration after ingestion of sucrose or fruits and fruit juices or after the ingestion of foods containing lactose will depend largely on the glucose content of these foods. That is, the glucose absorbed after digestion of carbohydrate-containing foods is largely responsible for raising the blood glucose concentration; other food constituents play only a minor role.

RELATIVE GLUCOSE AREA RESPONSES TO CARBOHYDRATE-CONTAINING FOODS

Over the past 90 years, several investigators have reported that the circulating glucose response to ingestion of different carbohydrate-containing foods was not the same, even though the amount of carbohydrate ingested in each food was similar (53–55). From the composition and known metabolism of the various carbohydrates discussed above, this should not be surprising. However, confirmation of the physiological basis for the differences was lacking. Therefore, we have studied these issues in a systematic fashion.

Data obtained in our laboratory (56,57) indicate that for sucrose, mixtures of glucose and fructose, or fruits or fruit juices containing these sugars, the serum glucose area response in untreated type 2 diabetic subjects was as might be predicted from the relative amounts of the sugars ingested and their known metabolism. The rate of rise in glucose concentration was just as fast after ingestion of sucrose as after ingestion of a mixture of fructose and glucose, confirming that sucrose hydrolysis was not rate limiting (56).

After ingestion of lactose, the glucose rise was just as fast as that after ingestion of glucose or a mixture of glucose and galactose, indicating that lactose hydrolysis was not rate limiting. The glucose area response was only modestly greater than when the amount of glucose in the lactose was ingested independently (49). A spectrum of glucose responses to starch-containing foods was obtained, indicating variability in rate and completeness of hydrolysis as expected (57). Nevertheless, the ordering of the responses to these foods was similar to that obtained in normal subjects by other investigators (58), and it was as might be predicted from the composition and preparation of the foods. A prepared cereal, corn flakes, which is composed largely of readily digestible corn starch, resulted in the greatest blood glucose response, and the increase in glucose concentration was essentially as fast as when pure glucose was ingested. Such data are compatible with glucose absorption, not starch digestion, being rate limiting for readily digestible starches. Ingested legumes, in which starch granules are difficult to disrupt, and a high-amylose corn starch that is known to be poorly digestible resulted in the smallest glucose responses (57).

It should be understood that in people with poorly controlled diabetes, where gluconeogenesis is expected to be greatly accelerated, the circulating glucose response to sugars and starches may not be greatly different.

Glycemic Index

The glucose response to carbohydrate-containing foods has been studied most extensively by Drs. Jenkins and Wolever and their associates. They have developed an ordering of glucose responses to a number of foods that they refer to as a "glycemic index" (58,59).

The glycemic index represents the blood glucose area above the fasting glucose concentration following the ingestion of 50-g carbohydrate portions of foods compared with the blood glucose area obtained with a 50-g carbohydrate portion of white bread as an index food in the same subjects. The glucose area response to the index food is considered to be 100%. The response to other foods is given as a percentage of that obtained with the index food. Normal subjects have been studied most extensively. However, nearly 600 foods have now been studied in people with diabetes receiving a variety of treatments and with varying degrees of insulin insufficiency (59,60).

In designing a dietary regimen for diabetic patients or in advising patients of the expected blood glucose response to a food, the concept of a list of foods and their glycemic indexes, or relative glucose area responses, is intuitively appealing. However, the glycemic index, as developed and used, has been criticized, and its utility in meal planning has been questioned (61–65). Some criticisms are as follows:

1. The reproducibility of the glucose response in the same subject has not been adequately studied for many foods. Current data would suggest considerable variability (60,62,66).
2. The time duration after a meal used to determine the glucose area was originally 2 h in normal subjects, but more recently, 1 h has

been used. In diabetic subjects, 3 h was used. For some foods, these times are too short if one wishes to accurately quantitate the response. This is particularly true in diabetic subjects, in whom the glucose concentration tends to remain elevated for a prolonged period of time. In fact, using any single time frame will lead to an under- or overestimation of the response for some foods. For accuracy, subjects should be studied until the glucose concentration returns to a basal level.

3. In people with untreated type 2 diabetes who are not given food over a 3- to 4-h period, there is a considerable decrease in glucose concentration (2). Therefore, merely using the blood glucose value before a food is ingested results in an underestimation of the glucose response (26,67). When people with more severe diabetes are not given food for that same period, blood glucose may rise (59).

4. It has not as yet been determined that the postmeal glucose area is linearly related to the quantity of each type of carbohydrate ingested. This could be important in mixed meals, where the quantities may vary. For example, we have obtained data in type 2 diabetic subjects that indicate a markedly curvilinear response to ingested fructose. When a conventional amount (15 g) was ingested, the glucose level did not increase or it actually decreased. However, with ingestion of 50 g of fructose, the glucose response was 30% of the response to 50 g of glucose (68).

5. The circulating glucose concentration clearly affects gastric motility and gastric emptying of both a glucose solution (69) and a mixed meal (70). At high glucose concentrations (>170 mg/dl), a dysmotility similar to diabetic gastroparesis is induced. Thus, the high and variable glucose concentration in people with diabetes is likely to affect the plasma glucose response to a food and cannot be predicted. A rapid gastric emptying rate in some people with diabetes has also been reported (71), and it occurs routinely when the blood glucose is low (69,72). It is estimated that the gastric emptying rate accounts for ~36% of the variance in glucose concentration after ingestion of a glucose load in people with type 2 diabetes (73).

6. The insulin response to the ingestion of foods was not determined. This would also affect the glucose response, particularly when mixed meals are ingested (26), and will vary with the severity of diabetes. Recently, the insulin area response to 1,000-kJ portions of 38 commonly ingested foods has been determined in healthy subjects. Based on the data obtained, an insulin index of foods has been generated (74). The value of this approach and its utility in people with diabetes remain to be determined.

7. The glycemic index was determined using the first meal of the day. The possible effect of the first meal on subsequent meal responses

needs to be determined if the information is to be useful in meal planning. It is known that the first meal can affect the glucose response to an identical meal ingested 4 h later (second meal effect) (75,76). When three identical meals are ingested 4 h apart, the glucose response to each succeeding meal is often different, and this may be sex related (77,78).

8. Lastly, it has been reported that mixed meals designed using the glycemic index data did not result in the postmeal glucose area responses that would be predicted for the individual foods included (61,63,79). This has been disputed, and data supporting the utility of the glycemic index have been reviewed (80,81).

In our opinion, the glycemic index is useful as an indictor of the general ordering of glucose responses to food. However, its accuracy is not great, and its overall utility remains to be determined. It also does not further our understanding of the physiological or pathophysiological principles that determine the glucose response to mixed meals. There are major interactions between foods in regard to hormone secretion, gastric emptying, and gut motility, as well as physical interactions between foods that may affect the digestion and absorption of nutrients and thus the blood glucose response. At present, our laboratory is attempting to learn more about these interactions and how they affect the blood glucose response to a meal.

Food Fiber

In recent years, there has been an increased interest in plant fiber as a dietary constituent. The American Diabetes Association has suggested that the fiber content in the diet for people with diabetes be increased from the current 10–20 g in the average American diet up to 20–35 g daily (23). This is the same as that recommended for the general population. However, the issue remains very controversial.

It has been well documented that mixing large amounts of guar gum and other viscous nonstarch polysaccharides with glucose or with carbohydrate-containing foods reduces the postprandial glucose response, presumably by slowing the absorption of glucose (82). However, the amounts required are not acceptable to most patients. A significant postprandial blood glucose–lowering effect of naturally occurring food fiber has not been well documented, and differences observed when foods with differing fiber contents are ingested are likely to be due to other factors, such as how readily the starch in a food can be digested. Overall, the best evidence suggests that dietary fiber is of only minor importance in postmeal glucose control (82).

Large amounts of plant fiber have been reported to lower serum cholesterol. Primarily LDL cholesterol is lowered; HDL is little changed. The fiber found in fruits and vegetables and the mucilaginous fibers, such as guar, or partially mucilaginous fibers, such as in oat bran, are most effective. These are viscous, water soluble, and colon fermentable. The mechanism by which this cholesterol lowering occurs is uncertain. It may be caused by decreased bile acid absorption (83). Whether food fiber is important in prevention of colon cancer remains an unanswered question (84).

CONCLUSION

For those foods in which the major carbohydrate present is sucrose and/or a mixture of glucose and fructose, the plasma glucose response is determined primarily by the relative proportion of glucose or potential glucose present. When ingested in conventional amounts, fructose has little effect on the plasma glucose concentration in normal people or people with type 2 diabetes. However, with severe insulin insufficiency, this may not be the case.

For those foods in which the major carbohydrate present is lactose, the plasma glucose response also is largely due to the glucose component of the lactose. Galactose contributes only modestly. The glucose response in people with poorly controlled diabetes (severe insulin insufficiency) has not been studied. Presumably the glucose response to the galactose component of lactose would be greater.

For those foods in which the major carbohydrate present is starch, the plasma glucose response will be determined by the composition of the starch, the source of the starch, and the preparation method used, i.e., the digestibility of the starch. This is likely to be quite variable, but the glucose area response to these foods has been grossly codified (60).

The nondigestible carbohydrate (both the nondigestible starch fractions and nonstarch polysaccharides, i.e., fiber) content of a meal has little effect on the plasma glucose response. However, it may result in a decrease in LDL cholesterol.

Overall, it is the amount of glucose absorbed from a meal that will largely determine the plasma glucose area response. However, the response will be modified by the gastric emptying rate, by intestinal motility, and by factors that affect glucose removal from the circulation, such as the insulin response, insulin resistance, etc.

In considering the plasma glucose response to a meal, the above generalizations are useful. However, considerable research in this area remains to be done, particularly in regard to the interaction of foods when ingested in mixed meals. In addition, the long-term metabolic consequences of diets varying in the amounts and types of food constituents need to be determined. In our opinion, it is premature to make specific dietary recommendations for people with diabetes. Until more information becomes available, there is little reason to advise people with diabetes that their diet be different than that of other family members or of their cultural group, unless the diet is nutritionally inadequate or is shown to accelerate development of atherosclerosis or other complications of diabetes.

In people with diabetes who require insulin, a thorough knowledge of the carbohydrate content of foods (this information is now available on all food labels) (85), their likely effect on blood glucose, and their effect on insulin requirements should be understood in a broad sense. Integration of this information into their glucose control regimen should prove useful. For people with type 1 diabetes, efforts to standardize the carbohydrate content in meals may also help reduce the variable blood glucose response to insulin injections. The latter is all too common in people whose ability to secrete insulin is nil.

REFERENCES

1. Nuttall FQ: Diet and the diabetic patient. *Diabetes Care* 6:197–207, 1983

2. Gannon MC, Nuttall FQ, Lane JT, Fang S, Gupta V, Sandhofer CR: Effect of twenty-four hours of starvation on plasma glucose and insulin concentrations in people with untreated non-insulin dependent diabetes mellitus. *Metabolism* 45:492–497, 1996

3. American Heart Association: Dietary guidelines for healthy American adults: a statement for physicians and health professionals by the Nutrition Committee, American Heart Association. *Circulation* 77:721A, 1988

4. Expert Panel on Detection, Evaluation, and Treatment of High Blood Cholesterol in Adults: Summary of the Second Report of the National Cholesterol Education Program (NCEP) Expert Panel on Detection, Evaluation, and Treatment of High Blood Cholesterol in Adults (Adult Treatment Panel II). *JAMA* 269:3015–3023, 1993

5. Chait A, Brunzell JD, Denke MA, Eisenberg D, Ernst ND, Franklin FA, Ginsberg H, Kotchen TA, Kuller L, Mullis RM, Nichaman MZ, Nicolosi RJ, Schaefer EJ, Stone NJ, Weidman WH: Rationale of the diet-heart statement of the American Health Association: Report of the Nutrition Committee. *Circulation* 88:3008–3029, 1993

6. Willett WC: Diet and health: what should we eat? *Science* 264:532–537, 1994

7. Katan MB, Grundy SM, Willett WC: Beyond low-fat diets. *N Engl J Med* 337:563–566, 1997

8. Connor WE, Connor SL: Should a low-fat, high-carbohydrate diet be recommended for everyone? The case for a low-fat, high-carbohydrate diet. *N Engl J Med* 337:562–563, 1997

9. Berry EM: Dietary fatty acids in the management of diabetes mellitus. *Am J Clin Nutr* 66:991S–997S, 1997

10. Reaven GM: Do high carbohydrate diets prevent the development or attenuate the manifestations (or both) of syndrome X? A viewpoint strongly against. *Curr Opin Lipidol* 8:23–27, 1997

11. The Diabetes Control and Complications Trial Research Group: The effect of intensive treatment of diabetes on the development and progression of long-term complications in insulin-dependent diabetes mellitus. *N Engl J Med* 329:977–986, 1993

12. U.K. Prospective Diabetes Study (UKPDS) Group: Intensive blood-glucose control with sulphonylureas or insulin compared with conventional treatment and risk of complications in patients with type 2 diabetes (UKPDS 33). *Lancet* 352:837–853, 1998

13. Purnell JQ, Brunzell JD: The central role of dietary fat, not carbohydrate, in the insulin resistance syndrome. *Curr Opin Lipidol* 8:17–22, 1997

14. Koskinen P, Manttari M, Manninen V, Huttenen JK, Heinonen OO, Frick MH: Coronary heart disease incidence in NIDDM patients in the Helsinki Heart Study. *Diabetes Care* 15:820–825, 1992

15. Sacks FM, Pfeffer MA, Moye LA, Rouleau JL, Rutherford JD, Cole TG, Brown L, Warnica J, Warnold JMO, Wun CC, Davis BR, Baunwald E, The Cholesterol And Recurrent Events (CARE) Trial Investigators: The effect of pravastatin on coronary events after myocardial infarction in patients with average cholesterol levels. *N Engl J Med* 335:1001–1009, 1996

16. Pyörälä K, Pedersen TR, Kjekshus J, Faergeman O, Olsson A, Thorgeirsson G, The Scandinavian Simvastatin Survival Study (4S) Group: Cholesterol lowering with simvastatin improves prognosis of diabetic patients with coronary heart disease: a subgroup analysis of the Scandinavian Simvastatin Survival Study (4S). *Diabetes Care* 20:614–620, 1997

17. Semenkovich CF, Heinecke JW: The mystery of diabetes and atherosclerosis: time for a new plot. *Diabetes* 46:327–334, 1997

18. Tattersall R: Targets of therapy for NIDDM. *Diab Res Clin Pract* 28:S49–S55, 1995

19. Barrett-Connor E: Does hyperglycemia really cause coronary heart disease? *Diabetes Care* 20:1620–1623, 1997

20. Lewis GF, Vranic M, Harley P, Giacca A: Fatty acids mediate the acute extrahepatic effects of insulin on hepatic glucose production in humans. *Diabetes* 46:1111–1119, 1997

21. Nuttall FQ: The high-carbohydrate diet in diabetes management. *Adv Intern Med* 33:165–184, 1988

22. Nuttall FQ, Gannon MC: Sucrose and disease. *Diabetes Care* 4:305–310, 1981

23. Franz MJ, Horton ES, Bantle JP, Beebe CA, Brunzell JD, Coulston AM, Henry RR, Hoogewerf BJ, Stacpoole PW: Nutrition principles for the management of diabetes and related complications. *Diabetes Care* 17:490–518, 1994

24. Hanover LM, White JS: Manufacturing, composition, and applications of fructose. *Am J Clin Nutr* 58:724S–732S, 1993

25. Slama G, Traynard PY, Desplangque N, Pudar H, Dhunputh I, Letanoux M, Bornet FR, Tchobroutsky G: The search for an optimized treatment of hypoglycemia: carbohydrates in tablets, solution, or gel, for the correction of insulin reactions. *Arch Intern Med* 150:589–593, 1990

26. Nuttall FQ, Gannon MC: Plasma glucose and insulin response to macronutrients in nondiabetic and NIDDM subjects. *Diabetes Care* 14:824–838, 1991

27. American Diabetes Association: Special Report: principles of nutrition and dietary recommendation for individuals with diabetes mellitus. *Diabetes* 28:1027–1030, 1979

28. Suarez FL, Savaiano DA, Levitt MD: A comparison of symptoms after the consumption of milk or lactose-hydrolyzed milk by people with self-reported severe lactose intolerance. *N Engl J Med* 333:1–4, 1995

29. Rosenthal SM, Zeigler EE: The effect of uncooked starches on the blood sugar of normal and of diabetic subjects. *Arch Intern Med* 44:344–350, 1929

30. Englyst HN, Cummings JH: Digestion of the carbohydrates of banana (musa paradisiaca sapientum) in the human small intestine. *Am J Clin Nutr* 44:42–50, 1986

31. Guilbot A, Mercier C: Starch: the polysaccharides. In *Molecular Biology*. Vol. 3. Aspinall GO, Ed. New York, Academic, 1985, pp. 209–282

32. Pauletig M: Digestibility of starches from various vegetable foods by the diastases from malt, pancreas and saliva. *Z Physiol Chem* 100:74–92, 1917

33. Würsch P, Del Vedovo S, Koellreuter B: Cell structure and starch nature as key determinants of the digestion rate of starch in legumes. *Am J Clin Nutr* 43:25–29, 1986

34. Read NW, Welch I, Austen CJ, Barnish C, Bartlett CE, Baxter AJ, Brown G, Compton ME, Hume KE, Storie I, Wording J: Swallowing food without chewing: a simple way to reduce postprandial glycemia. *Br J Nutr* 55:43–47, 1986

35. Englyst HN, Hudson GJ: The classification and measurement of dietary carbohydrates. *Food Chemistry* 57:15–21, 1996

36. Jenkins DJA, Wolever TMS, Taylor RH: The glycemic index of foods tested in diabetic patients: a new basis for carbohydrate exchange favoring the use of legumes. *Diabetologia* 24:257–264, 1983

37. Coniff RF, Shapiro JA, Seaton TB: Long-term efficacy and safety of acarbose in the treatment of obese subjects with non-insulin-dependent diabetes mellitus. *Arch Intern Med* 154:2442–2448, 1994

38. Brand-Miller JC, Colagiuri S: The carnivore connection: dietary carbohydrate in the evolution of NIDDM. *Diabetologia* 37:1280–1286, 1994

39. Castello A, Guma A, Sevilla L, Furiols M, Testar X, Palacin M, Zorzano A: Regulation of GLUT5 gene expression in rat intestinal mucosa: regional distribution, circadian rhythm, perinatal development and effect of diabetes. *Biochem J* 309:271–277, 1995

40. Niewoehner CB: Metabolic effects of dietary vs. parenteral fructose. *J Am Coll Nutr* 5:443–450, 1986

41. Niewoehner CB, Gilboe DP, Nuttall GA, Nuttall FQ: Metabolic effects of oral fructose in the liver of fasted rats. *Am J Physiol* 247:E505–E512, 1984

42. Radziuk J, MacDonald TJ, Rubenstein D: Initial splanchnic extraction of ingested glucose in normal man. *Metabolism* 27:657–669, 1978

43. Butler PC, Rizza RA: Contribution to postprandial hyperglycemia and effect on initial splanchnic glucose clearance of hepatic glucose

cycling in glucose-intolerant or NIDDM patients. *Diabetes* 40:73–81, 1991

44. Hems DA: Short-term hormonal control of liver glycogen metabolism. *Trends Biochem Sci* 2:241–244, 1977

45. Katz J, McGarry JD: The glucose paradox: is glucose a substrate for liver metabolism? *J Clin Invest* 74:1900–1909, 1984

46. Niewoehner CB, Nuttall FQ: Mechanism of stimulation of liver glycogen synthesis by fructose in alloxan diabetic rats. *Diabetes* 35:705–711, 1986

47. MacDonald I, Keyser A, Pacy D: Some effects in man of varying the load of glucose, sucrose, fructose or sorbitol on various metabolites in blood. *Am J Clin Nutr* 31:1305–1311, 1978

48. Niewoehner CB, Nuttall BQ, Nuttall FQ: Effects of graded intravenous doses of fructose on glycogen synthase in the liver of fasted rats. *Metabolism* 36:338–344, 1987

49. Ercan N, Nuttall FQ, Gannon MC, Redmon JB, Sheridan KJ: Effects of glucose, galactose and lactose on the plasma glucose and insulin response in persons with non-insulin-dependent diabetes mellitus. *Metabolism* 42:1560–1567, 1993

50. Niewoehner C, Neil B: Mechanism of delayed hepatic glycogen synthesis after an oral galactose load vs. an oral glucose load in adult rats. *Am J Physiol* 263:E42–E49, 1992

51. Williams CA, Phillips T, MacDonald I: The influence of glucose on serum galactose levels in man. *Metabolism* 32:250–256, 1983

52. Ionescu-Tirgoviste C, Popa E, Sintu E, Mihalache N, Cheta D, Mincu I: Blood glucose and plasma insulin responses to various carbohydrates in type 2 diabetes. *Diabetologia* 24:80–84, 1983

53. Labbe M: Tolerame comparee des divers hydrates de carbone par l'organisme des diabetiques. *Bull Mem Soc Med Hosp* 24:221–234, 1907

54. MacLean H: *Modern Methods in the Diagnosis and Treatment of Glycosuria and Diabetes.* London, Constable, 1924

55. Otto H, Bleyer G, Pehhartz M: Kehlenhydrataustausch nach biologischen Aquivalenten. In *Diatetik bei Diabetes Mellitus.* Bern, Switzerland, Verlag Hans Huber, 1983, pp. 41–51

56. Gannon MC, Nuttall FQ, Krezowski PA: The serum insulin and plasma glucose responses to milk and fruit products in type 2 (non-insulin dependent) diabetic subjects. *Diabetologia* 29:784–791, 1986

57. Krezowski PA, Nuttall FQ, Gannon MC, Billington CJ, Parker S: The insulin and glucose responses to various starch-containing foods in type 2 diabetic subjects. *Diabetes Care* 10:205–212, 1987

58. Jenkins DJA, Wolever TMS, Taylor RH: Glycemic index of foods: a physiological basis for carbohydrate exchange. *Am J Clin Nutr* 34:362–366, 1981

59. Wolever TMS, Katzman-Relle L, Jenkins AL, Vuksan V, Josse RG, Jenkins DJA: Glycemic index of 102 complex carbohydrate foods in patients with diabetes. *Nutr Res* 14:651–669, 1994

60. Foster-Powell K, Brand-Miller J: International tables of glycemic index. *Am J Clin Nutr* 62:871S–893S, 1995

61. Coulston AM, Hollenbeck CB, Reaven GM: Utility of studies measuring glucose and insulin responses to various carbohydrate-containing foods. *Am J Clin Nutr* 39:163–165, 1984

62. Gannon MC, Nuttall FQ: Factors affecting interpretation of postprandial glucose and insulin area. *Diabetes Care* 10:759–763, 1987

63. Calle-Pascual AL, Gomez V, Leon F, Bordiu E: Foods with a low glycemic index do not improve glycemic control of both type 1 and type 2 diabetic patients after one month of therapy. *Diabete Metab* 14:629–633, 1988

64. Marks V: Glycemic responses to sugars and starches. In *Dietary Starches and Sugars in Man: A Comparison*. New York, Springer-Verlag, 1989, pp. 151–167

65. Coulston AM, Reaven GM: Much ado about (almost) nothing. *Diabetes Care* 20:241–243, 1997

66. Wolever TMS: The glycemic index. *World Rev Nutr Diet* 62:120–185, 1990

67. Gannon MC, Nuttall FQ: Quantitation of the glucose area response to a meal. *Diabetes Care* 13:1095, 1990

68. Nuttall FQ, Gannon MC, Burmeister LA, Lane JT, Pyzdrowski KL: The metabolic response to various doses of fructose in type 2 diabetic subjects. *Metabolism* 41:510–517, 1992

69. Schvarcz E, Palmer M, Aman J, Horowitz M, Stridsberg M, Berne C: Physiological hyperglycemia slows gastric emptying in normal subjects and patients with insulin-dependent diabetes mellitus. *Gastroenterology* 113:60–66, 1997

70. Hasler WL, Soudah HC, Dulai G, Owyang C: Mediation of hyperglycemia-evoked gastric evoked slow-wave dysrhythmias by endogenous prostaglandins. *Gastroenterology* 108:727–736, 1995

71. Kong MF, Macdonald IA, Tattersall RB: Gastric emptying in diabetes. *Diabetic Med* 13:112–119, 1996

72. Schvarcz E, Palmer M, Aman J, Berne C: Hypoglycemia increases the gastric emptying rate in healthy subjects. *Diabetes Care* 18:674–676, 1995

73. Jones KL, Horowitz M, Carney BI, Wishart JM, Guha S, Green L: Gastric emptying in early non-insulin dependent diabetes mellitus. *J Nucl Med* 37:1643–1648, 1996

74. Holt SHA, Miller JCB, Petocz P: An insulin index of foods: the insulin demand generated by 1000-kj portions of common foods. *Am J Clin Nutr* 66:1264–1276, 1997

75. Collier GR, Wolever TMS, Jenkins DJA: Concurrent ingestion of fat and reduction in starch content impairs carbohydrate tolerance to subsequent meals. *Am J Clin Nutr* 45:963–969, 1987

76. Ercan N, Gannon MC, Nuttall FQ: Effect of added fat on the plasma glucose and insulin response to ingested potato given in various combinations as two meals in normal individuals. *Diabetes Care* 17:1453–1459, 1994

77. Ahmed M, Gannon MC, Nuttall FQ: Postprandial glucose, insulin, glucagon and triglyceride responses to a standard diet in normal subjects. *Diabetologia* 12:61–67, 1976

78. Nuttall FQ, Gannon MC, Wald JL, Ahmed M: Plasma glucose and insulin profiles in normal subjects ingesting diets of varying carbohydrate, fat and protein content. *J Am Coll Nutr* 4:437–450, 1985

79. Laine DC, Thomas W, Levitt MD, Bantle JP: Comparison of predictive capabilities of diabetic exchange lists and glycemic index of foods. *Diabetes Care* 10:3887–3394, 1987

80. Brand-Miller JC: Importance of glycemic index in diabetes. *Am J Clin Nutr* 59:747S–752S, 1994

81. Wolever TMS: The glycemic index: flogging a dead horse? *Diabetes Care* 20:452–456, 1997

82. Nuttall FQ: Dietary fiber in the management of diabetes. *Diabetes* 42:503–508, 1993

83. Marlett JA: Sites and mechanisms for the hypocholesterolemic actions of soluble dietary fiber sources. In *Dietary Fiber in Health and Disease*. New York, Plenum, 1997, pp. 109–121

84. Chapkin RS, Jiang YH, Davidson LA, Lupton JR: Modulation of intracellular second messengers by dietary fat during colonic tumor

development. In *Dietary Fat and Cancer*. New York, Plenum, 1997, pp. 85–96

85. Wheeler ML, Franz M, Heins J, Schafer R, Holler H, Bohannon B, Bantle JP, Barrier P: Food labeling. *Diabetes Care* 17:480–487, 1994

Dr. Nuttall is Chief, Metabolic/Endocrine Section, and Professor of Medicine, and Dr. Gannon is Director of the Metabolic Research Laboratory and Associate Professor of Food Science & Nutrition and of Medicine at the University of Minnesota, Minneapolis VA Medical Center, Minneapolis, MN.

7. Protein and Diabetes

MARY C. GANNON, PHD, AND FRANK Q. NUTTALL, MD, PHD

Highlights

- Ingested protein has minimal effects on the blood glucose concentration in people with type 2 diabetes, and when ingested with a mixed meal, protein may actually result in a small decrease in postprandial glucose levels.
- The small rise in blood glucose concentration after ingestion of protein is because dietary protein strongly stimulates insulin secretion in people with type 2 diabetes.
- In people with type 1 diabetes who are adequately treated with insulin, ingested protein also has only a modest effect on blood glucose concentration.
- In the American diet, the amount of protein ingested is 15–20% of food energy (calories). Evidence indicates that this amount of protein is not harmful.
- Additional research is needed to determine whether a diet containing a higher proportion of protein would be beneficial for people with diabetes.

INTRODUCTION

When dietary recommendations for the general population or for people with diabetes have been considered, the focus has been on the relative amounts and types of carbohydrates and fats to include in the diet (1–3). Protein content of the diet, both the type and the amount, has largely been ignored. Generally, protein has only been considered in the context of that necessary for maintenance of lean body mass, i.e., to maintain nitrogen balance, whether people have diabetes or not.

Minimal Protein Content of the Diet

Proteins are continuously being synthesized and degraded. The estimated turnover is ~280 g/day (4). The amino acids resulting from protein degradation can be recycled, i.e., reused for synthesis, but this is incomplete. Therefore, dietary protein is necessary for maintenance of lean body mass. The actual daily loss of protein through hair, nails, skin, gut wall, and various secretions is estimated to be ~6–8 g/day for a 70-kg man (~0.09–0.11 g/kg body wt/day) (5). This is considerably less than the 32 g/day (~0.45 g/kg body wt/day) losses reported to be required for replacement (6). In any regard, the minimal high-quality dietary protein requirement in adults may be quite low and less than previously thought. In addition, current data indicate that the efficiency with which amino acids are reutilized may be regulated by the amount of protein in the diet (4). The lower the protein content of the diet, the more efficiently it is utilized.

The recommended dietary protein allowance for adults is 0.8 g high-quality protein/kg body wt/day (6). This represents 56 g protein/day for a 70-kg man, or ~11% of energy from protein when consuming 2,000 kcal/day (8,200 kJ/day). In support of the daily dietary protein allowance recommended by the National Academy of Sciences, it has been reported that a 3,000 kcal/day diet consisting of 6% protein (i.e., 45 g protein) is adequate to maintain nitrogen balance in moderately active young males (5). More recently, Campbell et al. (7) reported that protein requirements are increased in the elderly (56–80 years of age) and recommended 1.0–1.25 g/kg body wt/day of high-quality protein for these individuals. All of these recommendations are generous and considerably in excess of minimal needs in normal people (6).

An increased loss of body protein with severe insulin deficiency has been known for millennia (8,9). In subjects with type 1 diabetes, withdrawal of insulin results in a 97% increase in protein loss (10). This represents the most severe form of insulin insufficiency. Unless severe insulin insufficiency is present, the protein requirement for people with diabetes has been considered to be similar to that for nondiabetic individuals (11). However, based on tracer studies indicating an increased leucine turnover, the minimum protein requirement is likely to be increased in most people with type 1 diabetes (12). If so, the reason protein malnutrition is not common is probably that the amount of dietary protein ingested by the average adult exceeds even the recommended daily allowance. That is, it is in large excess over minimal needs.

In summary, based on the few published studies, the dietary protein requirements for people with type 1 diabetes will depend on the degree of insulin insufficiency present, but the usual amount of protein present in a typical Western diet is sufficient for most people. The estimated amount of protein ingested by the general population (15–20% of energy as protein, or 1.1–1.4 g/kg body wt for a 70-kg person ingesting 2,000 kcal/day, i.e., 8,200 kJ/day) is considerably more than the minimum protein necessary even in people with diabetes and is greater than the 0.8 g/kg body wt/day recommended by the National Academy of Sciences (6).

In people with established renal insufficiency, with or without diabetes, a restriction in dietary protein has been considered desirable because it may modify the progression of the disease. This is controversial, and there is concern that protein deficiency will result (12–15). Whether protein should be restricted, and if so, how severely, remains to be determined. At present, there is also no evidence that restricting protein in the diet of people with diabetes will prevent or delay the onset of renal insufficiency.

Maximum Tolerated Protein Content of the Diet

It has been suggested that primitive humans routinely ingested a relatively high-protein diet. It has been estimated that during the Paleolithic period (~400,000–45,000 years ago), the diet consisted of 34% of food energy as protein (16). It has been estimated that in the pre-Neolithic period (20,000–12,000 years ago), the diet could have been ~50% protein if the proportion of dietary energy from animal sources was 80%, as was expected to be the case during part of the year in specific locations (17). In 1928, it was reported that the Baffin Island Eskimos ate between 4 and 8 lb of meat per day when food was plentiful. The only source of carbohydrate in the diet was the glycogen in the meat (18). This amount of meat would provide ~363–726 g protein/day! The *average* daily protein intake was calculated to be 280 g (44% of food energy). The traditional diet of Australian Aborigines (19) was reported to be very high in protein (up to 80% of energy) and low in carbohydrate. Thus, these data indicate that diets high in protein are likely to have been at least tolerated by humans.

In spite of the relatively high amounts of protein calculated to have been present in the diets of some groups, anecdotal information is available indicating that these diets are not readily acceptable. A diet composed mainly of lean meat, in quantities that would satisfy energy requirements, was avoided by members of the Lewis and Clark expedition because of untoward effects, even though food was in short supply (20). Weight-maintenance diets as high as 62% protein (~245 g, or 3.15 g/kg body wt) have been provided to Australian Aboriginal subjects with type 2 diabetes for a 2-week period (21). All subjects lost weight, suggesting a decrease in total food energy intake. Indeed, the authors state that 3 of 10 subjects on this diet averaged 653 kcal/day (2,677 kJ/day) less than their energy intake on the control diet, and they had to be eliminated from the study. Thus, it appears that a diet containing >40–45% protein is not acceptable to most people, except perhaps in an Inuit population. This is compatible with our own experience during a study in which meals consisting of 41% protein (4.0 g/kg body wt) were ingested by normal young subjects as three identical meals, 4 h apart (22). The volunteers were able to consume the three meals containing 41% protein during the day of the study, but they indicated that this amount of food was more than they were comfortable eating, even though the total energy content of the diet was not different than that of a standard, a high-fat, or a high-carbohydrate diet ingested by the same subjects (22). They also complained of malaise and lethargy after ingesting the high-protein diet.

In summary, the minimum amount of high-quality protein necessary to replace body stores is relatively small, and the amount of protein that can be tolerated without toxic effects is relatively large. The questions then are *1)* whether diets either relatively low or relatively high in protein compared with a typical Western diet (15–20% protein) are beneficial for people with diabetes and *2)* whether there are any untoward consequences of consuming such a diet. These questions cannot be answered in a definitive fashion at present. Evidence suggests that the amount of protein in the typical Western diet (~15–20%) is not harmful (23). However, whether greater amounts of protein would have untoward effects or be beneficial, in our opinion, is an important issue.

The latest position statement from the American Diabetes Association recommends ~10–20% of daily calories in the form of protein; 10% for people with overt nephropathy (24).

In this chapter, we briefly discuss the metabolic effects of protein ingestion in normal subjects and subjects with type 2 diabetes in an effort to indicate the likely physiological consequences of conventional or greater amounts of protein in the diet.

PROTEIN: DIGESTION, ABSORPTION, AND METABOLISM

Digestion of protein begins in the stomach, where pepsin enzymes hydrolyze some of the peptide bonds. The products of protein digestion in the stomach are polypeptides of various sizes. Next, the stomach contents are mixed with the alkaline secretions of the exocrine pancreas in the duodenum, which inactivates the pepsin enzymes. The presence of polypeptides in the duodenum stimulates the secretion of pancreatic enzymes. The pancreatic enzymes then catalyze the hydrolysis of large polypeptide chains into smaller peptides and free amino acids. The enzymatic hydrolysis of proteins in the stomach and intestine results in free amino acids and di- and tripeptides, which are absorbed via specific transporters on the luminal surface of the intestinal mucosal cells. In the mucosal cells, the di- and tripeptides are further hydrolyzed (25).

Some amino acids, particularly glutamine, glutamate, and aspartate, are metabolized primarily in the gut mucosa (26). The remaining amino acids are metabolized in the intestinal mucosal cells, then diffuse down a concentration gradient into the mucosal capillaries and are transported by the portal vein to the liver. In the liver, the amino acids—particularly the nonessential amino acids, i.e., those not required to replace body proteins—are largely deaminated (27). The amino group is condensed with CO_2 to form urea, which is then carried to the kidneys and excreted in the urine. The amount of urea excreted per day is an index of the amount of protein metabolized, although ~14% of newly synthesized urea is utilized by bacteria in the colon (28). Small amounts of amino acids are also metabolized (deaminated) in the kidney (29).

The carbon skeletons remaining after deamination can be converted to glucose. The resulting glucose may also then enter the circulation. This potential addition of glucose to the circulation is one reason why metabolism of dietary protein is of particular interest when making dietary recommendations for people with diabetes.

BLOOD GLUCOSE RESPONSE

Nondiabetic People and People with Type 2 Diabetes

Janney (30) calculated that ~3.5 g glucose could be produced for every gram of nitrogen excreted in the urine as the result of a beef protein meal. Beef protein is 16% nitrogen; thus, 1 g of nitrogen is excreted for every 6.25 g protein metabolized. Therefore, 3.5 g of glucose can be produced from 6.25 g protein. Theoretically then, 56% of ingested beef protein, by weight, can be converted to glucose. The range varies from 50 to 80%, depending on the specific protein ingested (30). However, as early as 1913, Jacobsen (31) reported that ingestion of egg white protein did not result in an increase in blood glucose concentration in normal people. Ingestion of protein and fat in the absence of carbohydrate also did not result in an increase in the blood glucose concentration in normal subjects (32).

In 1924, MacLean (33) fed 250 g of meat (~50 g protein) to a subject with type 2 diabetes whose fasting glucose concentration was ~280 mg/dl. Over the subsequent 5-h period of the study, there was no change in blood glucose concentration. When the same subject was given 25 g glucose, which is the theoretical amount of glucose that could be produced from the 50 g of protein in the 250 g of meat, there was a dramatic increase in glucose concentration. In fact, it increased to almost 600 mg/dl.

Subsequently, Conn and Newburgh (34) gave an enormous amount of beef to a normal young subject and a subject with type 2 diabetes. The subjects were each given 1.3 lb of beef, which was calculated to be 136 g of protein and was expected to result in the production of 68 g of glucose. Nevertheless, over the 8-h period of the study, the blood glucose concentration did not increase in either the normal subject or the person with diabetes. When the same subjects were given 68 g glucose, the glucose concentration was clearly increased in both.

More recently, data from many laboratories, including our own (35–39), indicate that the peripheral glucose concentration does not increase after protein ingestion in normal subjects or people with type 2 diabetes. Protein ingestion actually results in a small decrease in postprandial glucose concentration in people with type 2 diabetes (40).

People with Type 1 Diabetes

The blood glucose response to ingestion of protein by people with type 1 diabetes is more difficult to interpret because with less-than-ideal insulin treatment there is an increase in hepatic gluconeogenesis. This is likely to vary depending on the adequacy of insulin replacement. A modest rise in circulating glucose has been described (27,41). Also, the addition of 51 g of turkey protein to a standard mixed meal containing 25 g of protein (22% of food energy) resulted in a modest increase in the insulin infusion rate (~20%) required to keep the glucose concentration similar to that resulting from the standard meal in insulin-requiring subjects (42). The need for additional insulin was also prolonged after the meal. However, the amount of protein ingested was very large. In a short-term study, a synthetic diet was decreased from 12% of energy as protein to 0% protein, and nearly all of the protein was replaced by fat (43). This resulted in a decrease in insulin requirement in people with type 1 diabetes. Presumably this was due to a decreased production of glucose derived from the dietary protein.

In summary, these studies indicate that large amounts of dietary protein have the potential to contribute to glucose production and may increase the insulin requirement in people with type 1 diabetes.

Effects of Ingested Protein on Rate of Appearance of Glucose

It is known that the carbon skeleton of all of the amino acids derived from protein digestion, with the exception of leucine, can be used to synthesize glucose. As indicated previously, ingestion of 100 g of protein potentially can yield 50–80 g glucose, depending on the protein source. Indeed, infusion of a mixture of 18 amino acids has been reported to result in an 84% increase in endogenous glucose production in normal human subjects (44). However, when a direct catheterization technique was used, ingestion of 3 g lean beef/kg body wt did not result in an increased release of glucose from the splanchnic bed (liver and gut) in normal young subjects, even though most of the amino acids were removed in the splanchnic bed and presumably metabolized (27). In insulin-requiring diabetic subjects withdrawn from insulin, there was an increased release of glucose (27). Using a direct catheterization technique, protein feeding also did not increase hepatic glucose output or raise the blood glucose concentration in dogs (45).

Using an isotope dilution technique combined with determination of the urea formation rate, it was calculated that ingestion of 50 g of cottage cheese protein resulted in 34 g being deaminated over the 8 h of the study in normal young subjects. The amount of glucose produced and entering the circulation was only 9.7 g (38). Thus, the amount of glucose produced was considerably less than the amount theorized (~25 g).

We have also determined the effect of ingested beef protein on hepatic glucose production rate using an isotope dilution technique in people with untreated type 2 diabetes. Preliminary data indicate that of the 50 g protein ingested, only ~2.0 g could be accounted for by appearance of glucose in the circulation over the 8-h period of the study (46). That is, it was even less than that in normal subjects ingesting cottage cheese protein. Again, this is considerably less than the theoretical amount of 28 g of glucose (56% of the protein by weight). The fate of the remaining carbon skeletons remains unknown. These results were rather surprising because, as expected, the basal glucose production rate in the diabetic subjects was greater than that in normal young subjects (47,48).

In summary, the observation that ingested protein does not increase the glucose concentration and may even decrease it modestly is based on the observation that considerably less than the theoretical amount of glucose that can be produced from the protein actually is produced and enters the circulation. The small amount of glucose released into the circulation is matched by a corresponding increase in glucose utilization. However, this response requires that the ingested protein stimulate insulin secretion.

In people with severe insulin insufficiency, the rise in glucose concentration is most likely due to an increased conversion of ingested protein into glucose and to a decreased glucose removal rate. In people with type 2 diabetes, protein ingestion does not result in an increase in glucose concentration, and when ingested with glucose (40), fructose (39), or in a mixed meal (49,50), it may result in a smaller glucose rise because of an increased insulin secretion. Thus, an increase in protein in the diet for people with type 2 diabetes potentially could be beneficial if protein is substituted for readily digestible carbohydrate.

HORMONAL RESPONSE

Insulin

Insulin affects the circulating blood glucose concentration by several mechanisms. An increased insulin concentration results in a decrease in hepatic glucose production directly (51) because of decreases in glycogenolysis and gluconeogenesis. Insulin also stimulates an increase in glucose uptake and storage of glucose as glycogen in muscle. Insulin inhibits lipolysis in fat cells. As a result, the concentration of circulating nonesterified fatty acids (NEFAs) is decreased. In the presence of a low NEFA concentration, there is an increase in glucose utilization (oxidation). In addition, insulin inhibits the degradation of body proteins and lowers the concentration of many amino acids (52). Indirectly then, insulin could reduce gluconeogenesis in the liver by decreasing the amino acid substrate supply to the liver.

After protein ingestion by normal people and people with type 2 diabetes, there is an increase in circulating insulin (53,54). However, in normal subjects, the insulin response to ingested beef protein was only 28% of that to an equivalent amount of glucose (55). When normal subjects ingested protein with glucose, a synergistic effect on insulin secretion was reported (54), i.e., the sum of the individual responses was less than the response when they were ingested simultaneously. We could not confirm this. In a larger study, we found that when normal subjects ingested protein with glucose, the insulin area response was equal to the sum of the responses to glucose alone and protein alone (Figure 7.1), i.e., the effects were additive (55).

In obese people with type 2 diabetes, it was reported that insulin secretion in response to protein was much greater than in normal subjects (56). Subsequently, this greater insulin response was attributed to the obesity and not the diabetes (57). Although we have not studied obese people without diabetes, we have confirmed that in obese people with mild untreated type 2 diabetes, an increased insulin response to dietary protein is present compared with normal-weight young subjects. Indeed, the insulin response was equal to the response to the same amount (in grams) of glucose. When people with type 2 diabetes ingested 50 g glucose with 50 g protein, the insulin area response was also greater than the sum of the responses to the individual nutrients (40) (Figure 7.1). That is, a synergistic interaction on insulin secretion was present in obese people with mild untreated type 2 diabetes.

When obese people with mild untreated type 2 diabetes ingested 25-g amounts of proteins from seven different sources with 50 g glucose, a strong synergistic effect on insulin area response was again observed with each protein source (58). The insulin response was qual-

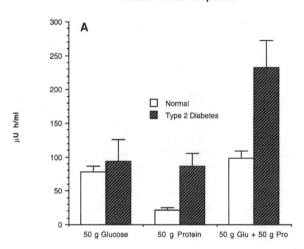

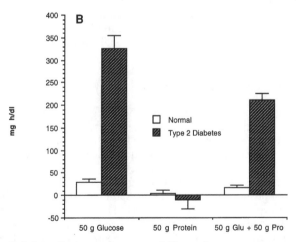

Figure 7.1 Insulin area response (*A*) or glucose area response (*B*) to ingestion of 50 g protein in the form of very lean beef, 50 g glucose, or 50 g glucose + 50 g protein by eight people without diabetes (open bars) and seven people with type 2 diabetes (hatched bars). Data for nondiabetic individuals are from Krezowski et al. (55). Data for individuals with type 2 diabetes are from Nuttall et al. (40).

itatively similar, although the proteins from some sources were more potent in increasing the insulin area response than others. The smallest insulin response was obtained with egg white; the largest response with cottage cheese. When compared with the ingestion of 50 g glucose alone, the responses were 190% and 360%, respectively. The small insulin response to egg white can be attributed to its relatively poor digestibility (59).

In summary, after ingestion of protein, the circulating insulin concentration is increased in both normal people and people with type 2 diabetes. In normal people, protein is a relatively weak insulin stimulator compared with glucose. In people with untreated type 2 diabetes, the protein and glucose are equipotent in stimulating insulin secretion. When protein was ingested with glucose, the insulin response was additive in normal subjects, but it was synergistic in people with untreated type 2 diabetes. When compared with glucose alone, the plasma glucose response was reduced after co-ingestion of glucose with any of the proteins studied except egg white. The reduction in glucose correlated with the increase in insulin for each protein source.

Ingestion of protein results in a decrease in NEFA concentration, presumably due to the rise in insulin concentration. The decrease is the same or greater than that resulting from the ingestion of a similar amount of glucose alone (37,58). This likely results in an increase in glucose oxidation, which could lower the glucose concentration. This would be in addition to an insulin-mediated decrease in glucose production in the liver and an increased uptake and storage of glucose as glycogen in skeletal muscle.

Glucagon

Glucagon stimulates an increase in hepatic glucose production due to an increase in glycogenolysis and an increase in gluconeogenesis. It antagonizes the effect of insulin in the liver. It does not antagonize the insulin-stimulated uptake of glucose in muscle or the insulin-mediated decrease in release of NEFA from fat cells.

In normal people, the plasma glucagon concentration increases after ingestion of protein (41,60–62). This response is considerably greater in people with type 1 (27) or type 2 (40,46,61) diabetes. After ingestion of glucose, the glucagon concentration decreases in both normal people and people with type 2 diabetes (63). When glucose is ingested with protein, the glucagon response is approximately the sum of the individual responses (37,55).

In people with type 1 or type 2 diabetes, both the glucagon and the insulin responses are exaggerated. The net effect on glucose output by the liver should depend on the ratio of insulin concentration to glucagon concentration, although the effect of glucagon may be transient (64,65).

Therefore, a question is, how does protein ingestion affect the amount of glucose produced by the liver?

DIETARY PROTEIN AND ATHEROSCLEROSIS

Protein generally is classified into one of two types: animal or plant. Meeker and Kesten (66) reported that rabbits developed atherosclerosis when fed a cholesterol-free diet containing 38% protein as casein. This effect was not observed when casein was replaced with soybean flour. This and other studies in animals established the concept that a difference in the two types of protein may be pathophysiologically significant (67). These data subsequently were confirmed by other studies in animals and humans (68). Clinical trials demonstrated a decrease in plasma cholesterol concentration when soy protein was substituted for animal protein in the diet of people with hypercholesterolemia (69–71). However, in normal cholesterolemic subjects, the results were highly variable (70). Generally, studies were done using artificial diets, and the plant protein used was not pure protein, i.e., it contained fiber, which could affect the results. Although atherosclerosis is more prevalent in populations consuming larger amounts of animal protein, these proteins frequently are ingested in association with fat.

It has been reported that the atherogenic and thrombogenic properties usually attributed to a diet high in animal protein are in fact due to the type and amount of fat and the amount of cholesterol in the diet. The major saturated fat in beef is stearic acid, which is readily converted to oleic acid, a monounsaturated fat that has been reported not to have atherogenic properties (72). Ulbricht and Southgate (73) developed an index of atherogenicity and thrombogenicity of various fat-containing foods. In this classification, lean beef and chicken are neither atherogenic nor thrombogenic. The authors point out that during the years of decreased coronary heart disease incidence in the U.S., there was little change in meat consumption, the direct use of beef fat increased, and the indirect use of beef fat in shortening and margarine increased (but butter consumption decreased by 50%). Their conclusion was that the incidence of coronary heart disease could not be attributed to any single factor in the diet.

In summary, interpretation of the studies relating dietary protein and atherosclerosis is complicated by the fact that ingestion of plant proteins generally is associated with an increased ingestion of dietary fiber, while ingestion of animal proteins is associated with an increased ingestion of dietary fat. Therefore, it is not possible to assess the effect of the type of dietary protein on atherosclerosis at present.

The prevalence of coronary heart disease is increased in people with type 2 diabetes. The insulin concentration is also often high and is part of the "metabolic syndrome," or "syndrome X." It has been postulated that insulin may be atherogenic. Therefore, the observation that dietary protein strongly stimulates a rise in insulin concentration in people with type 2 diabetes may be of concern. However, current evidence indicates that it is the insulin resistance and not the insulin concentration per se that is relevant to atherosclerosis (74).

MILK AND TYPE 1 DIABETES

It has been suggested that exposure to cow's milk early in life is associated with development of type 1 diabetes. A relationship between short periods, or absence, of breastfeeding and increased incidence of type 1 diabetes was first reported in 1984 on the basis of epidemiological data (75). Subsequently, evidence was presented suggesting that ingestion of cow's milk in early infancy was related to the production of specific antibodies (76). It was hypothesized that these antibodies were somehow related to the destruction of pancreatic β-cells in certain genetically susceptible individuals (77). Indeed, an association between cow's milk protein antibodies and type 1 diabetes was reported (78,79). However, more recent data dispute this (80). Scott et al. (81) have written a thoughtful review of the evidence supporting and contradicting the milk hypothesis. These authors point out that milk is but one of the suspected foods that may be involved in the autoimmune response that results in type 1 diabetes. They wisely suggest that infant feeding practices not be changed until data are available on the identity of foods that may induce diabetes, as well as on the timing, duration, and exposure of an individual to such foods.

CONCLUSION

The current data would suggest that protein from animal and/or plant sources in amounts currently being ingested in a typical Western diet is not harmful, even though these amounts are in considerable excess of the minimum amount required. A significant issue is whether increasing the protein content of the diet, from either plant or animal sources, should be encouraged for people with diabetes. An increase in dietary protein may be useful in the diet of people with type 2 diabetes because protein does not raise blood glucose concentration. Further, when people with type 2 diabetes ingest protein with carbohydrate, the circulating insulin concentration is greater than that when either macronutrient is ingested individually. An increase in dietary protein may also be useful for people with type 1 diabetes because protein raises the glucose concentration less and more slowly than comparable amounts of dietary carbohydrate. Theoretically then, an increase in protein with a decrease in carbohydrate content of the diet should result in a lower and more stable blood glucose concentration. However, long-term studies are necessary to determine whether there are any untoward effects of ingestion of a high-protein diet.

REFERENCES

1. American Heart Association: Dietary guidelines for healthy American adults: a statement for physicians and health professionals by the Nutrition Committee. *Circulation* 74:1465A–1468A, 1986

2. American Diabetes Association: Nutritional recommendations and principles for individuals with diabetes mellitus: 1987. *Diabetes Care* 10:126–132, 1987

3. American Institute for Cancer Research: *Food, Nutrition, and the Prevention of Cancer: A Global Perspective.* Washington, DC, American Institute for Cancer Research, 1997

4. Newby FD, Price SR: Determinants of protein turn-over in health and disease. *Mineral Electrolyte Metab* 24:6–12, 1998

5. Carpenter KJ: Protein requirements of adults from an evolutionary perspective. *Am J Clin Nutr* 55:913–917, 1992

6. Protein and amino acids. In *Recommended Dietary Allowances.* 10th ed. Washington, DC, National Academy Press, 1989, pp. 52–77

7. Campbell WW, Crim MC, Dallal GE, Young VR, Evans WJ: Increased protein requirements in elderly people: new data and retrospective reassessments. *Am J Clin Nutr* 60:501–509, 1994

8. Reed JA: Aretaeus, the Cappadocian. *Diabetes* 3:419–421, 1954

9. Frank LL: Diabetes mellitus in the text book of Old Hindu medicine. *Am J Gastroenterol* 27:76–95, 1957

10. Nair KS, Garrow JS, Ford C, Mahler RF, Halliday D: Effect of poor diabetic control and obesity on whole body protein metabolism in man. *Diabetologia* 25:400–403, 1983

11. Marsh PJ, Newburgh LH, Holly LF: The nitrogen requirement for maintenance of diabetes mellitus. *Arch Intern Med* 29:97–130, 1922

12. Hoffer LJ: Are dietary protein requirements altered in diabetes mellitus? *Can J Physiol Pharmacol* 71:633–638, 1993

13. Dullaart RP, Beusekamp BJ, Meijer S, van Doormaal JJ, Sluiter WJ: Long-term effects of protein-restricted diet on albuminuria and

renal function in IDDM patients without clinical nephropathy and hypertension. *Diabetes Care* 16:483–492, 1993

14. Henry RR: Protein content of the diabetic diet. *Diabetes Care* 17:1502–1513, 1994

15. Maroni BJ, Mitch WE: Role of nutrition in prevention of the progression of renal disease. *Annu Rev Nutr* 17:435–455, 1997

16. Eaton SB, Konner M: Paleolithic nutrition: a consideration of its nature and current implications. *N Engl J Med* 312:283–289, 1985

17. Ulijaszek SJ: Human dietary change. *Phil Trans R Soc Lond B* 334:271–279, 1991

18. Heinbecker P: Studies on the metabolism of Eskimos. *J Biol Chem* 80:461–475, 1928

19. O'Dea K, Spargo RM: Metabolic adaptation to a low carbohydrate-high protein ("traditional") diet in Australian Aborigines. *Diabetologia* 23:494–498, 1982

20. Speth JD, Spielmann KA: Energy source, protein metabolism, and hunter-gatherer subsistence strategies. *J Anthropol Archaeol* 2:1–31, 1983

21. O'Dea K, Traianedes K, Ireland P, Niall M, Sadler J, Hopper J, De Luise M: The effects of diet differing in fat, carbohydrate, and fiber, on carbohydrate and lipid metabolism in type 2 diabetes. *J Am Diet Assoc* 89:1076–1086, 1989

22. Nuttall FQ, Gannon MC, Wald JL, Ahmed M: Plasma glucose and insulin profiles in normal subjects ingesting diets of varying carbohydrate, fat and protein content. *J Am Coll Nutr* 4:437–450, 1985

23. Diet and Health Committee, Food and Nutrition Board, Commission on Life Sciences, National Research Council, National Academy of Sciences: Dietary intake and nutritional status: trends and assessment. In *Diet and Health: Implications for Reducing Chronic Disease Risk*. Washington, DC, National Academy Press, 1989, p. 62

24. American Diabetes Association: Nutrition recommendations and principles for people with diabetes mellitus (Position Statement). *Diabetes Care* 21 (Suppl. 1):S32–S35, 1998

25. Alpers DH: Digestion and absorption of carbohydrates and proteins. In *Physiology of the Gastrointestinal Tract*. 2nd ed. New York, Raven, 1987, pp. 1469–1487

26. Windmueller HG, Spaeth AE: Uptake and metabolism of plasma glutamine by the small intestine. *J Biol Chem* 249:5070–5079, 1978

27. Wahren J, Felig P, Hagenfeldt L: Effect of protein ingestion on splanchnic and leg metabolism in normal man and in patients with diabetes mellitus. *J Clin Invest* 57:987–999, 1976

28. Vilstrup H: Synthesis of urea after stimulation with amino acids: relation to liver function. *Gut* 21:990–995, 1980

29. Ganong WF: *Review of Medical Physiology.* Los Altos, CA, Lange Medical Publications, 1979

30. Janney NW: The metabolic relationship of the proteins to glucose. *J Biol Chem* 20:321–347, 1915

31. Jacobsen ATB: Untersuchungen über den Einfluß verschiedener Nahrungsmittel auf den Blutzucker bei normalen, zuckerkranken und graviden Personen. *Biochem Z* 56:471–494, 1913

32. Strouse S, Stein IF, Wiseley A: The accurate clinical study of blood sugar. *Bull Johns Hopkins Hosp* 26:211–215, 1915

33. MacLean H: *Modern Methods in the Diagnosis and Treatment of Glycosuria and Diabetes.* London, Constable, 1924

34. Conn JW, Newburgh LH: The glycemic response to isoglucogenic quantities of protein and carbohydrate. *J Clin Invest* 15:665–671, 1936

35. Nuttall FQ, Gannon MC: Plasma glucose and insulin response to macronutrients in nondiabetic and NIDDM subjects. *Diabetes Care* 14:824–838, 1991

36. Westphal SA, Gannon MC, Nuttall FQ: The metabolic response to glucose ingested with various amounts of protein. *Am J Clin Nutr* 52:267–272, 1990

37. Gannon MC, Nuttall FQ, Lane JT, Burmeister LA: Metabolic response to cottage cheese or egg white protein, with or without glucose in type 2 diabetic subjects. *Metabolism* 41:1137–1145, 1992

38. Khan MA, Gannon MC, Nuttall FQ: Glucose appearance rate following protein ingestion in normal subjects. *J Am Coll Nutr* 11:701–706, 1992

39. Gannon MC, Nuttall FQ, Grant CT, Ercan-Fang S, Ercan-Fang N: Stimulation of insulin secretion by fructose ingested with protein in people with untreated NIDDM. *Diabetes Care* 21:16–22, 1998

40. Nuttall FQ, Mooradian AD, Gannon MC, Billington CJ, Krezowski PA: Effect of protein ingestion on the glucose and insulin response to a standardized oral glucose load. *Diabetes Care* 7:465–470, 1984

41. Müller WA, Faloona FR, Aquilar-Parada F, Unger RH: Abnormal alpha-cell function in diabetes: response to carbohydrate and protein ingestion. *N Engl J Med* 283:109–115, 1970

42. Peters AL, Davidson MB: Protein and fat effects on glucose responses and insulin requirements in subjects with insulin-dependent diabetes mellitus. *Am J Clin Nutr* 58:555–560, 1993

43. Lariviére F, Chiasson JL, Schiffrin A, Taveroff A, Hoffer LJ: Effects of dietary protein restriction on glucose and insulin metabolism in normal and diabetic humans. *Metabolism* 43:462–467, 1994

44. Tappy L, Acheson K, Normand S, Schneeberger D, Thélin A, Pachiaudi C, Riou JP, Jéquier E: Effects of infused amino acids on glucose production and utilization in healthy human subjects. *Am J Physiol* 262:E826–E833, 1992

45. Ishida T, Chow J, Lewis RM, Kartley CJ, Entman M, Field JB: The effect of ingestion of meat on hepatic extraction of insulin and glucagon and hepatic glucose output in conscious dogs. *Metabolism* 32:558–567, 1983

46. Gannon MC, Nuttall FQ: The metabolic response to dietary protein in subjects with type 2 diabetes (Abstract). *J Am Coll Nutr* 16:478, 1997

47. Mitrakou A, Kelley D, Mokan M, Veneman T, Pangburn T, Reilly J, Gerich J: Role of reduced suppression of glucose production and diminished early insulin release in impaired glucose tolerance. *N Engl J Med* 326:22–29, 1992

48. Consoli A: Role of liver in pathophysiology of NIDDM. *Diabetes Care* 15:430–441, 1992

49. Gannon MC, Nuttall FQ, Westphal SA, Sheridan KJ, Fang S, Ercan-Fang N: Metabolic response to meals varying in CHO and starch content in subjects with NIDDM (Abstract). *Diabetologia* 40:A391, 1997

50. Gannon MC, Nuttall FQ, Westphal S, Sheridan KJ, Fang S, Ercan-Fang N: Acute metabolic response to high-carbohydrate, high-starch meals compared with moderate-carbohydrate, low-starch meals in subjects with type 2 diabetes. *Diabetes Care* 21:1619–1626, 1998

51. Maheux P, Chen YDI, Polonsky KS, Reaven GM: Evidence that insulin can directly inhibit hepatic glucose production. *Diabetologia* 40:1300–1306, 1997

52. Zinneman HH, Nuttall FQ, Goetz FC: Effect of endogenous insulin on human amino acid metabolism. *Diabetes* 15:5–8, 1966

53. Floyd JC, Fajans SS, Conn JW, Knopf RF, Rull J: Insulin secretion in response to protein ingestion. *J Clin Invest* 45:1479–1486, 1966

54. Rabinowitz D, Merimee TJ, Maffezzoli R, Burgess JA: Patterns of hormonal release after glucose, protein, and glucose plus protein. *Lancet* ii:454–457, 1966

55. Krezowski PA, Nuttall FQ, Gannon MC, Bartosh NH: The effect of protein ingestion on the metabolic response to oral glucose in normal individuals. *Am J Clin Nutr* 44:847–856, 1986

56. Berger S, Vongaraya M: Insulin response to ingested protein in diabetes. *Diabetes* 15:303–306, 1966

57. Fajans SS, Floyd JC, Pek S, Knopf RF, Jacobson M, Conn JW: Effect of protein meals on plasma insulin in mildly diabetic patients. *Diabetes* 18:523–528, 1969

58. Gannon MC, Nuttall FQ, Neil BJ, Westphal SA: The insulin and glucose responses to meals of glucose plus various proteins in type 2 diabetic subjects. *Metabolism* 37:1081–1088, 1988

59. Nuttall FQ, Gannon MC: Metabolic response to egg white and cottage cheese protein in normal subjects. *Metabolism* 39:749–755, 1990

60. Fujita Y, Gotto AM, Unger RH: Basal post-protein insulin and glucagon levels during a high and low carbohydrate intake and their relationships to plasma triglycerides. *Diabetes* 24:552–558, 1975

61. Raskin P, Aydin L, Yamamoto T, Unger RH: Abnormal alpha cell function in human diabetes. *Am J Med* 64:988–997, 1978

62. Ahmed M, Nuttall FQ, Gannon MC, Lamusga RF: Plasma glucagon and alpha-amino acid nitrogen response to various diets in normal humans. *Am J Clin Nutr* 33:1917–1924, 1980

63. Unger RH, Aguilar-Parada E, Muller WA, Eisentraut AM: Studies of pancreatic alpha-cell function in normal and diabetic subjects. *J Clin Invest* 49:837–848, 1970

64. Bomboy JD, Lewis SB, Lacy WW, Sinclair-Smith BC, Liljenquist JE: Transient stimulatory effect of sustained hyperglucagonemia on splanchnic glucose production in normal and diabetic man. *Diabetes* 26:177–184, 1977

65. Ferrannini E, DeFronzo RA, Sherwin RS: Transient hepatic response to glucagon in man: role of insulin and hyperglycemia. *Am J Physiol* 242:E73–E81, 1982

66. Meeker DR, Kesten HD: Experimental atherosclerosis and high protein diets. *Proc Soc Exp Biol Med* 45:543–545, 1940

67. Kritchevsky D: Dietary protein, cholesterol and atherosclerosis: a review of the early history. *J Nutr* 125:589S–593S, 1995

68. Carroll KK, Kurowska EM: Soy consumption and cholesterol reduction: review of animal and human studies. *J Nutr* 125:594S–597S, 1995

69. Sirtori CR, Agradi E, Conti F, Mantero O, Gatti E: Soybean-protein diet in the treatment of type 2 hyperlipoproteinemia. *Lancet* i:275–277, 1977

70. Carroll KK: Review of clinical studies on cholesterol-lowering response to soy protein. *J Am Diet Assoc* 91:820–827, 1991

71. Sirtori CR, Even R, Lovati MR: Soybean-protein diet and plasma cholesterol: from therapy to molecular mechanisms. *Ann NY Acad Sci* 676:188–201, 1993

72. Garg A, Bonanome A, Grundy SM, Zhang ZJ, Unger RH: Comparison of a high-carbohydrate diet with a high-monounsaturated-fat diet in patients with non-insulin dependent diabetes mellitus. *N Engl J Med* 319:829–834, 1988

73. Ulbricht TLV, Southgate DAT: Coronary heart disease: seven dietary factors. *Lancet* 338:985–992, 1991

74. Wingard DL, Barrett-Connor EL, Ferrara A: Is insulin really a heart disease risk factor? *Diabetes Care* 18:1299–1304, 1995

75. Borch-Johnsen K, Mandrup-Poulsen T, Zachau-Christiansen B, Joner G, Christy M, Kastrup K, Nerup J: Relation between breast-feeding and incidence rates of insulin-dependent diabetes mellitus. *Lancet* ii:1083–1086, 1984

76. Martin JM, Trink B, Daneman D, Dosch HM, Robinson B: Milk proteins in the etiology of insulin-dependent diabetes mellitus (IDDM). *Ann Med* 23:447–452, 1991

77. Dosch HM: The possible link between insulin dependent (juvenile) diabetes mellitus and dietary cow milk. *Clin Biochem* 26:307–308, 1993

78. Dahl-Jorgensen K, Joner G, Hanssen KF: Relationship between cows' milk consumption and incidence of IDDM in childhood. *Diabetes Care* 14:1081–1083, 1991

79. Virtanen SM, Saukkonen T, Savilahti E, Ylönen K, Räsänen L, Aro A, Knip M, Tuomilehto J, Akerblom HK, the Childhood Diabetes in Finland Study Group: Diet, cow's milk protein antibodies, and the risk of IDDM in Finnish children. *Diabetologia* 37:381–387, 1994

80. Norris JM, Beaty B, Kingensmith G, Yu L, Hoffman M, Chase P, Erlich HA, Hamman RF, Eisenbarth GS, Rewers M: Lack of association between early exposure to cow's milk protein and β-cell autoimmunity: Diabetes Autoimmunity Study in the Young (DAISY). *JAMA* 276:609–614, 1996

81. Scott FW, Norris JM, Kolb H: Milk and type 1 diabetes: examining the evidence and broadening the focus. *Diabetes Care* 19:379–383, 1996

Dr. Gannon is Director of the Metabolic Research Laboratory and Associate Professor of Food Science & Nutrition and of Medicine, and Dr. Nuttall is Chief, Metabolic/Endocrine Section, and Professor of Medicine, at the University of Minnesota, Minneapolis VA Medical Center, Minneapolis, MN.

8. Food Fats and Dyslipidemia

Jonathan Q. Purnell, MD, and John D. Brunzell, MD

Highlights

- Lipid abnormalities associated with greater risk for coronary heart disease in people with central obesity and type 2 diabetes include abnormalities in both total lipid levels and lipoprotein particle composition: elevated triglyceride, increased cholesterol in small dense LDL particles, and decreased HDL cholesterol.
- Restriction of saturated fat (≤10% of total daily calories) has a beneficial effect on lipid levels and insulin sensitivity in people with diabetes.
- Both low-fat (<30% of total daily calories), high-carbohydrate diets and diets enriched with monounsaturated fat improve glucose tolerance and lipid levels compared with diets high in saturated fat.
- Consuming a greater percentage of total calories from fat (both saturated and monounsaturated) has been associated with obesity, and dietary fat restriction has been shown to result in modest spontaneous weight loss. It is advisable to limit total fat intake to optimize weight management.

"The important issue for physicians is how to apply the knowledge gained from controlled in-depth metabolic studies on a small number of subjects to dietary advice aimed at ultimately reducing the severe and accelerated atherosclerotic cardiovascular disease in the diabetic patient."

—Ed Bierman, *Diabetes Care* 12:163, 1989

INTRODUCTION

Before 1971 (1), most expert advice on nutritional therapy for diabetes was to restrict dietary carbohydrates and, out of necessity, increase dietary fat intake to meet daily caloric needs. From epidemiological studies in the 1960s, however, coronary artery disease (CAD) risk in many different populations was shown to increase with increasing intake of total and saturated fat (2). As it became apparent that a leading cause of death in people with diabetes was CAD (3–5) and as a result of studies demonstrating that diets restricted in saturated fat improve glycemic control and lipid levels (see below), nutritional recommendations for people with diabetes called for reduction of total dietary fat intake to <30% of total daily calories and of saturated fats to <10% (6).

For most patients with type 1 diabetes, lipid levels are normal soon after instituting insulin therapy (7) and the above dietary recommendations for fat intake would apply. Centrally obese subjects with type 1 diabetes and those with type 2 diabetes, however, have a dyslipidemia consisting of increased triglyceride levels, reduced HDL cholesterol levels, and small dense LDL particles that does not normalize with improving glycemic control (8–12). This dyslipidemia is strongly associated with increased central (visceral) obesity (13–16), insulin resistance (11,17), and CAD (18,19). Controversy has arisen over recommending a low-fat, high-carbohydrate diet to these patients because of concern that this may worsen triglyceride and HDL abnormalities and ultimately increase CAD risk (20). This chapter attempts to address this controversy and offers professional caregivers treating patients with diabetes practical advice about dietary fat intake. The goals for nutritional therapy related to dietary fats for people with diabetes are to optimize glycemic control, to minimize the risk for weight gain, and most importantly, to reduce the risk for CAD.

DIABETIC DYSLIPIDEMIA AND DIETARY FATTY ACIDS

As mentioned above, the lipid abnormalities that characterize central obesity and type 2 diabetes include increased triglyceride levels, increased secretion of small very-low-density lipoprotein (VLDL) particles, decreased HDL cholesterol, and increased small dense LDL particles (8–12,21–25). Total and LDL cholesterol levels, on the other hand, are usually similar to those of the general population. In part because the National Cholesterol Education Program (NCEP) guidelines emphasize nutritional and pharmacological treatment based on LDL cholesterol levels (26), many practitioners may not recognize and treat lipid abnormalities associated with a greater risk for CAD in individuals with diabetes (27). Although some studies have suggested that triglyceride level is a good predictor of CAD risk in subjects with diabetes (28–30), reductions in total and LDL cholesterol remain a goal in patients with diabetes who have hyperlipidemia. In recent drug trials using HMG-CoA reductase inhibitors, reduction in total and LDL cholesterol resulted in reductions in CAD incidence and mortality in subjects with diabetes (31,32). Of note is that when medications from this group of drugs are used in subjects with diabetes, decreases in triglyceride levels and increases in HDL cholesterol are seen (32,33) and small dense LDL may be cleared (34).

As discussed below, different dietary fatty acids may have either detrimental (saturated fats) or beneficial (polyunsaturated or monounsaturated fats) effects on lipid levels in subjects with diabetes. Therefore, restriction of dietary saturated fat is a desirable goal of nutritional therapy for diabetes. Replacement of dietary saturated fat with carbohydrates or monounsaturated fat leads to improvement in lipid levels in subjects with diabetes, but controversy exists over whether carbohydrates should also be restricted.

Reduction in Saturated Fats

The conventional wisdom that diets for people with diabetes should be limited in carbohydrates and high in fat began to be questioned in the 1920s and 1930s, soon after the discovery of insulin. Joslin observed a high incidence of atherosclerosis in his patients with diabetes and suggested that treatment include normalization of serum cholesterol through restriction of fat- and cholesterol-rich foods (35). Soon thereafter, reports of decreased need for insulin and improved glucose control from limiting fat and increasing carbohydrate content in the diet began to appear (36–41). In addition, some of these investigators observed improvements in lipid levels on these low-fat, high-carbohydrate diets (38–40).

In an early controlled-feeding study of the effects on lipids of altering dietary fat and carbohydrate, Stone and Connor (42) studied 25 free-living subjects with insulin-treated diabetes randomized to receive either a diet high in total and saturated fat (42% total fat intake; 22% saturated fat; polyunsaturated-to-saturated fat [P/S] ratio of 0.8) or a diet low in fat and high in carbohydrates (20% total fat; 4% saturated fat; P/S ratio of 1; 64% carbohydrate) (42). After an average follow-up of 1 year, total cholesterol levels fell by 20% (250 mg/dl to 198 mg/dl, $P < 0.001$) and triglyceride levels fell 15% ($P < 0.1$) on the low-fat, high-carbohydrate diet, but remained unchanged on the high-fat diet. Other studies have confirmed reductions in cholesterol levels ranging from 9% to 29% when saturated fat is replaced with carbohydrates in subjects with diabetes (43–48). Two of these studies also included measurements of LDL and

HDL cholesterol and found that the reduction in total cholesterol on the low-fat, high-carbohydrate diet versus the high–saturated fat diet resulted from reductions in LDL but not HDL cholesterol (46,48). On the low-fat, high-carbohydrate diet, triglyceride levels in these studies improved when subjects had severe hypertriglyceridemia (43) and remained unchanged in the presence of modest hypertriglyceridemia (42,44,46–50).

In each of the above lipid studies and in others designed to measure glycemic control and insulin action, glucose control was improved or unchanged as a result of restricting dietary saturated fat and replacing it with carbohydrates (41,42,46,50–54). The debate, therefore, is not whether saturated fat should be limited to 10% or less of total caloric intake, as is currently recommended by the NCEP for the prevention of heart disease in those at greater risk of CAD (26), but what is the best alternative energy source for the patient with diabetes. Dietary protein is generally ~10–20% of total daily calories; this leaves roughly 70–80% of daily calories to be derived from a combination of polyunsaturated fats, monounsaturated fats, and carbohydrates.

Monounsaturated Fats Versus Carbohydrates

Coulston and colleagues (55,56) questioned the restriction of total fat to <30% of total daily caloric intake in patients with diabetes in two studies comparing lipids, glucose, and insulin levels in subjects with diabetes treated in a random crossover design with either a low-fat, high-carbohydrate diet (20% fat, 60% carbohydrate) or a high-fat diet (40% fat, although restricted in saturated fat, with a P/S ratio ≥1.0; 40% carbohydrate). Both studies were designed to maintain weight stability throughout (isocaloric diets), and at the end of each dietary intervention, both studies demonstrated no difference in fasting levels of glucose, insulin, total cholesterol, and LDL cholesterol between the two diets. Triglyceride levels, VLDL cholesterol, and postprandial excursions of glucose and insulin were higher and HDL cholesterol was lower, however, when subjects consumed the low-fat, high-carbohydrate diet compared with when they consumed the high-fat, low–saturated fat diet. Garg et al. (57) reported nearly identical effects on lipid levels and glycemic control when comparing a low-fat, high-carbohydrate diet (25% total fat, 60% carbohydrate) with a high-fat, low–saturated fat diet (50% total fat: 10% saturated, 33% monounsaturated, 7% polyunsaturated) in subjects with type 2 diabetes. Both groups of investigators argued from these results that diets high in fat, especially monounsaturated fat, were superior to low-fat, high-carbohydrate diets because they resulted in lower triglyceride levels, higher HDL levels, and lower postprandial excursions of glucose and insulin.

Since then, numerous investigators have studied the effect of a high–monounsaturated fat diet versus a low-fat, high-carbohydrate diet in subjects with type 2 diabetes (58–64). Each study included small numbers of subjects, required weight maintenance with isocaloric feedings, and lasted 6 weeks or less. The most consistent findings in these studies were higher triglyceride levels in subjects consuming the high-carbohydrate diet compared with when they were consuming a high–monounsaturated fat, low-carbohydrate diet (58,60–62,64). No difference in fasting blood glucose (58–62,64) or HDL cholesterol levels (58,59,61–64) was observed between subjects on the two diets. In the two studies that used clamp techniques to measure glucose disposal while subjects were on each diet, one demonstrated no significant differences in insulin sensitivity between the diets (60), whereas the other showed increased glucose disposal in subjects while consuming a high–monounsaturated fat diet compared with while they were consuming a low-fat, high-carbohydrate diet (62).

To address the shortcomings of using small numbers of subjects in the above studies, a large multicenter study comparing the effects of a low-fat, high-carbohydrate diet and a diet high in monounsaturated fat on lipids and glycemic control in 42 subjects with type 2 diabetes was published in 1994 (65). Fasting levels of lipids, glucose, insulin, and glycated hemoglobin, along with 24-h profiles of glucose and insulin, were compared at the end of 6 weeks on each diet in a randomized crossover design. At the end of the study period on each diet, no significant differences in fasting plasma glucose, fasting insulin, LDL cholesterol, or HDL cholesterol could be demonstrated. Consistent with the smaller studies, while subjects were on the low-fat, high-carbohydrate diet, plasma triglyceride and VLDL cholesterol levels were higher than while they were on the high–monounsaturated fat diet. Day-long plasma glucose and insulin excursions were also higher on the low-fat, high-carbohydrate diet. Despite these higher excursions of glucose and insulin, long-term glycemic control, as measured using glycated hemoglobin, was not different between the groups.

What can be reasonably concluded from this study is that when subjects with type 2 diabetes are maintained at a constant weight, consuming a diet either high in monounsaturated fat or high in carbohydrates results in similar glycemic control and similar levels of LDL and HDL cholesterol. On this protocol requiring weight stability, however, VLDL triglyceride and cholesterol is increased on the high-carbohydrate diet compared with the high–monounsaturated fat diet. This lipid finding deserves special attention because the authors of this study argue that this may worsen the CAD risk in these subjects. Whereas increased triglyceride levels in subjects with diabetes before dietary or pharmacological therapy is begun are a risk factor for CAD, as mentioned above, the hypertriglyceridemia in subjects with type 2 diabetes results from increased secretion of small VLDL particles (23,25), and it is these small VLDL particles that are thought to be atherogenic. This increased secretion of small VLDL results in increased levels of apolipoprotein B (apo B), the major structural apoprotein of VLDL (66). In addition, this triglyceride elevation accompanies a clustering of other metabolic abnormalities, including accumulation of visceral adiposity (13–16), worsened insulin resistance (11), small dense LDL (8–10,24), and decreased HDL (21,22,24). On the other hand, the increased triglyceride that results from a low-fat, high-carbohydrate diet is the result of an increased amount of triglyceride per VLDL particle, which produces larger, more buoyant particles (67,68). Apo B levels remain unchanged or slightly lower on the low-fat, high-carbohydrate diet, indicating that the VLDL particles are not accumulating in greater amounts (57,58). Finally, this increase in triglyceride level on a low-fat, high-carbohydrate diet is not the result of the clustering of adverse metabolic changes described above because these subjects do not develop more central obesity (they were weight stable during the duration of the studies) and glycemic control does not worsen. In fact, several therapies, including treatment with estrogens (69) and bile acid–binding resins (70), have been shown to lower LDL cholesterol, have beneficial effects on CAD risk, and yet result in increased triglyceride levels as a result of production of larger, more buoyant VLDL particles.

Long-term studies of subjects with diabetes consuming low-fat, high-carbohydrate and monounsaturated fat–enriched diets in a free-living setting with ad libitum access to food are needed to determine effects of these dietary interventions on glycemic control and risk for CAD. In the meantime, rather than limit the use of one diet or the other, several investigators have used the previous data to emphasize that *both* low-fat, high-carbohydrate diets and monounsaturated fat–enriched diets demonstrate improvements in glucose tolerance and lipid levels *compared with diets high in saturated fats* (59,71,72). Once saturated fats are restricted, therefore, nutritional intervention for subjects with type 2 diabetes using components of both diets is desirable. Given the multiethnic makeup of many clinics serving large numbers of patients with diabetes, having a variety of food choices will likely enhance adherence to recommendations.

Although studies of the effect of diets high in carbohydrate versus monounsaturated fat on cardiovascular disease outcomes in diabetes are not currently available, it is informative to compare the incidence of and mortality from CAD in subjects with diabetes in populations that consume different amounts of carbohydrate and fat. In Japan in the 1960s and 1970s, carbohydrate consumption was typically 60–70% and total fat intake <20% of total calories in people with diabetes (73,74). Compared with Japanese men with diabetes living in the U.S. and populations in other Western countries consuming a higher-fat diet (carbohydrate ~45%, total fat ~30–40% of total calories), native Japanese had not only a lower incidence of diabetes (74) but also a lower frequency of and mortality from vascular complications (74–76). Because differences other than dietary composition exist between nations that might affect risk factors for CAD, this argument certainly could not be offered as proof that high-carbohydrate diets are protective against heart disease in people with diabetes. At the very least, however, it could be reasonably concluded that high-carbohydrate diets do not worsen the risk for CAD and are, in fact, likely to be beneficial.

Polyunsaturated Fats

In contrast to the large number of studies evaluating the effect of monounsaturated fat on lipid levels and glycemic control in subjects with diabetes, much less has been reported on how dietary polyunsaturated fats affect these parameters. It has been suggested that polyunsaturated fats are less desirable than monounsaturated fats for people with diabetes because substituting polyunsaturated fats for saturated fats in the diets of nondiabetic subjects results in greater HDL lowering than does substituting monounsaturated fats (77). In what is perhaps the best study to date designed to test whether a diet high in total and polyunsaturated fat (total fat 38%, P/S 0.9) improves lipid levels and glucose control compared with a diet high in total and saturated fat (total fat 39%, P/S 0.3), 15 subjects with type 2 diabetes were sampled after 30 weeks on each diet in a randomized crossover design (78). On the high–polyunsaturated fat diet, total and LDL cholesterol levels were lower than on the high–saturated fat diet, but no differences in triglyceride levels, HDL cholesterol, apo B, fasting blood glucose, or long-term glycemic control (as measured by glycated hemoglobin) were found between the two diets. Other small studies comparing diets enriched with monounsaturated versus polyunsaturated fat (linoleic acid) are not conclusive as to the superiority of one or the other as a substitute for saturated fat (79,80).

On the basis of the evidence, it can be concluded that substituting polyunsaturated fat for saturated fat improves lipids and is therefore the more desirable choice. In practical terms, however, high–polyunsaturated fat diets are not recommended for subjects with diabetes. Because very little data are available from subjects who chronically consume >10% of calories as polyunsaturated fats, and given the potential effect of a high-fat diet in promoting weight gain and potentially worsening the metabolic abnormalities of people with diabetes (see below), emphasis should be placed on limiting both saturated and polyunsaturated fat to <10% of total caloric intake each.

Omega-3 (ω-3) Fatty Acids

A number of epidemiological studies have shown that populations consuming diets rich in fish have lower rates of CAD (81,82). Omega-3 (ω-3) fatty acids are a major constituent of cold-water fish oils and have been shown to reduce triglyceride levels, especially in people who are hypertriglyceridemic (83), through a mechanism thought to include reduction in VLDL secretion (84). In addition, ω-3 fatty acids may have beneficial effects on platelet activity and thrombogenicity (85). Because of the potential of these oils to improve both atherogenic and thrombogenic profiles in people at high risk for CAD, their effects on lipid levels, platelet activity, and clotting factors have been assessed in a number of trials. A few of these trials simply had subjects eat more fish. In the majority of interventions, however, subjects took supplemental daily doses of oil (in grams) with their usual meals.

Since the mid-1980s, there have been more than 25 dietary intervention trials of fish oil in subjects with type 1 and type 2 diabetes (see reviews by Malasanos et al. [86] and Prince et al. [87]). Meaningful conclusions from these studies about the effects of ω-3 fatty acids on lipids and glycemic control in diabetes are limited because of the small numbers of subjects, the heterogeneity of doses of oil, the limited duration of therapy, and the lack of adequate controls in many of them. Two recent studies, however, deserve mention (88,89). Using a placebo-controlled, double-blind design for extended follow-up, both studies evaluated the effect of supplementation on lipids and glycemic control in subjects with type 2 diabetes and hypertriglyceridemia.

In a study of 16 subjects by Connor et al. (88), either 15 g fish oil containing 6.0 g ω-3 fatty acids or 15 g olive oil were supplemented on a daily basis in a crossover design for 6 months on each treatment. Compared with treatment with olive oil, treatment with fish oil resulted in lower total triglyceride (260 mg/dl vs. 449 mg/dl, $P < 0.001$) and VLDL cholesterol (41 mg/dl vs. 72 mg/dl, $P < 0.001$), but higher LDL cholesterol (145 mg/dl vs. 117 mg/dl, $P < 0.001$). Glycemic control at follow-up, as assessed by fasting blood glucose and glycated hemoglobin (HbA_{1c}), was not different between the two treatment groups.

Rivellese et al. (89) randomized 16 subjects to receive either daily doses of 2.5 g ω-3 fatty acids for 2 months followed by 1.7 g ω-3 fatty acids for 4 more months (6-month total duration of ω-3 fatty acid supplementation) or 1 g olive oil as placebo. At the end of 6 months on each treatment, just as Connor et al. (88) had shown, levels of triglyceride and VLDL cholesterol were significantly lower, but LDL cholesterol was significantly higher in subjects on fish oil compared with baseline, with no change in lipid levels as a result of placebo use. Likewise, use of fish oil did not result in deterioration in fasting blood glucose or in HbA_{1c}. Additionally, Rivellese et al. (89) showed no change in insulin-mediated glucose disposal on either treatment using a euglycemic-hyperinsulinemic clamp.

While fish oil supplementation appears to be beneficial in lowering triglyceride levels in subjects with type 2 diabetes and hypertriglyceridemia, the accompanying rise in LDL cholesterol that has been demonstrated in the above studies and others (90–93) is worrisome. No study to date has determined whether this increase in LDL results from increases in intermediate-density lipoprotein or dense LDL particles (more atherogenic) or more buoyant LDL particles (less atherogenic). Certainly, nutritional advice to increase consumption of fish is reasonable given the evidence to date. If conventional medical therapy to lower triglyceride levels is not adequate, supplementation with fish oil might be considered. LDL cholesterol levels should be monitored closely, however, to ensure that significant elevations be managed appropriately.

FATS AND OBESITY

Epidemiological studies have demonstrated that obese subjects consume a greater percentage of their total calories as fat than do lean subjects (94–99), and it appears that this effect is seen with both higher saturated and higher monounsaturated fat intake (94,95,98). The finding from the cross-sectional studies mentioned above of an association between high dietary fat intake and obesity implies that weight stability or weight loss may be achieved by lowering the total fat content of the diet. A number of prospective studies have now demonstrated modest spontaneous weight loss when subjects are allowed to consume a low-fat, high-carbohydrate diet, as opposed to a high-fat diet, on an ad lib basis (subjects choose the amount and type of food and stop when they are full) through a voluntary reduction in caloric intake (100–108). Long-term studies have demonstrated that this weight loss is sustainable for up to 2 years of follow-up (100,104,105,108).

In the previous studies comparing the effects of low-fat, high-carbohydrate and high–monounsatureated fat intake on lipids in subjects with diabetes, isocaloric feedings were required to maintain weight stability. This is because weight change may have independent effects on lipids and glycemic control. Several investigators have now demonstrated that triglyceride levels are not increased in subjects who consume an ad lib low-fat diet and experience weight loss (100,105). Using a rigorous, prospective study design, Schaefer et al. (107) recently studied subjects on an isocaloric high-fat diet or an isocaloric low-fat, high-carbohydrate diet and then allowed them to consume their low-fat, high-carbohydrate calories on an ad lib basis. The increase in triglyceride and VLDL cholesterol levels in subjects consuming the isocaloric low-fat, high-carbohydrate diet was completely reversed when subjects were allowed to eat ad lib. Therefore, it is important to interpret results from isocaloric feeding studies with an understanding that total dietary fat intake may have an adverse effect on weight, which in turn may adversely affect lipid levels and glycemic control. Because central obesity is an important determinant of insulin resistance and the accompanying dyslipidemia characteristic of type 2 diabetes, it is advisable to limit total fat intake to optimize weight management.

CHYLOMICRONEMIA SYNDROME

Very high triglyceride levels can lead to accumulation of chylomicrons and to life-threatening pancreatitis (43,109). The presence of a triglyceride level >2,000 mg/dl, eruptive xanthoma, and lipemia retinalis in addition to pancreatitis has been termed the chylomicronemia syndrome and most often results when an individual with an inherited form of hypertriglyceridemia acquires a disorder, such as diabetes, that further increases triglyceride secretion and/or impairs removal of triglyceride-rich particles (109). To prevent onset of this syndrome, subjects with treated diabetes and triglyceride levels >1,000 mg/dl should have acute restriction of all types of dietary fat and treatment with a pharmacological agent, such as a fibric acid derivative, to reduce the risk of pancreatitis.

CURRENT DIETARY FAT INTAKE GUIDELINES AND THE PATIENT WITH DYSLIPIDEMIA

Primarily because of the controversy over the amount of dietary carbohydrate to recommend for subjects with diabetes, specific guidelines for the amount of total fat (which previously had been to limited to <30% of daily calories [6]) and carbohydrate were dropped in 1994 (110). Instead, after restriction of saturated fat to <10% of total daily calories, which remains the cornerstone of nutritional advice to optimize both lipid levels and glycemic control, clinicians are advised to vary the amount of fat and carbohydrate based on treatment goals (110). With 10–20% of calories derived from protein and ≤10% from polyunsaturated fats, that leaves 60–70% of calories to be divided between carbohydrates and monounsaturated fats. On one hand, because most subjects with type 2 diabetes are obese (centrally obese in particular), limitation of total fat, including monounsaturated fat, would be desirable to optimize weight management. On the other hand, because most centrally obese patients with type 2 diabetes also have elevated triglyceride levels, current recommendations would suggest an increase in monounsaturated fat and a limitation in carbohydrate intake. Unfortunately, this becomes confusing to clinician and patient alike and obscures the importance of limiting saturated fat. In other words, both low-fat, high-carbohydrate and low–saturated fat, high–monounsaturated fat diets result in improved lipids (including triglyceride levels) over those in a subject who typically consumes a high–saturated fat diet. Although metabolic ward studies using isocaloric feedings to maintain weight have shown that triglyceride levels tend to be higher on a low-fat, high-carbohydrate diet than on a high–monounsaturated fat diet, no evidence exists that the more buoyant, triglyceride-rich VLDL particles that result from high-carbohydrate feedings persist beyond 3 months (42,111,112) or are atherogenic. In fact, similar changes in triglyceride levels and VLDL particles are seen with the use of alcohol (113), estrogens in postmenopausal women (69), and bile acid resin binders (70), all of which are associated with decreased CAD risk. In addition, maintaining weight stability is difficult on a high-carbohydrate diet compared with that on an isocaloric high-fat diet, but the modest weight loss that occurs with ad lib consumption of high-carbohydrate diets may result in further improvements in metabolic risk factors for CAD.

The most recent position statement by the American Diabetes Association on the management of dyslipidemia in adults with diabetes suggests that an LDL cholesterol cutoff of >100 mg/dl be used to decide when to institute medical nutrition therapy (i.e., restrict saturated fats) and an exercise program (114). An argument could be made, however, that given the benefits of saturated fat restriction on lipids and glycemic control, all adult subjects with newly diagnosed diabetes should be advised to restrict total and saturated dietary fat. The level of LDL cholesterol at which to initiate drug therapy is more controversial.

SUMMARY

In patients with triglyceride levels >1,000 mg/dl, dietary intake of fat should be acutely restricted. In subjects without such high levels of triglyceride, nutritional recommendations about the dietary fat content should emphasize restriction of saturated fat to <10% of total daily energy needs to optimize lipid levels and glycemic control. Because central obesity is a strong risk factor for dyslipidemia and CAD, and because low-fat, high-carbohydrate diets allow spontaneous loss of modest amounts of weight and improvements in lipid levels, total fat should also be restricted to ≤30% of daily calories. It should be emphasized, however, that dietary advice is best given within the context of the patient's cultural background. For instance, a patient of Asian background might find it easy to limit saturated fat and continue with a high-carbohydrate diet. For a patient of Mediterranean origin whose intake of monounsaturated fat is higher, these guidelines may be liberalized, so long as emphasis is placed on restricting saturated fat and weight is followed over time to ensure stability. Although consumption of fish as part of a balanced meal plan is advisable, a definitive role for supplemental fish oil in the management of hyperlipidemic subjects with diabetes remains to be determined.

Future Areas of Research

Long-term follow-up studies are needed in subjects with diabetes in free-living settings with ad lib access to food to determine effects of high–monounsaturated fat, low-fat, high-carbohydrate, and supplementary fish oil intake on:

1. Total lipids, glucose control, and body weight
2. Heterogeneity of LDL particles and their distribution (dense versus buoyant)
3. CAD incidence and mortality

REFERENCES

1. Bierman EL, Albrink MJ, Arky RA, Connor WE, Dayton S, Spritz N, Steinberg D: Principles of nutritional and dietary recommendations for patients with diabetes mellitus: 1971. *Diabetes* 20:633–634, 1971

2. Keys A: Coronary heart disease in seven countries. *Circulation* 41:I186–I195, 1970

3. Garcia MJ, McNamara PM, Gordon T, Kannel WB: Morbidity and mortality in diabetics in the Framingham population: sixteen-year follow-up study. *Diabetes* 23:105–111, 1974

4. Stamler, J, Vaccaro O, Neaton JD, Wentworth D: Diabetes, other risk factors, and 12-yr cardiovascular mortality for men screened in the Multiple Risk Factor Intervention Trial. *Diabetes Care* 16:434–444, 1993

5. Koivisto VA, Stevens LK, Mattock M, Ebeling P, Muggeo M, Stephenson J, Idzior-Walus B, the EICS Group: Cardiovascular disease and its risk factors in IDDM in Europe. *Diabetes Care* 19:689–697, 1996

6. American Diabetes Association: Nutritional recommendations and principles for individuals with diabetes mellitus: 1986. *Diabetes Care* 10:126–132, 1987

7. Nikkila EA, Hormila P: Serum lipids and lipoproteins in insulin-treated diabetes: demonstration of increased high-density lipoprotein concentrations. *Diabetes* 27:1078–1085, 1978

8. Feingold KR, Grunfield C, Pang M, Doerrler W, Krauss RM: LDL subclass phenotypes and triglyceride metabolism in non-insulin-dependent diabetes. *Arterioscler Thromb* 12:1496–1502, 1992

9. Selby JV, Austin AM, Newman B, Zhang D, Quesenberry CP, Mayer EJ, Krauss RM: LDL subclass phenotypes and the insulin resistance syndrome in women. *Circulation* 87:381–387, 1993

10. Stewart MW, Laker MF, Dyer RG, Game F, Mitcheson J, Winocour PH, Alberti KGMM: Lipoprotein compositional abnormalities and insulin resistance in type II diabetic patients with mild hyperlipidemia. *Arterioscler Thromb* 13:1046–1052, 1993

11. Fujimoto WY, Abbate SL, Kahn SE, Hokanson JE, Brunzell JD: The visceral adiposity syndrome in Japanese-American men. *Obes Res* 2:364–371, 1994

12. Purnell JQ, Hokanson JE, Marcovina SM, Cleary PA, Steffes MW, Brunzell JD: Weight gain accompanying intensive diabetes therapy in type I diabetes is associated with higher levels of dense LDL cholesterol (Abstract). *J Invest Med* 44:180A, 1996

13. Kissebah AH, Vydelingum N, Murray RW, Evans DJ, Hartz AJ, Kalkhoff RK, Adams PW: Relation of body fat distribution to metabolic complications of obesity. *J Clin Endocrinol Metab* 54:254–260, 1982

14. Pouliot M, Despres J, Nadeau A, Moorjani S, Prud'homme D, Lupien PJ, Tremblay A, Bouchard C: Visceral obesity in men: associations with glucose tolerance, plasma insulin, and lipoprotein levels. *Diabetes* 41:826–834, 1992

15. Fujimoto WY, Newell-Morris LL, Grote MN, Bergstrom RW, Shuman WP: Visceral fat obesity and morbidity: NIDDM and atherogenic risk in Japanese American men and women. *Int J Obes* 15:41–44, 1991

16. Tchernof A, Lamarche B, Prud'homme D, Nadeau A, Moorjani S, Labrie F, Lupien PJ, Despres J-P: The dense LDL phenotype: association with plasma lipoprotein levels, visceral obesity, and hyperinsulinemia in men. *Diabetes Care* 19:629–637, 1996

17. Reaven GM, Chen YD, Jeppesen J, Maheux P, Krauss RM: Insulin resistance and hyperinsulinemia in individuals with small, dense low density lipoprotein particles. *J Clin Invest* 92:141–146, 1993

18. Gardner CD, Fortmann SP, Krauss RM: Association of small low-density lipoprotein particles with the incidence of coronary artery disease in men and women. *JAMA* 276:875–881, 1996

19. Stampfer MJ, Krauss RM, Ma J, Blanche PJ, Holl LG, Sacks FM, Hennekens CH: A prospective study of triglyceride level, low-density lipoprotein particle diameter, and risk of myocardial infarction. *JAMA* 276:882–888, 1996

20. Garg A: High–monounsaturated fat diet for diabetic patients: is it time to change the current dietary recommendations? *Diabetes Care* 17:242–246, 1994

21. Lopes-Virella MF, Stone PG, Colwell JA: Serum high density lipoprotein in diabetic patients. *Diabetologia* 13:285–291, 1977

22. Barrett-Connor E, Witztum JL, Holdbrook MJ: A community study of high density lipoproteins in adult noninsulin-dependent diabetics. *Am J Epidemiol* 117:186–192, 1983

23. Dunn FL, Raskin P, Bilheimer DW, Grundy SM: The effects of diabetic control on very low density lipoprotein triglyceride metabolism in patients with type II diabetes mellitus and marked hypertriglyceridemia. *Metabolism* 33:117–123, 1984

24. Haffner SM, Mykkanen L, Stern MP, Paidi M, Howard BV: Greater effect of diabetes on LDL size in women than in men. *Diabetes Care* 17:1164–1171, 1994

25. Cummings MH, Watts GF, Umpleby AM, Hennessy TR, Naoumova R, Salvin BM, Thompson GR, Sonksen PH: Increased hepatic secretion of very-low-density lipoprotein apolipoprotein B-100 in NIDDM. *Diabetologia* 38:959–967, 1995

26. NCEP Expert Panel: Summary of the Second Report of the National Cholesterol Education Program (NCEP) Expert Panel on Detection, Evaluation, and Treatment of High Blood Cholesterol in Adults. *JAMA* 269:3015–3023, 1993

27. Stern MP, Patterson JK, Haffner SM, Hazuda HP, Mitchell BD: Lack of awareness and treatment of hyperlipidemia in type II diabetes in a community survey. *JAMA* 262:360–364, 1990

28. Santen RJ, Willis PJ, Fajans SS: Atherosclerosis in diabetes mellitus: correlation with serum lipid levels, adiposity, and serum insulin levels. *Arch Intern Med* 130:833–843, 1972

29. West KM, Ahuja MMS, Bennett PH, Czyzky A, Mateo de Acosta O, Fuller JH, Grab B, Grabauskas V, Jarrett RJ, Kosaka K, Keen H, Krolewski AB, Miki E, Schliak V, Teuscher A, Watkins PJ, Stober JA: The role of circulating glucose and triglyceride concentrations and their interactions with other "risk factors" as determinants of arterial disease in nine diabetic population samples from the WHO multinational study. *Diabetes Care* 6:361–369, 1983

30. Fontbonne A, Eschwege E, Cambien F, Richard J-L, Ducimetiere P, Thibult N, Warnet JM, Claude J-R, Rosselin GE: Hypertriglyceridemia as a risk factor of coronary heart disease mortality in subjects with impaired glucose tolerance or diabetes. *Diabetologia* 32:300–304, 1989

31. Sacks FM, Pfeffer MA, Moye LA, Rouleau JL, Rutherford JD, Cole TG, Brown L, Warnica JW, Arnold JMO, Wun C, Davis BR, Braunwald E: The effect of pravastatin on coronary events after myocardial infarction in patients with average cholesterol levels. *N Engl J Med* 335:1001–1009, 1996

32. Pyorala K, Pedersen TR, Kjekshus J, Faergeman O, Olsson AG, Thorgeirsson G: Cholesterol lowering with simvastatin improves prognosis of diabetic patients with coronary heart disease. *Diabetes Care* 20:614–620, 1997

33. Garg A, Grundy SM: Lovastatin for lowering cholesterol levels in non-insulin-dependent diabetes mellitus. *N Engl J Med* 318:81–86, 1988

34. Zambon A, Brown BG, Hokanson JE, Brunzell JD: Hepatic lipase changes predict coronary disease progression/regression in the familial atherosclerosis treatment study (FATS). *Circulation* 94:I539, 1996

35. Joslin EP: *The Treatment of Diabetes Mellitus*. 4th ed. Philadelphia, Lea & Febiger, 1928, p. 252

36. Rabinowitch IM: Experiences with a high carbohydrate-low calorie diet for the treatment of diabetes mellitus. *Can Med Assoc J* 23:489–498, 1930

37. Singh I: Low-fat diet and therapeutic doses of insulin in diabetes mellitus *Lancet* i:422–425, 1955

38. Kempner W, Peschel RL, Schlayer C: Effect of rice diet on diabetes mellitus associated with vascular disease. *Postgrad Med* 24:359–371, 1958

39. Van Eck WF: The effect of a low fat diet on the serum lipids in diabetes and its significance in diabetic retinopathy. *Am J Med* 27:196–211, 1959

40. Ernest I, Linner E, Svanborg A: Carbohydrate-rich, fat-poor diet in diabetes. *Am J Med* 39:594–600, 1964

41. Brunzell JD, Lerner RL, Hazzard WR, Porte D, Bierman EL: Improved glucose tolerance with high carbohydrate feeding in mild diabetes. *N Engl J Med* 284:521–524, 1971

42. Stone DB, Connor WE: The prolonged effects of a low cholesterol, high carbohydrate diet upon the serum lipids in diabetic patients. *Diabetes* 12:127–132, 1963

43. Brunzell JD, Porte D, Bierman EL: Reversible abnormalities in postheparin lipolytic activity during the late phase of release in diabetes mellitus. *Metabolism* 24:1123–1137, 1975

44. Kiehm TG, Anerson TW, Ward K: Beneficial effects of a high carbohydrate, high fiber diet on hyperglycemic diabetic men. *Am J Clin Nutr* 29:895–899, 1976

45. Anderson JW, Ward K: High-carbohydrate, high fiber diets for insulin-treated men with diabetes mellitus. *Am J Clin Nutr* 32:2312–2321, 1979

46. Simpson RW, Mann JI, Eaton J, Moore RA, Carter R, Hockaday TDR: Improved glucose control in maturity-onset diabetes treated with high-carbohydrate-modified fat diet. *BMJ* 1:1753–1756, 1979

47. Hjollund E, Pedersen O, Richelsen B, Beck-Nielsen H, Sorensen NS: Increased insulin binding to adipocytes and monocytes and increased insulin sensitivity of glucose transport and metabolism in adipocytes from non-insulin-dependent diabetics after a low-fat/high starch/high fiber diet. *Metabolism* 32:1067–1074, 1983

48. Abbott WGH, Boyce VL, Grundy SM, Howard BV: Effects of replacing saturated fat with complex carbohydrate in diets of subjects with NIDDM. *Diabetes Care* 12:102–107, 1989

49. Anderson JW: Effect of carbohydrate restriction and high carbohydrate diets on men with chemical diabetes. *Am J Clin Nutr* 30:402–408, 1977

50. Simpson HCR, Lousley S, Geekie M, Simpson RW, Carther RD, Hockaday TDR, Mann JI: A high carbohydrate leguminous fibre diet improves all aspects of diabetic control *Lancet* i:1–5, 1981

51. Hales CN, Randle PJ: Effects of low-carbohydrate diet and diabetes mellitus on plasma concentrations of glucose, non-esterified fatty acid, and insulin during oral glucose tolerance tests. *Lancet* i:790–794, 1963

52. Brunzell JD, Lerner RL, Porte D, Bierman EL: Effect of a fat free, high carbohydrate diet on diabetic subjects with fasting hyperglycemia. *Diabetes* 23:138–142, 1974

53. Kolterman OG, Greenfield M, Reaven GM, Saekow M, Olefsky JM: Effect of a high carbohydrate diet on insulin binding to adipocytes and on insulin action in vivo in man. *Diabetes* 28:731–736, 1979

54. Bantle JP, Laine DC, Castle GW, Thomas JW, Hoogwerf BJ, Goetz FC: Postprandial glucose and insulin responses to meals containing different carbohydrates in normal and diabetic subjects. *N Engl J Med* 309:7–12, 1983

55. Coulston AM, Hollenbeck CB, Swislocki ALM, Chen Y-DI, Reaven G: Deleterious metabolic effects of high-carbohydrate,

sucrose-containing diets in patients with non-insulin-dependent diabetes mellitus. *Am J Med* 82:213–220, 1987

56. Coulston AM, Hollenbeck CB, Swislocki ALM, Reaven GM: Persistence of hypertriglyceridemic effect of low-fat high-carbohydrate diets in NIDDM patients. *Diabetes Care* 12:94–101, 1989

57. Garg A, Bonanome A, Grundy SM, Zhang ZJ, Unger RH: Comparison of a high-carbohydrate diet with a high-monounsaturated fat diet in patients with non-insulin-dependent diabetes. *N Engl J Med* 319:829–834, 1988

58. Rivellese AA, Giacco R, Genovese S, Patti L, Marotta G, Pacioni D, Annuzzi G, Riccardi G: Effects of changing amount of carbohydrate in diet on plasma lipoproteins and apolipoproteins in type II diabetic patients. *Diabetes Care* 13:446–448, 1990

59. Bonanome A, Visona A, Lusiani L, Beltramello G, Confortin L, Biffanti S, Sorgato F, Costa F, Pagnan A: Carbohydrate and lipid metabolism in patients with non-insulin-dependent diabetes mellitus: effects of a low-fat, high-carbohydrate diet versus a diet high in monounsaturated fatty acids. *Am J Clin Nutr* 54:586–590, 1991

60. Garg A, Grundy SM, Unger RH: Comparison of effects of high- and low-carbohydrate diets on plasma lipoproteins and insulin sensitivity in patients with mild NIDDM. *Diabetes* 41:1278–1285, 1992

61. Garg A, Grundy SM, Koffler M: Effect of high carbohydrate intake on hyperglycemia, islet function, and plasma lipoproteins in NIDDM. *Diabetes Care* 15:1572–1580, 1992

62. Parillo M, Rivellese AA, Ciardullo AV, Capaldo B, Giacco A, Genovese S, Riccardi G: A high-monounsaturated-fat/low carbohydrate diet improves peripheral insulin sensitivity in non-insulin-dependent diabetic patients. *Metabolism* 41:1373–1378, 1992

63. Rasmussen OW, Thomsen C, Hansen KW, Vesterlund M, Winther E, Hermansen K: Effects on blood pressure, glucose, and lipid levels of a high–monounsaturated fat diet compared with a high-carbohydrate diet in non-insulin-dependent diabetic (NIDDM) subjects. *Diabetes Care* 16:1565–1571, 1993

64. Campbell LV, Marmot PE, Dyer JA, Borkman M, Storlien LH: The high–monounsaturated fat diet as a practical alternative for NIDDM. *Diabetes Care* 17:177–182, 1994

65. Garg A, Bantle JP, Henry RR, Coulston AM, Griver KA, Raatz SK, Brinkley L, Chen YD, Grundy SM, Huet BA: Effects of vary-

ing carbohydrate content of diet in patients with non-insulin-dependent diabetes mellitus. *JAMA* 271:1421–1428, 1994

66. Zambon S, Manzato E, Solini A, Sambataro M, Brocco E, Sartore G, Crepaldi G, Nosadini R: Lipoprotein abnormalities in non-insulin-dependent diabetic patients with impaired extrahepatic insulin sensitivity, hypertension, and micoralbuminuria. *Arterioscler Thromb* 14:911–916, 1994

67. Ruderman NB, Jones AL, Krauss RM, Shafrir E: A biochemical and morphologic study of very low density lipoproteins in carbohydrate-induced hypertriglyceridemia. *J Clin Invest* 50:1355–1368, 1971

68. Melish J, Le N, Ginsberg H, Steinberg D, Brown WV: Dissociation of apoprotein B and triglyceride production in very-low-density lipoproteins. *Am J Physiol* 239:E354–E362, 1980

69. Walsh BW, Schiff I, Rosner B, Greenberg L, Ravnikar V, Sacks FM: Effects of postmenopausal estrogen replacement on the concentrations and metabolism of plasma lipoproteins. *N Engl J Med* 325:1196–1204, 1991

70. Angelin B, Leijd B, Hultcrantz R, Einarsson K: Increased turnover of very low density lipoprotein triglyceride during treatment with cholestyramine in familial hypercholesterolemia. *J Intern Med* 227:201–206, 1990

71. Milne RM, Mann JI, Chisholm AW, Williams SM: Long-term comparison of three dietary prescriptions in the treatment of NIDDM. *Diabetes Care* 17:74–80, 1994

72. Purnell JQ, Brunzell JD: The central role of dietary fat, not carbohydrate, in the insulin resistance syndrome. *Curr Opin Lipidol* 8:17–22, 1997

73. Hirata Y, Nakamura Y, Kaku M: Characteristics of the treatment of diabetics in Japan. In *Diabetes Mellitus in Asia, 1970*. Tsuji S, Wada M, Eds. Amsterdam, Excerpta Medica, 1970, pp. 216–220

74. Kawate R, Yamakido M, Nishimoto Y, Bennett PH, Hamman RF, Knowler WC: Diabetes mellitus and its vascular complications in Japanese migrants on the island of Hawaii. *Diabetes Care* 2:161–170, 1979

75. Kuzuya N, Kosaka K: Diabetes in Japan. In *Diabetes Mellitus in Asia, 1970*. Tsuji S, Wada M, Eds. Amsterdam, Excerpta Medica, 1970, pp. 11–21

76. Keen H, Jarrett RJ: The WHO multinational study of vascular disease in diabetes. 2. Macrovascular disease prevalence. *Diabetes Care* 2:187–195, 1979

77. Mattson FH, Grundy SM: Comparison of effects of dietary saturated, monounsaturated, and polyunsaturated fatty acids on plasma lipids and lipoproteins in man. *J Lipid Res* 26:194–202, 1985

78. Heine RJ, Mulder C, Popp-Snijders C, van der Meer J, van der Meer EA: Linoleic-acid-enriched diet: long-term effects on serum lipoprotein and apolipoprotein concentrations and insulin sensitivity in noninsulin-dependent diabetic subjects. *Am J Clin Nutr* 49:448–456, 1989

79. Vessby B, Karlstrom B, Boberg M, Lithell H, Berne C: Polyunsaturated fatty acids may impair blood glucose control in type 2 diabetic patients. *Diabetic Med* 9:126–133, 1992

80. Parfitt VJ, Desomeaux K, Bolton CH, Hartog M: Effects of high monounsaturated and polyunsaturated fat diets on plasma lipoproteins and lipid peroxidation in type 2 diabetes mellitus. *Diabetic Med* 11:85–91, 1993

81. Kromann N, Green A: Epidemiological studies in the Upernavik district, Greenland: incidence of some chronic diseases 1950–74. *Acta Med Scand* 208:401–406, 1980

82. Kromhout D, Bosschieter EB, Coulander CL: The inverse relation between fish consumption and 20-year mortality from coronary heart disease. *N Engl J Med* 312:1205–1209, 1985

83. Phillipson BE, Rothrock DW, Connor WE, Harris WS, Illingworth DR: Reduction of plasma lipids, lipoproteins, and apoproteins by dietary fish oils in patients with hypertriglyceridemia. *N Engl J Med* 312:1210–1216, 1985

84. Harris WS, Connor WE, Illingworth DR, Rothrock DW, Foster DM: Effects of fish oil on VLDL triglyceride kinetics in humans. *J Lipid Res* 31:1549–1558, 1990

85. Leaf A, Weber PC: Cardiovascular effects of n-3 fatty acids. *N Engl J Med* 318:549–557, 1988

86. Malasanos TH, Stacpoole PW: Biologic effects of omega-3 fatty acids in diabetes mellitus. *Diabetes Care* 14:1160–1179, 1991

87. Prince MJ, Deeg MA: Do n-3 fatty acids improve glucose tolerance and lipemia in diabetics? *Curr Opin Lipidol* 8:7–11, 1997

88. Connor WE, Prince MJ, Ullmann D, Riddle M, Hatcher L, Smith FE, Wilson D: The hypotriglyceridemic effect of fish oil in adult-

onset diabetes without adverse glucose control. *Ann NY Acad Sci* 683:337–340, 1993

89. Rivellese AA, Mafettone A, Iovine C, Di Marino L, Annuzzi G, Mancini M, Riccardi G: Long-term effects of fish oil on insulin resistance and plasma lipoproteins in NIDDM patients with hypertriglyceridemia. *Diabetes Care* 19:1207–1213, 1996

90. Haines AP, Sanders TAB, Imeson JD, Mahler RF, Martin J, Mistry M, Vickers M, Wallace PG: Effects of fish oil supplement on platelet function, homeostatic variables and albuminuria in insulin-dependent diabetics. *Thromb Res* 43:643–655, 1986

91. Mori TA, Vandongen R, Masarei JRL, Dunbar D, Stanton KG: Serum lipids in insulin-dependent diabetics are markedly altered by dietary fish oils. *Clin Exp Pharmacol Physiol* 15:333–337, 1988

92. Glauber H, Wallace P, Griver K, Brechtel G: Adverse metabolic effect of omega-3 fatty acids in non-insulin-dependent diabetes mellitus. *Ann Intern Med* 108:663–668, 1988

93. Westerveld HT, de Graaf JC, van Breugel HH, Akkerman JWN, Sixma JJ, Erkelens DW, Banga JD: Effects of low-dose EPA-E on glycemic control, lipid profile, lipoprotein (a), platelet aggregation, viscosity, and platelet and vessel wall interaction in NIDDM. *Diabetes Care* 16:683–688, 1993

94. Romieu I, Willett WC, Stampfer MJ, Colditz GA, Sampson L, Rosner B, Hennekens CH, Speizer FE: Energy intake and other determinants of relative weight. *Am J Clin Nutr* 47:406–412, 1988

95. Dreon DM, Frey-Hewitt B, Ellsworth N, Williams PT, Terry RB, Wood PD: Dietary fat:carbohydrate ratio and obesity in middle-aged men. *Am J Clin Nutr* 47:995–1000, 1988

96. George V, Tremblay A, Despres JP, Leblanc C, Bouchard C: Effect of dietary fat content on total and regional adiposity in men and women. *Int J Obes* 14:1085–1094, 1989

97. Miller WC, Linderman AK, Wallace J, Niederpruem M: Diet composition, energy intake, and exercise in relation to body fat in men and women. *Am J Clin Nutr* 52:426–430, 1990

98. Miller WC, Niederpruem MG, Wallace JP, Lindeman AK: Dietary fat, sugar, and fiber predict body fat content. *J Am Diet Assoc* 94:612–615, 1994

99. Maffeis C, Pinelli L, Schutz Y: Fat intake and adiposity in 8 to 11-year-old obese children. *Int J Obes* 20:170–174, 1996

100. Thuesen L, Henriksen LB, Engby B: One-year experience with a low-fat, low-cholesterol diet in patients with coronary artery disease. *Am J Clin Nutr* 44:212–219, 1986

101. Lissner L, Levitsky DA, Strupp BJ, Kalkwarf HJ, Roe DA: Dietary fat and the regulation of energy intake in human subjects. *Am J Clin Nutr* 46:886–892, 1987

102. Kendall A, Levitsky DA, Strupp BJ, Lissner L: Weight loss on a low-fat diet: consequence of the imprecision of the control of food intake in humans. *Am J Clin Nutr* 53:1124–1129, 1991

103. Prewitt TE, Schmeisser D, Bowen PE, Aye P, Dolecek TA, Langenberg P, Cole T, Brace L: Changes in body weight, body composition, and energy intake in women fed high- and low-fat diets *Am J Clin Nutr* 54:304–310, 1991

104. Sheppard L, Kristal AR, Kushi LH: Weight loss in women participating in a randomized trial of low-fat diets. *Am J Clin Nutr* 54:821–828, 1991

105. Kasim SE, Martino S, Kim P, Khilnani S, Boomer A, Depper J, Reading BA, Heilbrun LK: Dietary and anthropometric determinants of plasma lipoproteins during a long-term low-fat diet in healthy women. *Am J Clin Nutr* 53:146–153, 1993

106. Raben A, Jensen ND, Marckmann P, Sandstrom B, Astrup A: Spontaneous weight loss during 11 weeks' ad libitum intake of a low fat/high fiber diet in young, normal weight subjects. *Int J Obes* 19:916–923, 1995

107. Schaefer EJ, Lichtenstein AH, Lamon-Fava S, McNamara JR, Schaefer MM, Rasmussen H: Body weight and low-density lipoprotein cholesterol changes after consumption of a low-fat ad libitum diet. *JAMA* 274:1450–1455, 1995

108. Siggaard R, Raben A, Astrup A: Weight loss during 12 weeks' ad libitum carbohydrate-rich diet in overweight and normal-weight subjects at a Danish work site. *Obes Res* 4:347–356, 1996

109. Brunzell JD: Lipoprotein lipase deficiency and other causes of the chylomicronemia syndrome. In *The Metabolic and Molecular Bases of Inherited Disease.* 7th ed. Scriver CR, Beaudet AL, Sly WS, Valle D, Eds. New York, McGraw-Hill, 1995, pp. 1913–1932

110. Franz MJ, Horton ES, Bantle JP, Beebe CA, Brunzell JD, Coulston AM, Henry RR, Hoogwerf JB, Stacpoole PW: Nutrition principles for the management of diabetes and related complications (Technical Review). *Diabetes Care* 17:490–518, 1994

111. Ullmann D, Connor WE, Hatcher LF, Connor SL, Flavell DP: Will a high-carbohydrate, low-fat diet lower plasma lipids and lipoproteins without producing hypertriglyceridemia? *Arterioscler Thromb* 11:1059–1067, 1991

112. Rivellese AA, Auletta P, Marotta G, Saldalamacchia G, Giacco A, Mastrilli V, Vaccaro O, Riccardi G: Long term metabolic effects of two dietary methods of treating hyperlipidemia. *BMJ* 308:227–231, 1994

113. Kervinen K, Savolainen MJ, Kesaniemi YA: Multiple changes in apoprotein B containing lipoproteins after ethanol withdrawal in alcoholic men. *Ann Med* 23:407–413, 1991

114. American Diabetes Association: Management of dyslipidemia in adults with diabetes (Position Statement). *Diabetes Care* 21 (Suppl. 1):S36–S39, 1998

Dr. Purnell is Acting Instructor and Dr. Brunzell is Professor of Medicine in the Division of Metabolism, Endocrinology and Nutrition at the University of Washington School of Medicine, Seattle, WA.

9. Sugar Alternatives and Fat Replacers

MAGGIE POWERS, MS, RD, CDE

Highlights

- A variety of sugar alternatives—high-intensity sweeteners, polyols (sugar alcohols), and natural sweeteners—are used alone or in sweetener blends.
- Fat replacers are made from carbohydrate, protein, or fat (or combinations).
- Sugar alternatives and fat replacers on the market are assumed to be safe for consumption because they either must be FDA (Food and Drug Administration) GRAS (Generally Recognized as Safe) food ingredients or must receive FDA approval.
- Support for using foods containing sugar alternatives and fat replacers as part of a healthful eating plan needs to be part of diabetes care.

INTRODUCTION

Sugar alternatives and fat replacers are used to decrease the sugar and fat contents of specific foods. Food products containing these ingredients may also be lower in calories than the traditional or regular foods. However, foods containing these ingredients are not always lower in calories, nor are they always sugar- and fat-free. Food label claims (Table 9.1) and the "Nutrition Facts" section of the label are important guides to using foods with these ingredients.

The American Diabetes Association and The American Dietetic Association have stated that these ingredients are acceptable for use by people with diabetes because they are safe for all populations; have the potential to reduce carbohydrate, fat, and calorie intake; and do not raise blood

Table 9.1 Definitions of Words Used for Nutrient Content Claims

Calories	■ Calorie free	■ <5 calories per serving
	■ Low calorie	■ ≤40 calories per serving; if the serving is <30 g or <2 tablespoons, per 50 g of the food
	■ Reduced or fewer calories	■ At least 25% fewer calories per serving than reference food
	■ Light, lite	■ Has one-third fewer calories or 50% less fat per reference amount; if more than half the calories are from fat, fat content must be reduced by 50% or more
Sugar	■ Sugar free	■ <0.5 g of sugar per serving
	■ Reduced sugar	■ At least 25% less sugar per serving than reference food
Fat	■ Fat free	■ <0.5 g of fat per serving
	■ Low fat	■ ≤3 g of fat per serving; if the serving is <30 g or <2 tablespoons, per 50 g of the food
	■ Reduced or less fat	■ At least 25% less fat per serving than reference food

Adapted from Stehlin D: A little "lite" reading. In *FDA Consumer Special Report: Focus on Food Labeling.* Washington, DC, U.S. Govt. Printing Office, May 1993, p. 32.

glucose levels at all or any more than other ingredients that contain carbohydrate (1–6).

Sugar alternatives and fat replacers may be used differently than commonly thought and may adjust the carbohydrate or fat content of a food in unexpected ways. Rarely is a simple substitution made. The properties that sugar and fat (Table 9.2) contribute to a food are intertwined with other ingredients, and recipe adjustments are required when an ingredient is substituted (7). Flavor, texture, and functionality issues must be addressed (8). Complementary ingredients are used that increase stability, shelf-life, and taste of the final food.

Sweetener blends will differ depending on other ingredients and desired characteristics. Some blends have a synergistic effect that results in less overall sweetener being used and an improved taste profile (9). Sweetener blends are made with caloric sweeteners as well as sugar alternatives.

The number of Americans using products with these ingredients (sugar-free, low-calorie, and/or reduced-fat products) has doubled in the past 12 years (10). A 1998 survey found that 178 million (90%) adult

Table 9.2 Role of Sugar and Fat in Foods

Sugar Provides	Fat Provides
Sweetness	Flavor carrier/taste enhancer
Structure and texture (crystalline properties)	Rich and creamy mouth-feel
	Emulsification
Bulk/volume	Aeration
Carmelization/browning	Heat stability
Lower freezing point	Moistness and tenderness (humectancy)
Moistness and tenderness (humectancy)	Aroma precursors

From Powers and Warshaw (7).

Americans use such products, whereas 78 million (45%) did in 1986. The 1998 survey also showed that more adults use reduced-fat products (85%) than use reduced-calorie/sugar products (73%).

Despite the increased availability and use of sugar alternatives and fat replacers, there is a continuing rise in obesity and total caloric intake in Americans (11). Furthermore, although the percentage of calories from fat in the American diet decreased from ~40–42% in the late 1950s and 1960s to ~34% in 1994, actual fat intake has increased from ~81 g/day in the late 1970s to ~83 g/day in the early 1990s (11). Fat contributes proportionately less energy to the American diet, however, because total energy intake has increased from an average 1,989 kcal/day in the late 1970s to 2,095 kcal/day in the early 1990s. This increase in calories is composed of a fuel mix that is relatively lower in fat (4). There was also an ~25% increase in all types of sweeteners consumed between 1966 and 1987 to 152 lb per capita per year. Refined cane and beet sugar consumption declined, whereas corn sweetener and noncaloric sweetener consumption increased (12).

The clinical question then becomes, How and when are sugar alternatives and fat replacers effective in achieving health goals? This chapter provides background information on these food products and guidelines for their use to help achieve health goals.

SUGAR ALTERNATIVES

Sugar alternatives are sweet ingredients that are used to replace some or all of the common mono- and disaccharides in a food. There are currently four high-intensity sugar alternatives approved by the Food and Drug Administration (FDA) for use in the U.S.: acesulfame K, aspartame, saccharin, and sucralose. Other sugar alternatives, namely polyols (sugar alcohols), are on the Generally Recognized As Safe (GRAS) list through FDA. Still more sugar alternatives, such as stevioside and glycyrrhizen, which are natural food substances, are receiving some interest.

High-Intensity Sweeteners

High-intensity sweeteners are so sweet that only very small amounts are needed to provide a sweet taste. It is a great challenge for food scientists and technologists to reformulate recipes to account for the absence of sugar's bulk/volume, as well as its caramelization/browning, structure/ texture, and moistness/tenderness properties. Even when a high-intensity sweetener is used simply as a tabletop sweetener, consideration is given to its volume. Bulking ingredients are added to the packet and granular forms. The additional ingredients—maltodextrin, dextrose, and/or lactose—add minimal calories. The amount of lactose, if added, is so small that it is not expected to be a concern for those with lactose intolerance.

Their negligible calories and subsequent lack of effect on blood glucose levels make high-intensity sweeteners of great interest to people with diabetes. A food may contain other ingredients that need to be accounted for in a meal, so the food label is still a "must read" even when the food contains a high-intensity sweetener. The "total carbohydrate" line in the Nutrition Facts section of the food label guides the person with diabetes on how the food can be incorporated into a meal plan.

Sweeteners approved by the FDA as food additives are assigned an accepted daily intake (ADI). The ADI is 100 times smaller than the largest amount of an ingredient that a person could consume on a daily basis without experiencing any physiological effects (Table 9.3).

Acesulfame K. Acesulfame K (acesulfame potassium) was discovered in 1967 at Hoechst in Germany. It was approved for use in Europe in 1983 and was brought to the U.S., where the FDA approved it in 1988. With the brand name Sunett, it is marketed by Nutrinova (Hoechst Food Ingredients) only to the food industry. It is approved for use in over 90 countries and is in over 4,000 products. Several companies do produce tabletop sweeteners containing acesulfame K, including Sweet One and Swiss Sweet.

Acesulfame K is the potassium salt of an organic substance that is not metabolized and is excreted by the kidneys with no tissue accumulation (13,14). The potassium component is minimal (20% by weight; 10 mg/packet of sweetener, equivalent sweetness of 2 tsp sucrose) and is not a concern for people limiting their potassium intake. The properties

**Table 9.3 Accepted Daily Intakes (ADIs) of
High-Intensity Sweeteners**

	ADI (mg/kg body wt)	Average amount (mg) in 12-oz can of soda*	Cans of soda to reach ADI for 60-kg (132-lb) person	Amount (mg) in packet of sweetener	Packets to reach ADI for 60-kg (132-lb) person
Acesulfame K	15	40†	25†	50	18
Aspartame	50	200	15	35	86
Saccharin	5‡	140	2	40	7.5
Sucralose	5	70	4.5	5	60

*Fountain drinks may have different amounts and may contain a sweetener blend. †Based on most typical blend with 90 mg aspartame. ADIs are independent. With this sweetener blend, it takes 35 cans to reach the ADI of aspartame. ‡Set by JECFA.

of the sulfa atom found in the sweetener are quite different from sulfa drugs and products containing sulfites. Therefore, it is not expected to cause any allergic reaction in people allergic to sulfites or sulfa drugs; there have been no reports of allergic reactions in over 10 years of use. Acesulfame K is very stable and retains its sweetness at high temperatures. The ADI has been set at 15 mg/kg body wt/day.

Acesulfame K is 200 times sweeter than sucrose and has a sweetness that is quickly perceived. Its July 1998 approval for use in liquid beverages means that it will now be used in over 20 food categories, including tabletop sweeteners, candy, baked goods, chewing gum, ice cream, syrup, dry beverage and dessert mixes, and of course, liquid beverages.

In liquid beverages, acesulfame K is most often blended with aspartame to provide a taste profile almost identical to that of sucrose. The multi-sweetener blend improves stability and extends shelf-life while using less total sweetener (9). Because of the synergistic properties of the blend, up to 40% less sweetener is used.

Aspartame. Aspartame was discovered in 1965 at G.D. Searle and Company. Its FDA approval was an uphill climb following the 1972 saccharin ban. In 1981, it was approved for use as a tabletop sweetener, with subsequent approvals in a number of food categories, including the 1983 approval for use in carbonated beverages, which account for 70% of its consumption. In 1996, it received approval as a general-purpose sweetener, which eliminates the need for future approvals in individual food categories. Aspartame is approved for use in over 100 countries and more than 6,000 products. It is sold as NutraSweet by Monsanto and also is available from Holland Sweetener.

When consumed, aspartame is metabolized to the amino acids aspartic acid and phenylalanine and to methanol, all of which are excreted at suggested intake levels. Those with phenylketonuria (PKU) need to be aware of the phenylalanine content. All foods that contain aspartame alert consumers that the product contains phenylalanine. The ADI for aspartame is 50 mg/kg body wt/day.

Some researchers have felt that the methanol that is released on breakdown of aspartame is a concern, as might be a subsequent metabolite, formate. However, no measurable blood levels of methanol (at intakes of 34 mg/kg) or changes in blood formate levels (at intakes of 200 mg/kg) have been seen (15,16). Methanol levels returned to normal within 24 h after the larger doses were ingested.

In 1996, a paper was published suggesting that aspartame was linked to a rise in brain tumors (17). The FDA reviewed the National Cancer Institute's database on cancer incidence in the U.S. and found no association between the use of aspartame and the increased incidence of brain tumors. Brain and central nervous system cancers began increasing in 1973 and continued to increase through 1985. Since 1985, the trend line for these cancers has flattened, with the incidence slightly decreasing from 1991 to 1993 (18). Aspartame was not introduced into the U.S. food supply until 1981 and was not used in soft drinks until 1983, making it difficult to correlate it as a factor in the statistics. FDA did review this question in its original review of the sweetener and recently reaffirmed its position (18).

Consumers occasionally report adverse reactions to aspartame that need to be carefully evaluated. Double-blind studies of those reporting reactions and other research comparing reactions to aspartame versus a placebo have not documented any connection (19,20). The Centers for Disease Control and Prevention (CDC) conducted an evaluation of consumer complaints related to aspartame ingestion and spoke to more than 500 people who reported complaints. The CDC summarized that there were no symptoms clearly related to aspartame consumption. The CDC did add that some individuals may have an "unusual sensitivity" (21). Health professionals can use detailed food and environmental diaries and possibly elimination studies if questions are raised.

Aspartame is 180–220 times sweeter than sucrose. Its sweetness profile shows a delayed onset, yet a long-lasting effect. Special care must be taken when using aspartame in baked products at home because it begins to break down at elevated temperatures. It can still be used in many other foods and can be added to heated foods at the end of the cooking process. An encapsulated form of aspartame is available to the food industry that enables the aspartame to be contained until the end of the heating process to ensure an adequate sweetness.

Saccharin. Saccharin (300 times sweeter than sucrose) has been around for over a century, having been discovered in 1879. In 1958, it was classified as a GRAS substance. In 1972, its status reverted to interim use; it was removed from the GRAS list because of its potential link to bladder cancer. In 1977, a ban was proposed, but soon a moratorium was placed on the ban. This moratorium has been extended seven times, and saccharin is available in the U.S. on an interim basis as a food additive. It is available in over 100 countries.

Saccharin is available in three forms: sodium salt, calcium salt, and the acid form. The salt forms contain minimal salt, so they are not a concern to those limiting sodium. It is excreted unchanged by the kidneys. Unlike other sugar alternatives, the amount of saccharin in a food must be listed on the food package in the U.S. The food label must also state, "Use of this product may be hazardous to your health. This product contains saccharin, which has been determined to cause cancer in laboratory animals." This is in spite of additional research confirming that saccharin is safe (22–24).

Some consumers prefer the taste of saccharin to that of other sweeteners despite the common statement that it has a "bitter" taste. Others unknowingly choose saccharin-flavored beverages, as diet fountain soft drinks contain a saccharin-aspartame blend. (This may change with additional sugar alternative approvals.) Saccharin adds stability to products and is considered sweeter by some. The U.S. does not have an ADI for saccharin because it is not a food additive, but the World Health Organization's Joint Expert Committee of Food Additions (JECFA) has set an ADI of 5 mg/kg body wt/day.

Sucralose. Sucralose was discovered in England in 1976. In 1987, McNeil Specialty Products Company submitted a petition to the FDA for approval of sucralose in 15 food categories. Approval was received in April 1998 (25). McNeil Specialty Products has a license agreement with Tate & Lyle to manufacture and market sucralose. It is approved for use in over 30 countries and in over 400 products. It will be marketed under the brand name Splenda.

Sucralose is made from sugar through a patented, multi-step process that selectively replaces three hydrogen-oxygen groups on the sugar molecule with three chlorine atoms. The body does not recognize this structure as a carbohydrate, and sucralose does not affect normal carbohydrate metabolism, including insulin secretion and glucose/fructose absorption. The majority is eliminated unchanged in the feces. About 15% is absorbed through the small intestine, then eliminated in the urine within 24 h. The ADI has been set at 5 mg/kg body wt/day.

Sucralose is 600 times as sweet as sucrose. It is very stable and can be used in foods that require an extended heating process. Under certain conditions, it may hydrolyze to its two monosaccharide derivatives,

4-cholorogalactose and 1,6-dichlorofrucose. If this does occur, evaluation studies on these products have shown that they pose no health problem. Some of the foods it will be found in include baked goods and baking mixes, beverages and beverage bases, frozen dairy desserts and mixes, chewing gums, and processed fruit and fruit juices

Pregnancy and high-intensity sweeteners. The use of high-intensity sweeteners is often a question when a woman with diabetes becomes pregnant or when a woman is diagnosed with gestational diabetes. Research shows that these sugar alternatives are safe during pregnancy, and there have been no complications related to their use in general practice.

The phenylalanine component of aspartame has been evaluated to determine if it could possibly reach neurotoxic levels in the fetus. It was found that the maximum maternal plasma phenylalanine concentration occurring after ingestion would be less than that occurring after ingestion of protein meals, making it highly unlikely that customary intakes could raise fetal levels to a neurotoxic range (26). Multigenerational rat studies with acesulfame K and sucralose have shown no adverse effects on fertility, number of animals per litter, birth weight, mortality, or fetal development (25,27). Saccharin, likewise, has not been shown to cause any negative effects, but it can cross the placenta and may remain in fetal tissue because of slow fetal clearance (28).

How questions about the use of high-intensity sweeteners are addressed varies from clinician to clinician. The issue should be discussed and should not be passed off lightly leaving the woman confused. If these sweeteners are decreased in or eliminated from the diet, appropriate substitutions should be made. It should be clear that a can of diet soda should not simply be replaced with a can of regular soda or fruit juice because the added carbohydrate can affect glycemic control. Also, in the discussion, the practitioner should be sensitive to the woman's situation if raising doubts about any sweeteners' safety (7). It can be a very stressful pregnancy if a woman worries about the condition of her fetus because she consumed a sugar alternative.

Polyols

Polyols (sugar alcohols) are often less sweet than sugar, yet give a sweet taste and add bulk to a food. They may be used for either or both of these properties, making the term sugar alternative sometimes inappropriate. Advantages are that they are incompletely absorbed, resulting in fewer calories being consumed (about 2 kcal/g), and have a lower glycemic effect than other nutritive sweeteners or bulking agents. However, consuming high amounts of sugar alcohols may result in gastric discomfort, including gas, bloating, abdominal cramps, and osmotic diarrhea.

Polyols include isomalt, lactitol, maltitol, mannitol, sorbitol, xylitol, and hydrogenated starch hydrolysate (HSH) mixtures. They can be found in certain plants, but are manufactured from mono-, di-, or polysaccharides for use as food ingredients. They are typically odorless, have a taste similar to sucrose, and have no aftertaste. Polyols are produced by modifying the originating carbohydrate, adding hydrogen to the basic sugar. During the manufacturing process, some polyols can be produced in different forms to match a food product. For example, sorbitol can be made in crystalline or syrup form. The composition of an HSH can vary, as can its form, so that it provides the best sweetness and additional properties for a particular food product.

Sorbitol and mannitol require label warnings when daily consumption of a food might reach 50 g or 20 g, respectively, that state, "Excess consumption may have a laxative effect." Some people may have side effects from smaller amounts or from a cumulative amount from a variety of food sources. This is critical information to explain to consumers, especially to people with diabetes, who may have an added interest in such products. Small children have been shown to have afebrile diarrhea with intakes ≥0.5 g/kg body wt (29).

Sorbitol from food sources does not contribute to the sorbitol pathway that leads to neuropathies and retinal changes (30). Ingested sorbitol is not available once it has been metabolized in the liver; sorbitol found in the nerves and eyes is a result of the reduction of glucose to the sugar alcohol sorbitol by the enzyme aldose reductase.

Sweeteners Awaiting Approval

Alitame. Alitame is extremely sweet, being 2,000 times as sweet as sucrose. In 1986, Pfizer, Inc., submitted a petition for FDA approval of alitame as a food additive in 16 food categories. It is approved for use in four other countries.

Cyclamate. Cyclamate is only 30 times as sweet as sucrose and was often blended with saccharin until it was banned in 1970. Abbott Laboratories submitted a petition in 1973 that included 400 toxicological reports showing it did not cause cancer, but the petition was turned down in 1980. Another petition was submitted in 1982 and is pending. The Cancer Assessment Committee of the FDA concluded that cyclamate was not carcinogenic, as did the National Academy of Sciences (31,32). It is approved for use in over 50 other countries.

Natural Sweeteners

Although many of the polyols are found naturally, they are manufactured for use as sweeteners and bulking agents. Several "natural" sweeteners are receiving interest from manufacturers and consumers. Examples are steviodose and glycyrrhizen.

Steviodose is an extract from the leaves of a South American shrub and is 300 times as sweet as sucrose. Its approval is pending in the U.S., but it is used in Japan.

Glycyrrhizen is found in the roots of an Asian and European shrub and is commonly know as licorice. It is 50–100 times as sweet as sucrose and is approved for use in the U.S. as a natural flavoring on the GRAS list, but it does not have approval as a low-calorie sweetener. Most licorice candy in the U.S. is flavored with anise oil. Large doses of candy and chewing tobacco sweetened with glycyrrhizen have been reported to produce headaches, lethargy, sodium and water retention, excessive excretion of potassium, high blood pressure, and heart failure (33).

FAT REPLACERS

The health emphasis placed on reducing fat consumption has led to the development of new ingredients to replace fat and to the increased use of "old" ingredients in new ways. The goal of a fat replacer is to reduce the amount of fat in a food product, thus also reducing its calorie content. Fat replacers have a lot to live up to: taste, texture, mouth-feel, smell, and satiety are just some of the properties that fat adds to a food. Interestingly, carbohydrates have comprised the majority of fat replacers to date. Other fat replacers are derived from protein or fat. All three categories will be described; an overview is provided in Table 9.4.

Carbohydrate-Based

Most carbohydrate-based fat replacers have been used in foods for a number of years, yet the intense interest in reducing fat in food has dramatically expanded their recent use. Manufacturers have even modified carbohydrates to tailor the resulting fat replacers for a specific use. The resulting foods are often labeled low-fat or reduced-fat and may have a higher carbohydrate content than the traditional foods.

The nutrient adjustment may affect how a person with diabetes uses the new food. For example, 2 Tbsp of regular salad dressing has 18 g fat and 2 g carbohydrate, while the fat-free version has 0 g fat and 11 g carbohydrate. When converting to food exchanges, the product goes from 2 fat servings to 1 carbohydrate serving. There are three subcategories of carbohydrate-based fat replacers:

Carbohydrate polymers. Carbohydrate polymers primarily add thickness to a food and give a desirable creamy mouth-feel when fat is decreased or omitted. The polymers are derived from cereals, grains, and/or starches and hold up three times their weight in water.

Hydrocolloids. Hydrocolloids is the group name for gums, gels, and fibers. They also create thickness and add structure to foods. Consumers

Table 9.4   Fat Replacers: Identification, Use in Foods, and Regulatory Status

Category	Trade Names	How Identified on Food Label	Types of Foods Used In	Role in Foods and Calorie Content
Carbohydrate-based polymers	Maltrin, Lycadex, Paselli Excell, Stelar, N-Oil, Sta-Slim, Oatrim	Maltodextrin, corn syrup solid, hydrolyzed corn-starch starch, modified food starch, polydextrose	Frozen desserts, cheese, baked goods, sauces, dressings, sour cream, yogurt, baked bread, meats, and poultry	Gelling, thickening, stabilizing, increasing shelf-life, anti-staling; adds creaminess and texture; decreases calories, 1 kcal/g when hydrated in product
Hydrocolloids: gums, gels, and fibers	Slendid, Viscarin, Sactarin, Gelcarin, Fibrex, Avicel, Novagel, Rohodigel, Uniguar, Pycol, Jaquar	Pectin, carrageenan, sugar beet fiber or powder, cellulose gel, locus bean gum, xanthan gum, guar gum	Yogurt, sour cream, salad dressings, bakery products, frozen desserts, cheese spreads, sauces	Binds water, texturizes, thickens, stabilizes, provides mouth-feel of fat; decreases calories, 0–0.5 kcal/g
Polyols (sugar alcohols)/bulking ingredients	Lycasin, Hystar, Neosor, Litesse, Sta-Lite	Hydrogenated starch hydrolysate (HSH), hydrogenated glucose syrup, sorbitol, maltitol syrup, polydextrose	Baked goods, confections, chewing gum, frozen dairy desserts, gelatins, puddings, sauces, salad dressings, meat-based products	Adds bulk, aids in retaining moisture, texturizes, lowers freezing point, inhibits crystallization; decreases calories compared with fat, 1–4 kcal/g

Protein-based	Simplesse, K-Blazer, Lita, Dairy-Lo, Veri-lo	Microparticulated egg white and milk protein, whey protein concentrate	Cheese, butter, mayonnaise, salad dressings, sour cream, bakery products, spreads	Provides mouth-feel of fat; cannot be used in fried foods; 1.3 kcal/g; ingredients being developed may have higher calories
Fat-based	Caprenin, Olean, salatrim, emulsifiers (e.g., polyglyceroles-ters)	Caprenin, olestra; others being developed not yet determined as to listing	Salatrim: chocolate and confections, cookies and crackers; Olestra: savory snack foods (e.g., chips) and crackers	Acts very similar to "fat," provides creamy texture; Caprenin and salatrim have 5 kcal/g because of decreased absorption; olestra has 0 kcal/g because it is not absorbed

From Warshaw et al. (6).

can purchase these and use them to modify home recipes. Ingredients include pectin, bran fiber, applesauce, and pureed prunes.

Polyols/bulking ingredients. These polyols are the same as those that can be used as sugar alternatives. Because they are frequently less sweet than sucrose, their sweetness becomes less important in foods that need a bulking agent.

Protein-Based

Protein-based fat replacers provide the creamy, smooth mouth-feel of fat. They are relatively new and are designed specifically as fat replacers. The first ingredient in this category, microparticulated protein, was approved for use in 1990 in selected food categories. To produce this ingredient, either egg white or whey protein is heated and blended at high temperatures to produce microscopic particles that recreate the mouth-feel of fat. A whey protein concentrate is also available for use in certain foods. People allergic to egg white or cow's milk should look for this ingredient on the food label. These fat replacers have specific uses because heat coagulates the protein and causes the ingredients to lose their creaminess, making them unsuitable for some foods (fried, baked).

Fat-Based

Fat-based fat replacers have been around for a while, but new ingredients in this category are now emerging and others are under development.

Emulsifiers have been used for quite some time. They are produced by replacing triglycerides in vegetable oils and may or may not contain some starch. Even when no starch is added, they reduce fat and calories in a food because less is used. They can also be designed to complement a particular food and can retain moisture, reduce fat content, reduce calories, match or reduce the cost of fats, aid aeration, increase volume, soften the crumb if used in bakery products, and/or increase the whippability and air incorporation in a cake batter (34).

Sucrose polyesters (SPEs) are synthesized by esterifying sucrose with long- and short-chain fatty acids from vegetable oil sources that may be saturated or unsaturated (8). Different properties are created by changing the degree of esterification and the type of fatty acid. Olestra, the only SPE currently approved for use by FDA, is a chain of sucrose molecules with six to eight fatty-acid side chains. It is too large to be hydrolyzed by the enzymes in the digestive tract. It dramatically reduces calories because it is not absorbed, providing 1.3 kcal/g versus 9 kcal/g from fat. Some users may experience abdominal cramping and loose stools, but reports indicate that this occurs rarely (34). Proctor and Gamble, the makers of olestra, are seeking to change the required advisory label about this.

Salatrim is the generic name for modified triglycerides that provide the properties of natural fat, but at a reduced energy value. Salatrim is an acronym for "short- and long-chain acid triglyceride molecules," which describes its chemical structure. Because of this change, salatrim provides only 5 kcal/g instead of the 9 kcal/g of a typical fat.

Caprenin and Trailblazer are two other fat-based fat replacers that have 5 kcal/g and are being used in select foods. They are composed of fatty acids, with one of the fatty acids being poorly absorbed, thus reducing available calories (35).

HEALTHFUL USE OF THESE INGREDIENTS

How can people with diabetes use these ingredients to their benefit? The answer is carefully and wisely and with support from their health care team. Some research shows that covert substitution of lower-calorie or lower-fat foods does not decrease total calorie intake (36–38). Yet other research shows that changes can occur when consumers are knowledgeably involved in the change (39,40). To help your clients achieve success in reducing or modifying their caloric, fat, and/or sugar intake, follow these three suggestions:

1. *Provide very specific suggestions to each client as to what food choices can help him/her improve nutritional intake.* A verbal dictate to cut back on calories, carbohydrate, or fat or a written handout does not solve application issues, nor does it provide needed knowledge or support. A thorough assessment of current eating habits, lifestyle factors that affect food choices, knowledge of available food products (changes/variations in carbohydrate, fat, and calorie content), and how they are best used is required to provide acceptable guidance (41). Become familiar with food products and trends, food preparation, meal planning, food content, and glycemic effects of individual foods and meals or else refer clients to a registered dietitian for assessment and medical nutrition therapy, which will usually include diabetes and blood glucose education.

2. *Provide consistent follow-up to resolve knowledge and application questions.* Initial food plans may not be applicable to certain lifestyle situations or obtain desired results, and this will not be discovered until the client is using information in that setting. Medical nutrition therapy requires follow-up similar to *1)* counseling therapies to discuss, support, and adjust behavior change and *2)* medical therapies to monitor clinical parameters and adjust nutrition therapy as needed.

3. *Collaborate with others on the health care team to provide support and reinforcement.* Diabetes care crosses many disciplines, and pro-

viders can give positive reinforcement on all aspects of care. If the client senses skepticism about any aspect of care, the education and support can become so diluted that the client does not deem nutrition therapy and/or food intervention worthwhile. Positive, reinforcing support reduces barriers to care.

REFERENCES

1. American Diabetes Association: Nutrition recommendations and principles for people with diabetes mellitus (Position Statement). *Diabetes Care* 21 (Suppl. 1):S32–S35, 1998
2. American Diabetes Association: Role of fat replacers in diabetes medical nutrition therapy (Position Statement). *Diabetes Care* 21 (Suppl. 1):S64–S65, 1998
3. The American Dietetic Association: Use of nutritive and non-nutritive sweeteners (Position Statement). *J Am Diet Assoc* 98:580–587, 1998
4. The American Dietetic Association: Fat replacers (Position Statement). *J Am Diet Assoc* 98:463–468, 1998
5. Franz MJ, Horton ES, Bantle JP, Beebe CA, Brunzell JD, Coulston AM, Henry RR, Hoogwerf BJ, Stacpoole PW: Nutrition principles for the management of diabetes and related complications (Technical Review). *Diabetes Care* 14:490–518, 1994
6. Warshaw H, Franz M, Powers MA, Wheeler M: Fat replacers: their use in foods and role in diabetes medical nutrition therapy (Technical Review). *Diabetes Care* 19:1294–1301, 1996
7. Powers MA, Warshaw HS: Low-calorie sweeteners and fat replacers: the ingredients, use in foods, and diabetes management. In *Handbook of Diabetes Medical Nutrition Therapy*. Powers MA, Ed. Gaithersburg, MD, Aspen, 1996, pp. 375–398
8. Harrigan KA, Breene WM: Fat substitutes: sucrose polyesters and other synthetic oils. In *Low-Calorie Foods Handbook*. Altshul AM, Ed. New York, Marcel Dekker, 1993, pp. 181–209
9. Powers M: Sweetening our foods: blending sweeteners. *Diabetes Educ* 20:243–244, 1994
10. Calorie Control Council: *National Consumer Survey, 1998*. Atlanta, GA, Calorie Control Council, 1998
11. Kuczmarski RJ, Flegal KM, Campbell SM, Johnson CL: Increasing prevalence of overweight among US adults: the National Health and Nutrition Examination Surveys, 1960–1991. *JAMA* 272:205–211, 1994
12. Senauer B, Asp E, Kinsey J: *Food Trends and the Changing Consumer*. St. Paul, MN, Eagan, 1991, p. 28

13. Volz M, Christ O, Eckert HG, Herok J, Kellner HM, Rupp W: Kinetics and biotransformation of acesulfame-K. In *Acesulfame-K.* Mayer DG, Kemper FN, Eds. New York, Marcel Dekker, 1991, pp. 7–26

14. Renwick AF: The fate of intense sweeteners in the body. *Food Chem* 16:281–285, 1985

15. Stegink LD, Brummel MC, McMartin K, Martin-Amat G, Filer LJ Jr, Baker GL, Tephly TR: Blood methanol concentrations in normal adult subjects administered abuse doses of aspartame. *J Toxicol Environ Health* 7:281–290, 1981

16. Stegink L, Filer LJ: Effects of aspartame ingestion on plasma aspartame, phenylalanine, and methanol concentrations in normal adults. In *The Clinical Evaluation of a Food Additive.* Tschanz C, Butchko H, Stargel W, Kotsonis F, Eds. New York, CRC, 1996

17. Olney JW, Farber MB, Spitznagel E, Robins LN: Increasing brain tumor rates: is there a link to aspartame? *J Neuropathol Exp Neurol* 55:1115–1123, 1996

18. Food and Drug Administration: FDA statement on aspartame. Washington, DC, FDA, 18 November 1996 (report no. FDA/USD-HHS T96–75)

19. Garriga M, Berkebile C, Metcalfe D: A combined single-blind, placebo controlled study to determine the reproducibility of hypersensitivity reactions to aspartame. *J Allergy Immunol* 87:821–827, 1991

20. Nehrling JK, Kobe P, McLane MP, Olson RE, Kamath S, Horwitz DL: Aspartame use by persons with diabetes. *Diabetes Care* 8:415–417, 1985

21. Food and Drug Administration: CDC evaluation of aspartame complaints. Washington, DC, FDA, 1 November 1984 (report no. FDA/USDHHS T84–77)

22. Morgan R, Wong O: A review of epidemiological studies on artificial sweeteners and bladder cancer. *Food Chem Toxicol* 23:529–533, 1985

23. Risch H: Dietary factors and the incidence of cancer of the urinary bladder. *Am J Epidemiol* 127:1179–1191, 1988

24. Council on Scientific Affairs: Saccharin: review of safety issues. *JAMA.* 254:2622, 1985

25. *Federal Register* 63:16417–16433, 1998

26. Stegink LD, Filer LF, Baker GL: Effect of aspartame and aspartate loading upon plasma and erythrocyte free amino acid levels in normal adult volunteers. *J Nutr* 107:1837–1845, 1977

27. World Health Organization Expert Committee on Food Additives: *Toxicological Evaluation of Certain Food Additives and Food Contaminants.* Geneva, World Health Organization, 16:11–27, 1981; 18:12–14, 1983

28. Pitkin R, Reynolds W, Filer LJ: Placental transmission and fetal distribution of saccharin. *Am J Obstet Gynecol* 111:280–286, 1971
29. Payne ML, Craig WJ, Williams AC: Sorbitol is a possible risk factor for diarrhea in young children. *J Am Dietetic Assoc* 97:532–534, 1997
30. Geil PB: Complex and simple carbohydrates in diabetes therapy. In *Handbook of Diabetes Medical Nutrition Therapy*. Powers MA, Ed. Gaithersburg, MD, Aspen, 1996, pp. 303–319
31. Cancer Assessment Committee: *Scientific Review of the Long-Term Carcinogenic Bioassays Performed on the Artificial Sweetener Cyclamate*. Washington, DC, Center for Food Safety and Applied Nutrition, Food and Drug Administration, 1984
32. National Academy of Sciences/National Research Council: *Evaluation of Cyclamate for Carcinogenicity*. Washington, DC, National Academy Press, 1985
33. Tyler VE: *The Honest Herbal*. Binghamton, NY, Pharmaceutical Products Press, 1993
34. Frye AM, Setser CS: Bulking agents and fat substitutes. In *Low-Calorie Foods Handbook*. Altschul AM, Ed. New York, Marcel Dekker, 1993, pp. 211–251
35. Peters JC, Holcombe BN, Hiller LK, Webb DR: Caprenin 3: absorption and caloric value in adult humans. *J Am Coll Toxicol* 10:357–367, 1991
36. Foltin RW, Fischman MW, Moran TH, Rolls BJ, Kelly TH: Caloric compensation for lunches varying in fat and carbohydrate content by humans in a residential laboratory. *Am J Clin Nutr* 52:969–980, 1990
37. Rolls BJ, Pirraglia PA, Jones MB, Peters JC: Effects of olestra, a non-caloric fat substitute, on daily energy intakes in lean men. *Am J Clin Nutr* 56:84–92, 1992
38. Mattes RD, Caputo FA: Caloric compensation to convert manipulations of dietary fat and carbohydrate intake. *Am J Clin Nutr* 53: Abstract 67, 1991
39. Kanders BS, Lavin PT, Kowalchuk M, Blackburn GL: Do aspartame (AMP) sweetened foods and beverages aid in long-term control of body weight? *Am J Clin Nutr* 51: Abstract 38, 1990
40. Powers MA: Diabetes medical nutrition therapy: the challenge of access. *Diabetes Spectrum* 9:119–121, 1996
41. American Diabetes Association: *A Guide to Fitting Foods with Sugar Substitutes and Fat Replacers into Your Meal Plan*. Alexandria, VA, American Diabetes Association, 1998

Ms. Powers is the president of Powers and Associates, Inc., a firm specializing in innovative nutrition and health communications, in St. Paul, MN.

10. Micronutrients and Diabetes

Marion J. Franz, MS, RD, LD, CDE

Highlights

- Dietary Reference Intake (DRI) is a new approach for determining nutrient requirements. DRIs are reference values that are quantitative estimates of nutrient intakes to be used for planning and assessing diets for healthy people. They consist of four reference intakes: Recommended Dietary Allowance (RDA), Estimated Average Requirement (EAR), Adequate Intake (AI), and Tolerable Upper Intake Level (UL).
- Many micronutrients are intimately involved in carbohydrate and/or glucose metabolism as well as with insulin release and sensitivity. This information, however, is frequently extrapolated beyond what the research intends or supports.
- Supplements are defined as any product that is intended to supplement the diet. Dietary supplements contain one or more of the following: vitamin, mineral, herb or other botanical, or amino acid. Although often sold as food, supplements are used more like drugs. Unlike drugs, however, they do not have to be proven effective or safe before being marketed.
- At present, there is no justification for routine supplementation of vitamins and minerals for people with diabetes. There are, however, select groups of people who may benefit, such as patients in poor glycemic control and deficient in water-soluble micronutrients. In the future, antioxidant supplements, particularly vitamin E, may be proven to play a role in preventing oxidative damage to tissues and may be recommended for use.

INTRODUCTION

Surveys show that more than half of the U.S. adult population take dietary supplements and that in 1996 alone, consumers spent more than $6.5 billion on dietary supplements (1). This is an increase from dietary supplement sales of $3.3 billion in 1990. It is not surprising then that consumers with diabetes ask questions about micronutrients and supplements: "Are there any vitamins or minerals that I should take because I have diabetes?" "Will they help my diabetes?" "Does the Food and Drug Administration approve vitamin and mineral supplements?" "Are they safe?" "Can their claims be trusted?" And the list of questions goes on and on.

This chapter should help health professionals answer some of these questions. It reviews requirements for micronutrients, including the new Food and Nutrition Board approach to requirements for nutrients; the relationship of micronutrients to carbohydrate/glucose metabolism and/or insulin, specifically focusing on four micronutrients—chromium, magnesium, nicotinamide, and vitamin E; and the way supplements are regulated (or not regulated) by the Food and Drug Administration (FDA). An American Diabetes Association (ADA) technical review paper addresses issues related to individual vitamins and minerals and their relationship to diabetes (2). Much of this chapter's content has been adapted from an article published in *Diabetes Spectrum* (3).

REQUIREMENTS FOR MICRONUTRIENTS: DIETARY REFERENCE INTAKES

Before addressing the role of vitamins and minerals in diabetes, it is helpful to review requirements for micronutrients and how they are determined. Vitamins and minerals are substances required in very small amounts to promote essential biochemical reactions in cells. Together, vitamins and minerals are called micronutrients. At low nutrient levels (deficiency), dependent biological functions are impaired. In contrast, very high intakes can result in toxicity and decreased absorption of other micronutrients because of competitive inhibition.

Micronutrients are specific in their functions, and most cannot be made by the body or be replaced by chemically similar elements. They must come from food or supplements. Very small amounts of micronutrients are needed for optimal performance, yet lack of a micronutrient for a prolonged period can result in disease seemingly disproportionate to the amount missing. For example, although only small amounts of vitamins are needed, lack of vitamin C results in scurvy, lack of thiamin in beriberi, and lack of niacin in pellagra.

Several factors make determining exact individual requirements for micronutrients difficult. First, metabolism and utilization of micronutrients are homeostatically regulated, making requirements and the effect of supplementation dependent on an individual's nutritional status. For example, if intake of a particular micronutrient is low, absorption is increased, and when intake is adequate, excess nutrient is excreted in the feces and in small amounts in the urine.

Assessment of micronutrient status is difficult. It is assumed that levels of micronutrients in body fluids (plasma) reflect tissue and intracellular status and, therefore, that decreased serum levels indicate suboptimal status. However, plasma levels generally do not reflect intracellular status. Correlations between plasma levels and tissue status, especially in marginal deficiencies, are not always apparent.

Furthermore, metabolism and utilization of nutrients in general is highly integrated with other nutrients, hormones, and physiological factors. With excessive (or deficient) intakes of a particular micronutrient, the balance of this highly orchestrated scheme is disrupted, which leads to a cascade of effects. For example, calcium use is affected by a high protein intake, phosphorus and vitamin D intakes, and parathyroid hormone. Changes in any of these factors have an impact on calcium requirements.

Requirements for micronutrients have been based on the 10th edition of the Recommended Dietary Allowances (RDAs) (4). However, the RDAs, published since 1941 by the Food and Nutrition Board of the Institute of Medicine, National Academy of Sciences, are being replaced by a new approach, Dietary Reference Intakes (DRIs). The DRIs are being developed by the Food and Nutrition Board in partnership with Health Canada and Canadian scientists and represent a comprehensive effort to include current concepts about the role of nutrient and food components in long-term health, going beyond the need to prevent deficiency diseases (5). DRIs are reference values that are quantitative estimates of nutrient intakes to be used for planning and assessing diets for healthy people. They consist of four reference intakes: RDA, Adequate Intake (AI), Tolerable Upper Intake Level (UL), and Estimated Average Requirement (EAR). Figure 10.1 illustrates the DRIs.

The four primary uses of the DRIs are for assessing intakes of individuals, assessing intakes of population groups, planning diets for individuals, and planning diets for groups. RDAs and AIs may both be used as goals for individual intakes, whereas EARs may be used to examine the possibility of inadequacy and ULs the possibility of overconsumption for individuals. EARs are also used as guides to limit individual intake and to set goals for the mean intake of groups or of a specific population, as well as for the assessment of inadequate intakes within a group.

Two reports providing DRIs for nutrients have been released. These include DRIs for calcium and its related nutrients—phosphorus, mag-

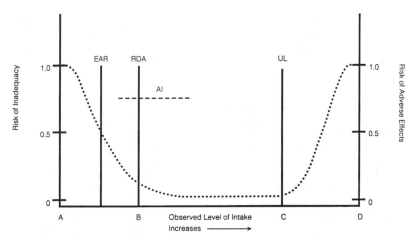

Figure 10.1 DRIs. EAR is the intake at which the risk of inadequacy is 0.5 (50%). RDA is the intake at which the risk of inadequacy is very small—only 0.02–0.03 (2% to 3%). AI does not bear a consistent relationship to EAR or RDA because it is set without being able to estimate the requirement. At intakes between RDA and UL, the risks of inadequacy and of adverse effects are both close to 0. UL is the highest level of daily nutrient intake that is likely to pose no risks of adverse effects. A dashed line is used for AI because the actual shape of the curve has not been determined experimentally. The distances between points A and B, B and C, and C and D may differ much more than is depicted in this figure. Thus, the AI might be greater or less than the RDA, if it were known. From Yates et al. (5).

nesium, vitamin D, and fluoride—and for folate, the B vitamins, and choline (6,7). The report on vitamins C and E, β-carotene, and selected other compounds is due in 1999, while at least three additional groups of nutrients are slated for review over the next 3–4 years. These groups include trace elements; vitamins A and K; electrolytes and fluids; macronutrients, including energy; and other food components, such as phytoestrogens, fiber, and other phytochemicals found in foods such as tea and garlic, assuming adequate data relating these compounds to risk of chronic disease and to health are available.

The DRI terms will not be used on food labels anytime soon. The term used on food labels is Daily Value (DV) and is derived from the 1968 RDAs. The FDA has stated that it will not change the term DV on food labels, but that the values may be adjusted. Table 10.1 summarizes the definitions for the various reference values.

Recommended Dietary Allowance (RDA)

The RDA is the average daily dietary intake level of a nutrient that is sufficient to meet the nutrient requirements of nearly all (97–98%) healthy individuals in a particular life stage (life stage considers age and, when applicable, pregnancy or lactation) and gender group (5). This is quite similar to past descriptions of RDAs, but past RDAs served as goals for individuals, not for groups. The RDA includes a generous safety factor related to a bell-shaped curve. The majority of the population actually requires only approximately two-thirds of the RDA. This is in contrast to energy requirements, which are based on average needs.

Estimated Average Requirement (EAR)

The process for setting the RDA depends upon being able to set the EAR. The EAR is the amount of nutrient that is estimated to meet the

---

Table 10.1 Terms for Nutrient Requirements

- **Dietary Reference Intakes (DRIs):** An umbrella term for RDAs, AIs, EARs, and ULs (see below).
- **Recommended Dietary Allowance (RDA):** The average daily dietary intake level of a nutrient that is sufficient to meet the nutrient requirements and decrease the risk of chronic disease of nearly all (97–98%) healthy individuals of a specified age and sex.
- **Adequate Intake (AI):** Same requirement as the RDA, but lacking enough scientific evidence to set an RDA. It is a recommended daily intake based on observation or experimentally determined approximation of nutrient intake for a group (or groups) of healthy people.
- **Tolerable Upper Intake Level (UL):** The highest level of daily nutrient intake that is likely to pose no risks of adverse health effects to almost all individuals. Total intake from food, fortified food, and supplements should not exceed this amount or the risk of adverse health effects increases.
- **Estimated Average Requirement (EAR):** The amount that is estimated to meet the optimal nutrient needs of half the individuals in a specified group. It is used to assess adequacy of intakes of population groups and, along with knowledge of the distribution of requirements, to develop RDAs.
- **Daily Value (DV):** This is not a new term, but it will continue to be the term used for nutrient levels on food and supplement labels. DVs are derived from RDAs (or AIs) in order to represent both sexes and most age-groups.

nutrient requirements of half the healthy individuals in a life stage and gender group (5). When selecting the EAR, reduction of disease risk is considered, along with many other health parameters. No RDA is proposed if it is determined that an EAR cannot be set. This differs from previous determinations of RDAs. The EAR is used to assess adequacy of intakes of population groups.

Adequate Intake (AI)

An AI is provided instead of an RDA when sufficient scientific evidence is not available to calculate an EAR. The AI is a recommended daily intake level based on observed or experimentally determined approximations of nutrient intake by a group of healthy people (5). The primary use of the AI is as a goal for the nutrient intake of individuals. For example, in the new revisions, an AI, not an RDA, is used to determine individual needs for calcium and vitamin D.

Tolerable Upper Intake Level (UL)

The UL is the highest level of nutrient intake that is likely to pose no risks or adverse health effects to almost all individuals in the general population. As intake increases above the UL, the risk of adverse effects increases. The UL is not intended to be a recommended level of intake. There is no established benefit for healthy individuals if they consume nutrient intakes above the RDA or AI (5). The UL applies to chronic daily use. It is useful because of the increased interest in availability of fortified foods and the increased use of dietary supplements.

REQUIREMENTS FOR MICRONUTRIENTS IN DIABETES

The literature on the micronutrient status of people with diabetes contains conflicting reports depending on the population studied and caused by uncertainties in methodologies (2,8). Adequately controlled studies that establish the role of trace elements in the pathogenesis of carbohydrate intolerance are not available. Although animal studies have suggested that deficiencies in many of the trace elements—including zinc, chromium, magnesium, copper, manganese, and vitamin B_6—may lead to glucose intolerance, evidence for their role in the pathogenesis of glucose intolerance in humans is not available.

Many of the studies are done in animals in the laboratory, where diet can be manipulated easily in comparison to the diet of free-living subjects. The results of animal studies should not be extrapolated to humans without studies in humans as well.

One of the problems with human studies in individuals with diabetes is that trace-metal and water-soluble vitamin urinary losses are increased during uncontrolled hyperglycemia with glycosuria and that therefore the effect of the response to micronutrients may be dependent on the degree of glucose intolerance. Furthermore, in some studies, the initial glucose tolerance varies from normal to glucose intolerant to diabetes. Results from all of these subjects may be combined, which would minimize the effects of a micronutrient.

Often, the effect of micronutrients on insulin secretion is biphasic. Low concentrations of the vitamin may stimulate insulin secretion, and high concentrations may have an inhibitory effect.

In human studies, the amount of the micronutrient being studied in the diet eaten is often unknown. For example, studies have reported beneficial effects of chromium on glucose and/or lipid metabolism in subjects eating varied diets with unknown chromium contents. To further confuse the role of micronutrients and diabetes, serum or tissue content of certain elements—copper, manganese, iron, and selenium—can be higher in people with diabetes than in nondiabetic control subjects. On the other hand, serum ascorbic acid, B vitamin group, and vitamin D may be lower in individuals with diabetes, whereas vitamins A and E have been reported to be normal or increased.

Regardless of the research problems, many micronutrients are intimately involved in carbohydrate and/or glucose metabolism as well as in insulin release and sensitivity. Unfortunately, this information is frequently extrapolated far beyond what the research intends or supports.

MICRONUTRIENTS, CARBOHYDRATE/GLUCOSE, AND INSULIN

Table 10.2 summarizes research related to micronutrients, their effects on carbohydrate and/or glucose metabolism, and the known effects of supplementation related to diabetes (9–88). Four micronutrients will be reviewed briefly below: chromium, magnesium, nicotinamide, and vitamin E. For additional information and a summary of other vitamins and minerals, see the technical review by Mooradian et al. (2).

Chromium

Elemental chromium's biologically active complex is glucose tolerance factor (GTF), whose structure is composed of nicotinic acid, elemental chromium, and the amino acids glutamic acid, glycine, and cysteine. GTF has a role in glucose homeostasis. In laboratory animals, chromium deficiency is associated with an increase in blood glucose,

Table 10.2 Effects of Vitamins and Minerals on Carbohydrate and/or Glucose Metabolism or Insulin and the Effects of Supplementation in Diabetes

Nutrient (Reference)	Effect on Carbohydrate/Glucose Metabolism or Insulin	Effect of Supplementation
Chromium (9–24)	One of several molecules making up glucose tolerance factor, which appears to potentiate insulin action—receptor binding and intracellular transport.	Supplementation may improve glycemic control in patients with Cr deficiency and impaired glucose tolerance; in a study done in China, at high levels (1,000 µg) Cr picolinate improved HbA_{1c}, glucose, insulin, and cholesterol levels in subjects with type 2 diabetes.
Magnesium (25–41)	Modulates glucose transport across cell membranes and is a cofactor in enzymatic pathways involved in glucose oxidation. Glycosuria may lead to excessive urinary losses of Mg.	Patients at high risk should have Mg status assessed and be supplemented with oral magnesium chloride (of dependable potency and bioavailability) if deficiency is demonstrated.
Zinc (42–51)	Insulin stored as inactive Zn crystals in β-cells.	Moderate Zn deficiency may occur frequently in people with type 2 diabetes, but supplementation has not been shown to be beneficial or to have an effect on diabetes management.
Copper (48–51)	Plasma levels higher in patients with retinopathy, hypertension, or macrovascular disease. Without complications, values are normal.	Supplementation not recommended because of high levels in patients with complications.
Manganese (48,52,53)	No evidence of altered Mn states in patients with diabetes.	Supplementation has not shown a glucose-lowering effect.

Iron (54,55)	Fe excess with hemochromatosis is associated with glucose intolerance.	Role of Fe deficiency in glucose control is minor.
Vitamin A (56–59)	No correlation between vitamin A and HbA_{1c} levels, although vitamin A plays a role in regulation of insulin secretion.	In rat studies, supplementation did not alter blood or urine glucose levels.
Niacin (nicotinic acid) (60,61)	As a drug, lowers cholesterol, VLDL, and TG and elevates HDL.	In drug form, leads to deterioration of glycemic control.
Nicotinamide (62–68)	A clinical trial is underway in Europe and Canada using pharmacological doses of nicotinamide to determine whether type 1 diabetes can be prevented or the onset delayed.	In pharmacological doses may offer protection to pancreatic β-cells against toxic or immune-mediated damage.
Thiamin (69)	Daily requirements dependent on amount of carbohydrate consumed.	Supplementation has no demonstrated effect on diabetes management.
Pyridoxine, Vitamin B_6 (70–72)	Deficiency in animals and humans has been associated with glucose intolerance and impaired secretion of insulin and glucagon. Poor glucose control may decrease levels of vitamin B_6.	Supplementation has no demonstrated benefits on glucose metabolism. Has been used to treat diabetic neuropathy, but better medications are available to treat neuropathy. Megadoses are associated with toxic effects including neuropathy.
Vitamin C (73–78)	Has a chemical structure similar to glucose. Tissue stores are depleted by chronic hyperglycemia. Large doses have the potential to interfere with glucose for blood glucose monitoring.	Potential for inhibition of protein glycosylation by competing with glucose for binding to proteins. Supplementation (500 mg/day) did not affect blood glucose levels.

(Continued)

Table 10.2 Effects of Vitamins and Minerals on Carbohydrate and/or Glucose Metabolism or Insulin and the Effects of Supplementation in Diabetes (*Continued*)

Nutrient (Reference)	Effect on Carbohydrate/Glucose Metabolism or Insulin	Effect of Supplementation
Vitamin D (70–82)	Patients with diabetes found to have reduced bone mass and mineral content.	Supplementation has no demonstrated effect on diabetes management.
Vitamin E (83–85), Tocopherols	Potent antioxidant, and people with diabetes may have higher requirements for antioxidants.	Usefulness unproven; potential benefit as antioxidant. Vitamin E has decreased LDL oxidation but has not consistently reduced protein glycosylation in people with type 2 diabetes.
Vanadium Vanadate (86–88)	In animal studies, pharmacological levels improved glucose tolerance.	Ubiquitous in air, soil, water, and foods. The biological effects of vanadium are pharmacological; therefore, vanadium should be considered as a drug rather than a supplement.

Adapted from Franz (3).

cholesterol, and triglycerides. GTF acts as a cofactor for insulin and may facilitate insulin–membrane receptor interaction. However, GTF lowers plasma glucose only in the presence of insulin (fed state) and not in 24-h–fasting animals (9).

Most chromium supplements are poorly absorbed. Chromium picolinate appears to be absorbed better because it incorporates picolinic acid, a natural mineral transporter produced in the liver and kidney. Picolinic acid binds with ingested metals, such as chromium, iron, and zinc, and is necessary to move them quickly and effectively into the body cells where they are needed.

Because no methods exist to determine chromium deficiency, the prevalence of a deficiency is unknown. In a study comparing people with diabetes to those without diabetes, Rabinowitz et al. (10) studied chromium in hair, serum, urine, and red blood cells and could not identify a deficiency of chromium in either group. Deficiency in people with diabetes is assumed to be the same as in the general population, in which it is assumed that most people are not chromium deficient. If a deficiency did exist, it would be in the middle-aged or elderly population and would be manifested by insulin resistance and lipid profile derangements (11).

Although severe chromium deficiency can lead to glucose intolerance, its role in the pathogenesis of clinically apparent diabetes is not significant (2). In two patients on total parenteral nutrition over a 6-month and a 5-year period, respectively, chromium deficiency was implicated in glucose intolerance (12,13). In another study, chromium picolinate supplements were reported to have a beneficial effect on serum triglyceride levels but no effect on glucose control (14).

At this time, there is no RDA or AI for chromium. Usual intake is 25 μg/1,000 kcal, and this appears to meet needs. A range of safe and adequate intake is reported to be 50–200 μg/day (4).

In the majority of healthy adults studied, chromium did not improve glucose tolerance. In three double-blind crossover studies in people with diabetes, chromium supplementation failed to improve glucose and lipid levels (15–17). If chromium does have an effect, the response may depend on the degree of glucose intolerance. Anderson et al. (18) studied the effects of supplementing chromium in individuals consuming controlled chromium-deficient diets. In subjects with elevated blood glucose levels but not diabetes (100–200 μg/dl at 90-min glucose tolerance test), blood glucose levels responded to 200 μg supplemental chromium. However, in subjects with low blood glucose levels, the supplements increased blood glucose levels, and in subjects with diabetes, the supplement had no effect on blood glucose levels.

Recent evidence from China has suggested a role for chromium supplementation. Individuals with type 2 diabetes were randomly divided into three groups and supplemented with 1,000 μg or 200 μg chromium as chromium picolinate or a placebo. In all three groups, fasting, 2-h glucose concentrations, and HbA_{1c} values decreased, but the decreases in the subjects receiving 1,000 µg supplemental chromium were much larger. Fasting and 2-h insulin concentrations were also lower in the two groups receiving the chromium supplement, although the control group's values also decreased. Total cholesterol decreased in the group receiving the 1,000-µg supplement. There were no significant effects of supplemental chromium on HDL cholesterol, triglycerides, or weight [19]. It appears that the mechanism of action of chromium on the control of blood glucose concentrations is the potentiation of insulin action. In the presence of chromium in a useable form, lower levels of insulin are required.

Trivalent chromium, the form of chromium found in foods and nutrient supplements, is considered one of the least toxic nutrients. The conservative estimate of safe intake has a much larger safety factor for trivalent chromium than for almost any other nutrient [20]. Although Anderson et al. [21] demonstrated a lack of toxicity of chromium chloride and chromium picolinate in rats at several thousand times the upper limit of the estimated safe and adequate daily dietary intake for humans (based on body weight), in an animal study, chromium picolinate used in very large amounts was shown to cause severe chromosome damage [22,23].

Before chromium supplements can be recommended in the U.S., double-blind crossover studies in people with diabetes with known dietary intake of chromium, using chromium supplements that may be better absorbed than older supplements, need to be undertaken. Until newer research contradicts older studies [24], it is assumed that chromium functions as a nutrient, not as a therapeutic agent, and that it benefits only individuals with marginal glucose intolerance whose signs and symptoms are due to marginal or overt chromium deficiency.

Magnesium

Magnesium is intimately involved in a number of important biochemical reactions that take place in the body, particularly processes that involve the formation and use of high-energy phosphate bonds (adenosine triphosphate [ATP]). It is a cofactor in over 300 enzymatic reactions. Magnesium also modulates glucose transport through the membranes and is a cofactor in several enzymatic systems involving glucose oxidation [2]. Magnesium deficiency may increase insulin resistance or may be its result [25].

Magnesium is unevenly distributed in the body. Approximately 50–60% is in the skeleton; nearly 50% is in the muscle, primarily skeletal and cardiac muscle, and soft tissues; and only ~1% is in the extracellular compartment, such as serum or interstitial body fluids. Serum magnesium measures only 0.3% of total body magnesium and does not provide a sensitive index of magnesium deficiency.

Low levels of magnesium have been associated with hypertension, cardiac arrhythmias, congestive heart failure, retinopathy, and insulin resistance (26–31). Data relating magnesium deficiency to causes of human diseases are limited. In the absence of prospective studies, it is possible that decreased magnesium levels may represent a marker rather than a cause of disease (32).

Magnesium concentrations remain remarkably constant in people without diabetes. However, people with diabetes appear to be prone to developing magnesium deficiency, which is reflected by low plasma or serum magnesium levels (33–37), but this is not a consistent finding (30). Magnesium deficiency in diabetes is most likely the result of increased urinary magnesium losses secondary to chronic glycosuria, although short-term improvement in glycemic control has not been shown to restore the serum magnesium levels (32). Hwang et al. (38) demonstrated that insulin, via its receptor, produces a dose- and time-dependent increase in free magnesium levels and that therefore, it is possible that the reduced intracellular free magnesium levels in hypertension and type 2 diabetes result from a decrease of insulin action on magnesium transport. Diuretic drugs may further increase magnesium loss and thus aggravate cardiovascular problems.

An increase in platelet reactivity can enhance the risks of vascular disease. In a short-term study, Nadler et al. (36) demonstrated that people with type 2 diabetes have intracellular magnesium deficiency and that oral magnesium supplementation could increase intracellular levels toward normal. In addition, magnesium supplementation markedly reduced platelet aggregation in response to known agonists of platelet aggregation.

A number of short-term studies on the effects of dietary magnesium supplements have reported improvements in glucose control and insulin sensitivity (37,39–41). Paolisso and associates (39,40) reported that glucose- and arginine-induced insulin secretion, as well as insulin sensitivity, were significantly improved by 3 g/day of magnesium supplements for 3 weeks.

The ADA consensus statement on magnesium supplementation in the treatment of diabetes (32) concluded that until accurate indexes of magnesium deficiency are available, routine evaluation of magnesium status in otherwise healthy individuals with diabetes is not recommended. However, in patients at risk for magnesium deficiency, measuring serum magnesium is appropriate. This includes patients with congestive heart failure or acute myocardial infarction, ketoacidosis, ethanol abuse, long-term parenteral nutrition, potassium or calcium deficiency, chronic use of certain drugs (e.g., diuretics, aminoglycosides, or digoxin), or pregnancy. In such patients with documented hypomagnesemia, oral magnesium chloride of dependable potency and bioavailability should be administered until the serum magnesium level is normalized or the condition producing the hypomagnesium is reversed. In patients at increased risk, but in whom no deficiency can be demonstrated clinically, magnesium supplementation is not recommended. The implementation of newer ion-selective electrodes or phosphate nuclear magnetic resonance assays for ionized or free intracellular magnesium may extend our understanding of magnesium deficiency.

Well-designed prospective studies demonstrating safety and beneficial results of magnesium replacement therapy have not been performed. Furthermore, adequate dietary magnesium intake can generally be achieved by a nutritionally balanced meal plan (32).

Nicotinamide

Nicotinamide and nicotinic acid (niacin), both soluble B group vitamins, are chemically very similar, but the two vitamins differ in their effects when administered in pharmacological doses. Nicotinamide, an amide of nicotinic acid, is a precursor of nicotinamide adenine dinucleotide (NAD), a coenzyme involved in a wide variety of energy-transfer processes within the cell. In animal studies, nicotinamide has been shown to offer protection to pancreatic β-cells against a variety of toxic or immune-mediated insults. Current experience also suggests that when nicotinamide is administered in pure form, there are virtually no detectable harmful acute physiological or biochemical changes, even at high doses (62). In contrast, nicotinic acid (niacin) is a lipid-lowering agent and vasodilator and leads to insulin resistance and glucose intolerance.

Initial trials of nicotinamide in patients with newly diagnosed type 1 diabetes produced conflicting results. Some reported no benefit, while others reported that nicotinamide protected pancreatic β-cell function in newly diagnosed type 1 diabetic patients and improved metabolic control (63–65).

At the University of Rome in 1989, 36 patients with type 1 diabetes were studied (23 were given 200 mg daily of nicotinamide plus insulin; 13 control subjects were given insulin alone). Patients given nicotinamide were reported to have increased C-peptide levels, lower glycated hemoglobin levels, and lower insulin requirements at 6 months and 1 year after diagnosis (63).

In France, 26 type 1 patients who were post-honeymoon but still had C-peptide levels were given 3 g/day of nicotinamide or a placebo for 9 months in a randomized double-blind study. Fasting and stimulated C-peptide levels were higher in the treated group than in the placebo group. The C-peptide response to a meal test gradually declined in the placebo group, but it remained stable in the nicotinamide group (64).

Additional evidence has demonstrated the safety and efficacy of nicotinamide as an adjunct to insulin in the early phase of type 1 diabetes to protect and improve residual C-peptide secretion, but only in patients who are diagnosed after puberty (66).

Nicotinamide has been reported to protect or strengthen the pancreatic β-cells by making them more resistant to autoimmune destruction in newly diagnosed type 1 diabetes, resulting in improved metabolic control. Toxins, including endogenous cytokines, are known to cause DNA strand breaks in islet β-cells, thus stimulating nuclear poly (ADP-ribose) synthetase for repair and depleting NAD levels. Intracellular NAD falls, and proinsulin synthesis is inhibited. Nicotinamide, a poly (ADP-ribose) synthetic inhibitor, has been shown in animal models to induce islet β-cell regeneration.

Two clinical trials in the U.S. could not demonstrate that nicotinamide preserved β-cell function in patients with early type 1 diabetes (65,67). A possible explanation for the disappointing results in humans may pertain to the dosages, which were ~10 times smaller than those used in animal studies. Furthermore, nicotinamide's use in pre–type 1 diabetes has produced more promising results.

Based on the results of pilot studies, including an intervention study in New Zealand using nicotinamide treatment in children tested for islet cell antibodies (ICAs) that reported a 50% reduction in the development of type 1 diabetes during a 5-year period (68), an intervention trial has been launched. The trial, called the European-Canadian Nicotinamide Diabetes Intervention Trial (ENDIT), involves centers in 18 European countries and in Canada. The ENDIT hypothesis is that the rate of type 1 diabetes can be substantially reduced with the use of pharmacological doses of nicotinamide.

Approximately 3,000 individuals between 5 and 40 years old are being screened to identify a sufficient number of those who are ICA positive and have normal glucose tolerance. The primary outcome will be the incidence of type 1 diabetes in 5 years, with a 3-year interim analysis planned to determine early support for the hypothesis (62).

Vitamin E

Endogenous antioxidants, such as vitamin E, vitamin C, and carotenoids, scavenger free radicals to prevent or limit peroxidative damage. Free radicals are toxic compounds generated in the process of normal metabolism that contain one or more unpaired electrons. Unpaired electrons have a strong affinity for electrons from other molecules. Because of their reactive nature, free radicals can initiate a chain of oxidative events leading to toxic cellular damage. Free radicals have been reported to initiate or promote aging, atherosclerosis, cancer, cataracts, and other chronic diseases. Antioxidants are compounds that are able to neutralize reactive free electrons. Supplementation with antioxidants such as vitamin E and β-carotene has been reported to reduce susceptibility of LDL cholesterol to oxidation. A controlled clinical study that tested the effect of the antioxidant β-carotene reported an increased incidence of lung cancer in Finnish men who took β-carotene compared with those who did not. As a result, the use of β-carotene as an antioxidant has fallen out of favor (59).

The major antioxidant for LDL appears to be α-tocopherol. When vitamin E was added to plasma, a linear increase in the oxidative resistance of LDL was noted as tocopherol levels increased. Studies also have suggested that vitamin E supplementation improves nonoxidative glucose metabolism in people with type 2 diabetes (83,84). Increased lipid peroxidation may also accelerate protein glycation and raises the possibility that these two processes, glycation and lipid peroxidation, may be mutually reinforcing. Therefore, it has been suggested that antioxidants such as vitamin E may be useful not only in preventing lipid oxidation but also in decreasing protein glycation.

A double-blind, crossover study by Paolisso et al. (84) in subjects with type 2 diabetes randomly taking a placebo or 900 mg/day of vitamin E reported that supplementation significantly reduced lipid, plasma glucose, and HbA$_{1c}$ levels, but did not affect β-cell response to glucose. Reaven et al. (85) also studied men with type 2 diabetes randomly assigned to either 1,600 IU/day of vitamin E or placebo for 10 weeks after a 4-week placebo period. In the vitamin E treatment group, vitamin E content in plasma and LDL increased significantly and decreased the susceptibility of LDL to oxidation in comparison with placebo. Despite a greater percentage increase in vitamin E content in small dense LDL, it remained substantially more susceptible to oxidation than did buoyant LDL. The investigators suggested that dense LDL may gain less protection against oxidation from antioxidant supplementation than does larger, more buoyant LDL. Glycemic indexes and lipid levels, however, did not change significantly in either group during the study.

Additional studies are needed to determine whether more potent antioxidants or other antioxidants, such as vitamin C, might inhibit glycation (78). Furthermore, Paolisso et al. (84) stress that in their study, a pharmacological dose of vitamin E was used, and no studies have investigated the possible effect of body storage of vitamin E in connection with long-term supplementation. Therefore, vitamin E at the dosage used in their study should not be taken routinely without careful monitoring of liver and renal functions.

Whether sufficient levels of vitamin E can be administered to humans to affect oxidized lipoprotein levels and reduce their atherogenic potential remains to be proven (2). For people with cardiovascular disease, the benefits of taking vitamin E in amounts no greater than 400 IU a day—although not completely proven—probably outweigh the risks. At higher doses (>1,080 IU), vitamin E can cause side effects that include bleeding, especially for people on blood-thinning medications, and gastrointestinal complaints.

Furthermore, the benefit vitamin E offers against cardiovascular disease is much less than that gained from exercise and healthful eating. Research consistently shows that diets high in fruits and vegetables are beneficial. Foods have beneficial compounds, such as phytochemicals, about which we know little. Supplements, even if proven helpful, can not replace a healthful diet.

DEFINITION AND REGULATION OF SUPPLEMENTS

The FDA defines *dietary supplement* as any product (other than tobacco) that is intended to supplement the diet. Dietary supplements contain one or more of the following: vitamin, mineral, herb or other botanical, amino acid, or other dietary substance (which could include phytochemicals, concentrates, metabolites, extracts, or combinations of any of the above) (89). Medical foods are exempt from this definition and are defined as foods used under medical supervision and intended for the specific dietary management of a disease or condition for which distinctive nutritional requirements, based on recognized scientific principles, are established by medical evaluation. Examples are enteral and parental products (89).

New categories of foods, called nutriceuticals or functional foods, are under development. These are foods and beverages with added or engineered health-promoting properties. They may provide a health benefit beyond the traditional nutrients they contain and may provide medical-health benefits, including the prevention and/or treatment of diseases. Some examples would include orange juice fortified with antioxidants and calcium, peanut butter with eight essential vitamins and minerals, yogurt with added vitamins, bars made from resistant starch, and so forth. They differ from fortified foods, which provide nutrients at a specific percentage of the RDAs to help prevent particular nutritional-deficiency diseases. Nutriceuticals do not address nutritional-deficiency diseases, but may address chronic diseases with other underlying causes (90). Tremendous growth in the functional food (or nutriceutical) market is evidenced by an estimated income in 1996 of $80 billion (which is about the size of the U.S. pharmaceutical market) to a potential $250 billion in annual sales (91).

Dietary supplements, although often sold as foods, are used more like drugs. However, unlike drugs, they do not have to be proven effective before being marketed. A drug is formally defined as a substance used as—or in the preparation of—a medication, and the FDA has clear premarket jurisdiction over these substances. Because dietary supplements consist of nutrient extracts of natural herbs and commonly eaten foods, they are considered to be GRAS (Generally Recognized As Safe) (92).

Supplements are designed to cure deficiencies, but do not further improve normal status unless proven to be useful as therapeutic agents. If they are to be used as therapeutic agents, their efficacy should be proven by the same stringent testing required of drugs.

Although the FDA is responsible for ensuring that supplements are safe for human consumption, the FDA cannot step in until damage or harm is documented. Under the Nutrition Labeling and Education Act of 1990, it was proposed that supplements should be required to meet the same requirements as conventional foods to qualify for a health claim and that they should follow the same labeling requirements. However, a Dietary Supplement Act, Title II of Prescription Drug User Free Act of 1992, prohibited the FDA from taking action against supplements for unauthorized health claims until at least December 1993 (93,94). Finally, in October 1994, Congress passed the Dietary Supplement Health and Education Act (DSHEA) (89), a compromise between the supplement industry and the original intent of the Nutrition Labeling and Education Act of 1990.

There are several key provisions of DSHEA. This act allows supplements to bypass the premarket FDA regulations for drugs or food additives. Supplement manufacturers or companies that sell supplements do not have to prove their products are effective or safe before they go to market. Instead, the burden of proof for an unsafe supplement is placed on the FDA. The FDA can intervene only after an illness or injury occurs. After complaints are received, the FDA is required to prove that the supplement causes harm when taken "as directed" on the label before a product can be restricted. Herbal remedies also may be sold without any knowledge of their mechanism of action (95).

Supplements must have the same type of nutritional labeling found on foods, and they cannot carry claims that mention a specific disease unless the claims are backed by solid scientific evidence. The new law does allow labels on vitamins, minerals, herbs, amino acids, and other supplements to make claims about maintaining a healthy body. To protect consumers, the law requires that supplement packages let shoppers know that these types of claims "have not been evaluated by the Food and Drug Administration" and are "not intended to diagnose, cure, or prevent any disease." The law also prohibits point-of-sale information, such as an article or book chapter supporting a dietary supplement claim, without prior FDA review (96).

Finally, the standards used to prepare and package supplements are left up to the company. Therefore, one cannot be sure of the product's purity or of the amount of the active ingredients in a supplement, even from one package to the next of the same product.

SUMMARY

Until reliable studies document the therapeutic benefits of large dosages of vitamins such as antioxidants, the best approach is to supplement with micronutrients only when a specific deficiency state is documented (2). Patients also should be educated concerning the toxicity of megadoses of micronutrients. The toxic effects of megadoses range from simple urticaria to serious neurological disorders and even death. Food is favored over supplements because food contains additional nutrients, including phytochemicals. Phytochemicals are compounds that occur naturally in foods and may have important health benefits. Researchers are just beginning to learn what role phytochemicals play in nutrition and health.

The first step in identifying a deficiency is an evaluation of the nutritional state, including the individual's food and eating habits, food preferences, and overall health status. Healthy adults can get all the necessary nutrients from foods, but certain high-risk groups, such as growing and developing children and youths, women during pregnancy and lactation, individuals eating <1,200 kcal/day, elderly individuals, especially those with low socioeconomic status, patients in intensive care units or long-term nursing facilities, and total vegetarians, may benefit from a vitamin-mineral supplement.

At present, there is no justification for routine supplementation of vitamins and minerals for people with diabetes (2). However, there are select groups of people who may benefit, such as patients with diabetes in poor glycemic control, who are more likely to have deficiencies in magnesium, zinc, and water-soluble vitamins.

Vitamin-mineral supplements should not be substituted for a healthful diet. However, there is probably no harm in taking a multiple vitamin-mineral supplement with dose levels no higher than 100% of the RDA. Doses above that do not give extra protection, but they do increase the risk of toxic side effects. Furthermore, it is likely that the response to supplements is determined by nutritional state, so only people with micronutrient deficiencies will respond favorably.

Synthetic vitamins are the same as so-called natural vitamins. Generic brands and synthetic vitamins are generally less expensive and are equally effective.

Micronutrients are intimately involved in the metabolism of carbohydrates and other nutrients and with the body's use of glucose and insulin. However, without clinical trials to prove efficacy, laboratory studies, often done in animals, are frequently extrapolated to clinical practice.

Supplements of micronutrients cure deficiencies; they are not therapeutic agents unless proven to be efficacious. In the future, antioxidants, especially vitamin E, may be proven to play a role in scavenging free radicals and therefore in limiting or preventing oxidative damage to tissues and may be recommended for use.

REFERENCES

1. Kurtzweil P: An FDA guide to dietary supplements. *FDA Consumer* 32:28, 1998

2. Mooradian AD, Faila M, Hoogwerf B, Isaac R, Maryniuk M, Wylie-Rosett J: Selected vitamins and minerals in diabetes mellitus (Technical Review). *Diabetes Care* 17:464–479, 1994

3. Franz MJ: Micronutrients, glucose metabolism, metabolic control, and supplements. *Diabetes Spectrum* 11:70–78, 1998

4. Food and Nutrition Board, Institute of Medicine, National Academy of Sciences: *Recommended Dietary Allowances*. 10th ed. Washington, DC, National Academy Press, 1989

5. Yates AA, Schlicker SA, Suitor CW: Dietary Reference Intakes: the new basis for recommendations for calcium and related nutrients, B vitamins, and choline. *J Am Diet Assoc* 98:699–706, 1998

6. Food and Nutrition Board, Institute of Medicine, National Academy of Sciences: *Dietary Reference Intakes for Calcium, Phosphorus, Magnesium, Vitamin D, and Fluoride*. Washington, DC, National Academy Press, 1997

7. Food and Nutrition Board, Institute of Medicine, National Academy of Sciences: *Dietary Reference Intakes for Thiamin, Riboflavin, Niacin, Vitamin B-6, Folate, Vitamin B-12, Pantothenic Acid, Biotin, and Choline*. Washington, DC, National Academy Press, 1998

8. Mooradian AD, Morley JE: Micronutrient status in diabetes mellitus. *Am J Clin Nutr* 45:877–895, 1987

9. Truman RW, Doisy RJ: Metabolic effects of the glucose tolerance factor (GTF) in normal and genetically diabetic mice. *Diabetes* 26:820–826, 1977

10. Rabinowitz MB, Levin SR, Gonick JE: Comparisons of chromium status in diabetic and normal men. *Metabolism* 29:355–364, 1980

11. Abraham AS, Brooks BA, Eylath U: The effects of chromium supplementation on serum glucose and lipids in patients with and without non-insulin-dependent diabetes. *Metab Clin Exp* 41:768–771, 1992

12. Jeejeeboy KN, Chu RC, Marliss EB, Greenberg GR, Bruce-Robertson A: Chromium deficiency, glucose intolerance, and neuropathy reversed by chromium supplementation, in a patient receiving long-term total parenteral nutrition. *Am J Clin Nutr* 30:531–538, 1977

13. Freund H, Atamian S, Fischer JE: Chromium deficiency during total parenteral nutrition. *JAMA* 241:496–498, 1979

14. Lee NA, Reasner CA: Beneficial effect of chromium supplementation on serum triglyceride levels in NIDDM. *Diabetes Care* 17:1449–1452, 1994

15. Rabinowitz MB, Gonick HC, Levin SR, Davidson MB: Effect of chromium and yeast supplements on carbohydrate and lipid metabolism in diabetic men. *Diabetes Care* 6:319–327, 1983

16. Sherman L, Glennon JA, Brech WJ, Klomberg GH, Gordon ES: Failure of trivalent chromium to improve hyperglycemia in diabetes mellitus. *Metabolism* 17:439–442, 1968

17. Uusitupa MIJ, Kumpulainen JT, Voutilainen E: Effect of inorganic chromium supplementation on glucose intolerance, insulin response and serum lipids in noninsulin-dependent diabetics. *Am J Clin Nutr* 38:404–410, 1983

18. Anderson RA, Polansky MM, Bryden NA, Canary JJ: Supplemental-chromium effects on glucose, insulin, glucagon, and urinary chromium losses in subjects consuming controlled low-chromium diets. *Am J Clin Nutr* 54:909–916, 1991

19. Anderson RA, Cheng N, Bryden NA, Polansky MM, Cheng N, Chi J, Feng J: Elevated intakes of supplemental chromium improve glucose and insulin variables in individuals with type 2 diabetes. *Diabetes* 46:1786–1791, 1997

20. Mertz W, Abernathy CO, Olin SS: *Risk Assessment of Essential Elements*. Washington, DC, ILSI Press, 1994, pp. xix–xxviii

21. Anderson RA, Bryden NA, Polansky MM: Lack of toxicity of chromium chloride and chromium picolinate. *J Am Coll Nutr* 16:273–279, 1997

22. Stearns DM, Belbruno JJ, Wetterhahn KE: A prediction of chromium (III) accumulation in humans from chromium dietary supplements. *FASEB J* 15:1650–1657, 1995

23. Stearns DM, Wise JP, Patierno SR, Wetterhahn KE: Chromium (III) picolinate produces chromosome damage in Chinese hamster ovary cells. *FASEB J* 15:1643–1648, 1995

24. Liu VJK, Morris JS: Relative chromium response as an indicator of chromium status. *Am J Clin Nutr* 31:972–976, 1978

25. Alzaid A, Dinneen S, Moyer T, Rizza R: Effects of insulin on plasma magnesium in non-insulin dependent diabetes mellitus: evidence for insulin resistance. *J Clin Endocrinol Metab* 80:1376–1381, 1995

26. Whelton PK, Klag MJ: Magnesium and blood pressure: review of the epidemiologic and clinical trial experience. *Am J Cardiol* 63:26G–30G, 1989

27. Resnick LM: Hypertension and abnormal glucose homeostasis: possible role of divalent ion metabolism. *Am J Med* 87 (Suppl. 6A):17–22, 1989

28. Shattock MJ, Hearse DJ, Fry CH: The ionic basis of the anti-ischemic and anti-arrhythmic properties of magnesium in the heart. *J Am Coll Nutr* 6:27–33, 1987

29. McNair P, Christiansen C, Madsbad S, Lauritzen E, Faber O, Binder C, Transbøl I: Hypomagnesemia, a risk factor in diabetic retinopathy. *Diabetes* 27:1075–1077, 1978

30. Yajnik CS, Smith RF, Hockaday TDR, Ward NI: Fasting plasma magnesium concentrations and glucose disposal in diabetes. *Br Med J* 288:1032–1034, 1984

31. Paolisso G, Scheen A, D'Onofrio E, Lefebvre P: Magnesium and glucose homeostasis. *Diabetologia* 33:511–514, 1990

32. American Diabetes Association: Magnesium supplementation in the treatment of diabetes (Consensus Statement). *Diabetes Care* 15:1065–1067, 1992

33. Mather HM, Nisbet JA, Burton GH, Pasten GJ, Bland JM, Bailey PA, Pilkington TRE: Hypomagnesium in diabetes. *Clin Chim Acta* 95:235–242, 1979

34. Sjogren A, Floren CH, Nilsson A: Magnesium, potassium, and zinc deficiency in subjects with type II diabetes mellitus. *Acta Med Scand* 224:461–465, 1988

35. McNair P, Christensen MS, Christiansen C, Modshod S, Transbol IB: Renal hypomagnesaemia in human diabetes mellitus: its relations to glucose homeostasis. *Eur J Clin Invest* 12:81–85, 1982

36. Nadler JL, Malayan S, Luong H, Shaw S, Natarajan RD, Rude RK: Intracellular free magnesium deficiency plays a key role in increased platelet reactivity in type II diabetes mellitus. *Diabetes Care* 15:835–841, 1992

37. Lima JDL, Cruz T, Pousada JC, Rodrigues LE, Barbosa K, Cangucu V: The effect of magnesium supplementation in increasing doses on the control of type 2 diabetes. *Diabetes Care* 21:682–686, 1998

38. Hwang DL, Yen CF, Nadler JL: Insulin increases intracellular magnesium transport in human platelets. *J Clin Endocrinol Metab* 76:549–553, 1993

39. Paolisso G, Passariello N, Pizza G, Marrazzo G, Giunta R, Sgambato S, Varricchio M, D'Onofrio F: Dietary magnesium supplements improve β-cell response to glucose and arginine in elderly non-insulin dependent diabetic subjects. *Acta Endocrinol* 121:16–20, 1989

40. Paolisso G, Sgambato S, Pizza G, Passariello N, Varricchio M, D'Onofrio F: Improved insulin response and action by chronic magnesium administration in aged NIDDM subjects. *Diabetes Care* 12:265–269, 1989

41. Paolisso G, Sgambato S, Gambardella A, Pizza G, Tesauro P, Varricchio M, D'Onofrio F: Daily magnesium supplements improve glucose handling in elderly subjects. *Am J Clin Nutr* 55:1161–1167, 1992

42. Arquilla ER, Packer S, Tarmas W, Miyamoto S: The effect of zinc on insulin metabolism. *Endocrinology* 103:1440–1449, 1978

43. Kinlaw WB, Levine AS, Morley HE, Silvis SE, McClain CJ: Abnormal zinc metabolism in type II diabetes mellitus. *Am J Med* 75:273–277, 1983

44. Niewoehner CB, Allen JI, Boosalis M, Levine AS, Morley JE: The role of zinc supplementation in type II diabetes mellitus. *Am J Med* 81:63–68, 1986

45. Mooradian AD, Norman DC, Morley JE: The effect of zinc status on the immune function in diabetic rats. *Diabetologia* 31:703–707, 1988

46. Hallbook T, Lanner E: Serum-zinc and healing of venous leg ulcers. *Lancet* ii:780–782, 1972

47. Blostein-Fujii A, DiSilvestro RA, Frid D, Katz C, Malarkey W: Short-term zinc supplementation in women with non-insulin-dependent diabetes mellitus: effects on plasma 5'-nucleotidase activities, insulin-like growth factor I concentrations, and lipoprotein oxidation rates in vitro. *Am J Clin Nutr* 66:639–642, 1997

48. Walter RM, Uriu-Hare JY, Olin KL, Oster MH, Anawalt BD, Critchfield JW, Keen CL: Copper, zinc, manganese, and magne-

sium status and complications of diabetes mellitus. *Diabetes Care* 14:1050–1056, 1991

49. Martin Mateo MC, Bustamante J, Gonzalez Cantalapiedra MA: Serum zinc, copper and insulin in diabetes mellitus. *Biomedicine* 29:56–58, 1978

50. Failla ML, Kiser RA: Hepatic and renal metabolism of copper and zinc in the diabetic rat. *Am J Physiol* 244:E115–E121, 1983

51. Lau AL, Failla ML: Urinary excretion of zinc, copper and iron in the streptozotocin-diabetic rat. *J Nutr* 114:224–233, 1984

52. Everson GJ, Shrader RE: Abnormal glucose tolerance in manganese deficient guinea pigs. *J Nutr* 94:89–94, 1968

53. Bond JS, Failla ML, Unger DF: Elevated manganese concentration and arginase activity in livers of streptozotocin-induced diabetic rats. *J Biol Chem* 258:8004–8009, 1983

54. Dandona P, Hussain MA, Varghese Z, Politis D, Flynn DM, Hoffbrand AV: Insulin resistance and iron overload. *Ann Clin Biochem* 20:77–79, 1983

55. Salonen JT, Nyyssonen K, Korpela H, Tuomilehto J, Seppanen R, Salonen R: High stored iron levels are associated with excess risk of myocardial infarction in Eastern Finnish men. *Circulation* 86:803–811, 1992

56. Chertow BS, Baker GR: The effects of vitamin A on insulin release and glucose oxidation in isolated rat islets. *Endocrinology* 103:1562–1572, 1979

57. Basu TK, Tze WJ, Leichter J: Serum vitamin A and retinol-binding protein in patients with insulin-dependent diabetes mellitus. *Am J Clin Nutr* 50:329–333, 1989

58. Facchini F, Coulston A, Reaven GM: Relation between dietary vitamin intake and resistance to insulin-mediated glucose disposal in healthy volunteers. *Am J Clin Nutr* 63:946–949, 1996

59. Hennekens CH, Buring JE, Manson JE, Stampfer M, Rosner B, Cook NR, Belanger C, LaMotte F, Gaziano JM, Ridker PM, Willett W, Peto R: Lack of effect of long-term supplementation with beta carotene on the incidence of malignant neoplasms and cardiovascular disease. *N Engl J Med* 334:1145–1149, 1996

60. Garg A, Grundy SM: Nicotinic acid as therapy for dyslipidemia in noninsulin-dependent diabetes. *JAMA* 264:723–726, 1990

61. Henkin Y, Oberman A, Hurst DC, Segrest JP: Niacin revisited: clinical observations on an important but underutilized drug. *Am J Med* 91:239–246, 1991

62. Gale EAM: Theory and practice of nicotinamide trials in pre-type 1 diabetes. *J Pediatr Endocrinol Metab* 9:375–379, 1996

63. Pozzilli P, Visalli N, Ghirlanda G, Manna R, Andreani D: Nicotinamide increases C-peptide secretion in patients with recent onset type I diabetes. *Diabetic Med* 6:568–572, 1989

64. Vague P, Picq R, Bernal M, Lassmann-Vague V, Vialettes B: Effect of nicotinamide treatment on the residual insulin secretion in type I diabetic patients. *Diabetologia* 32:316–321, 1989

65. Lewis CM, Canafax DM, Sprafka JM, Barbosa JJ: Double-blind randomized trial of nicotinamide on early-onset diabetes. *Diabetes Care* 15:121–123, 1992

66. Pozzilli P, Visalli N, Signore A, Baroni NG, Buzzetti R, Cavallo MG, Boccuni ML, Fava D, Gragnoli C, Andreani D, Lucentini L, Matteoli MC, Crino A, Cicconetti CA, Teodonio C, Paci F, Amoretti R, Pisano L, Pennafina MG, Santopadre G, Marozzi G, Multari G, Suppa MA, Campea L, DeMattia GC, Cassone M, Faldetta G, Marietti G, Perrone F, Greco AV, Ghirlanda G: Double blind trial of nicotinamide in recent-onset IDDM (the IMDIAB III study). *Diabetologia* 38:848–852, 1995

67. Chase HP, Butler-Simon N, Garg S, McDuffie M, Hoos SL, O'Brien D: A trial of nicotinamide in newly diagnosed patients with type I (insulin-dependent) diabetes mellitus. *Diabetologia* 33:444–446, 1990

68. Elliott RB, Pilcher CC, Stewart A: The use of nicotinamide in the prevention of type I diabetes. *Ann NY Acad Sci* 696:333–334, 1993

69. Saito N, Kimura M, Kuchiba A, Itokawa Y: Blood thiamine levels in outpatients with diabetes mellitus. *J Nutr Sci Vitaminol* 33:421–430, 1987

70. Rao RH, Vigg BL, Jaya Rao KS: Failure of pyridoxine to improve glucose tolerance in diabetics. *J Clin Endocrinol Metab* 50:198–200, 1980

71. Solomon LR, Cohen K: Erythrocyte O_2 transport and metabolism and effects of vitamin B_6 therapy in type II diabetes mellitus. *Diabetes* 38:881–886, 1989

72. Kaplan WE, Abourizk NN: Diabetic peripheral neuropathies affecting the lower extremity. *J Am Podiatry Assoc* 71:356–362, 1981

73. Schorah CJ, Bishop N, Wales JK, Hansbro PM, Habibzadeh N: Blood vitamin C concentrations in patients with diabetes mellitus. *Int J Vitam Nutr Res* 58:312–318, 1988

74. Mooradian AD: The effect of ascorbate and dehydroascorbate on tissue uptake of glucose. *Diabetes* 36:1094–1097, 1987

75. Cox BD, Butterfield WJH: Vitamin C supplements and diabetic cutaneous capillary fragility. *Br Med J* 3:205, 1975

76. Davie SJ, Gould BJ, Yudkin JS: Effect of vitamin C on glycosylation of proteins. *Diabetes* 41:167–173, 1992

77. Cunningham JJ, Mearkle PL, Brown RG: Vitamin C: an aldose reductase inhibitor that normalizes erythrocyte sorbitol in insulin-dependent diabetes mellitus. *J Am Coll Nutr* 13:344–350, 1994

78. Som S, Basu S, Mukherjee D, Deb S, Choudhury PR, Mukherjee S, Chatterjee SN, Chatterjee IB: Ascorbic acid metabolism in diabetes mellitus. *Metabolism* 30:572–577, 1981

79. Hui SL, Epstein S, Johnston CC Jr: A prospective study of bone mass in patients with type I diabetes. *J Clin Endocrinol Metab* 60:74–80, 1985

80. Auwerx J, Dequeker J, Bouillon R, Geusens P, Nijs J: Mineral metabolism and bone mass at peripheral and axial skeleton in diabetes mellitus. *Diabetes* 37:3–12, 1988

81. Levin ME, Boisseau VC, Avioli LV: Effects of diabetes mellitus on bone mass in juvenile and adult-onset diabetes. *N Engl J Med* 294:241–245, 1976

82. Ishida H, Seino Y, Matsukura S, Ikeda M, Yawata M, Yamashita G: Diabetic osteopenia and circulating levels of vitamin D metabolites in type 2 diabetes. *Metabolism* 34:797–801, 1985

83. Ceriello A, Giugliano D, Quatraro A, Donzella C, Diplao G, Lefebvre PJ: Vitamin E reduction of protein glycosylation in diabetes: new prospect for prevention of diabetic complications? *Diabetes Care* 14:68–72, 1991

84. Paolisso G, D'Amore A, Galzzerano D, Balbi V, Giugliano D, Varricchio M, D'Onofrio F: Daily vitamin E supplements improve metabolic control but not insulin secretion in elderly type II diabetic patients. *Diabetes Care* 16:1433–1437, 1993

85. Reaven PD, Herold DA, Barnett J, Edelman S: Effects of vitamin E on susceptibility of low-density lipoprotein and low-density lipoprotein subfractions to oxidation and on protein glycation in NIDDM. *Diabetes Care* 18:807–816, 1995

86. Harland BF, Harden-Williams BA: Is vanadium of human nutritional importance yet? *J Am Diet Assoc* 94:891–894, 1994

87. Schechter Y: Insulin-mimetic effects of vanadate. *Diabetes* 39:1–5, 1990

88. Subodh V, Cam MC, McNeill JH: Nutritional factors that can favorably influence the glucose/insulin system: vanadium. *J Am Coll Nutr* 17:11–18, 1998

89. *Dietary Supplement Health and Education Act of 1994.* Public Law 103-417

90. Hunt JR: Nutritional products for specific health benefits—foods, pharmaceuticals, or something in between? *J Am Diet Assoc* 94:151–153, 1994

91. Sloan AE: America's appetite '96: the top 10 trends to watch for and work on. *Food Technol* 54–71, July 1996

92. About supplements. *FDA Consumer* 18–19, May 1993

93. Food and Drug Administration: Regulation of dietary supplements. *Federal Register* 58:33692, 1993

94. Food and Drug Administration: Food labeling: mandatory status of nutrition labeling and nutrient content, revision, format for nutrition label. *Federal Register* 58:2151, 1993

95. Angell M, Kassirer JP: Alternative medicine—the risks of untested and unregulated remedies. *N Engl J Med* 339:839–841, 1998

96. Porter DV: Dietary Supplement Health and Education Act of 1994: P.L. 103-417. *Nutrition Today* 30:89–94, 1995

Ms. Franz is Director of Nutrition and Professional Education at the International Diabetes Center, Institute for Research and Education, HealthSystem Minnesota, Minneapolis, MN.

11. Alcohol and Diabetes

Marion J. Franz, MS, RD, LD, CDE

Highlights

- Acute alcohol ingestion has minimal effects on blood glucose levels in people with type 1 or type 2 diabetes. However, in people with type 1 diabetes, late-onset hypoglycemia has been reported.
- Light-to-moderate alcohol intakes have been associated with lower levels of insulin resistance and enhanced insulin-mediated glucose uptake in type 2 diabetes.
- Chronic use of light-to-moderate alcohol also has been associated with decreased coronary heart disease, presumably by raising HDL cholesterol levels. However, alcohol consumption and diabetes are also associated with hypertriglyceridemia.
- Under normal circumstances and when diabetes is well controlled, blood glucose levels will not be affected by the moderate use of alcohol: no more than two drinks per day for men and no more than one drink per day for women. People using insulin should only consume alcohol with food, and because of the danger of hypoglycemia, no food should be omitted. For people with type 2 diabetes, alcohol calories are best substituted for fat calories.

INTRODUCTION

In the most recent report on sources of nutrients in U.S. adults from 1989 to 1991, alcohol accounted for 2.5% of nutrient energy (1), compared with ~5% in the previous report (2). It is unknown whether this change is due to decreased intake or to methodological differences.

Nearly two-thirds of the adult American population are reported to drink alcoholic beverages, whereas one-third claim to be abstainers (3). People with diabetes no doubt fall into both categories; however, if people with diabetes choose to drink alcoholic beverages, they need to know what effect it can have on blood glucose control and how to do it safely. This chapter will review the literature on the use of occasional, moderate amounts of alcohol. It will not deal with chronic abuse or alcoholic liver disease. For a review of these issues, see Lieber (4).

The alcohol in beverages is ethanol (ethyl alcohol, C_2H_5OH), which is the intoxicating molecule present in distilled spirits (hard liquor), wine, and beer. It is the byproduct of the oxidation of sugars for energy by yeast enzymes (fermentation). The term alcohol will be used in this article. One drink, or an alcoholic beverage, is commonly defined as 12 oz of beer, 5 oz of wine, or 1.5 oz (one jigger) of distilled spirits, each of which contains ~1 oz (~15 g) of alcohol.

The American Diabetes Association (ADA) nutrition recommendations caution that the same precautions regarding the use of alcohol that apply to the general public also apply to people with diabetes (5). The ADA guidelines support the *Dietary Guidelines for Americans* (6), which recommends no more than two drinks per day for men and no more than one drink per day for women. Abstention from alcohol should be advised for people with a history of alcohol abuse or for pregnant women. Reduction of or abstention from alcohol intake is also advisable for individuals with diabetes with other medical problems, such as pancreatitis, dyslipidemia, especially elevated triglycerides, or neuropathy (5).

ABSORPTION AND METABOLISM OF ALCOHOL

Alcohol is absorbed by a process of simple diffusion across the gastrointestinal mucosa of the stomach, duodenum, and jejunum. It is the only substance that can be absorbed through the walls of the stomach into the bloodstream. With the ingestion of food, especially high-fat food, fewer alcohol molecules diffuse from the stomach into the capillaries. However, no matter how much food is present, when alcohol arrives in the duodenum, it is absorbed quickly and completely.

The liver is the major organ for alcohol metabolism. Only 2–10% of the alcohol absorbed is eliminated via the kidneys and lungs; the rest must be oxidized in the body, principally in the liver (7). The liver metabolizes alcohol slowly, at an average rate of ~0.1 g/kg body wt/h. Therefore, an average 70-kg man will require ~2 h to metabolize the alcohol in 12 oz of beer or 2.5–3 h to metabolize the alcohol in 2 oz of whiskey. People who drink routinely appear to adapt so as to metabolize alcohol somewhat more rapidly.

The only way for the body to dispose of alcohol is to oxidize it. Although the liver is the chief site, it has been reported that the gastric mucosa may contribute to alcohol metabolism as well. This effect varies with sex, being decreased in women and in men who are chronic alcoholics (8). The total quantity of alcohol and the rate of ingestion determine its effect. Time between alcohol ingestion is essential so that the liver can oxidize it. Excessive alcohol that the liver cannot metabolize immediately enters the general circulation, where it becomes a part of all body fluids and enters into cells. It has a special affinity for the brain and quickly reaches the brain cells. At first this results in a state of euphoria, often accompanied by release of inhibitions. Although alcohol is a depressant, the initial feeling is just the opposite because it lifts the barriers of self-control.

The concentration of alcohol in the breath and urine is proportional to the concentration of unmetabolized alcohol circulating in the blood. Instruments that measure breath alcohol content operate on this principle.

The hepatocyte contains three pathways for ethanol metabolism, each located in a different subcellular compartment: *1)* the alcohol dehydrogenase (ADH) pathway in the cytosol (the soluble fraction of the cell); *2)* the microsomal ethanol-oxidizing system (MEOS) located in the endoplasmic reticulum; and *3)* catalase, located in the peroxisomes. All three pathways result in the production of acetaldehyde, a highly toxic metabolite (4).

ADH Pathway

Alcohol is oxidized to acetaldehyde and acetate and then to energy. The major pathway for ethanol disposition involves ADH, an enzyme that catalyzes the conversion of ethanol to acetaldehyde. This pathway determines the action and speed of alcohol metabolism. If the limited number of ADH molecules in the liver cells are occupied, excess alcohol molecules will enter the general circulation and return to the liver when ADH molecules are free to process them. The conversion of alcohol to acetaldehyde in the liver requires ADH and the coenzyme nicotinamide adenine dinucleotide (NAD^+), which is then reduced to NADH. The oxidation of acetaldehyde requires acetaldehyde dehydrogenase as well as NAD. Acetate that is released into the bloodstream completes oxidation in other tissues. Alcohol oxidation is an effective source of energy because it is coupled with the synthesis of adenosine triphosphate (ATP) (Figure 11.1).

The hepatic oxidation of alcohol generates an excess of reducing equivalents in the form of NADH and alters the redox state of the organism; affects many additional biochemical reactions; and is linked to hypoglycemia, hyperlipemia, fatty liver, lactic acidemia, hyperuricemia, and ketosis (9).

Ethanol $\xrightarrow[\text{NAD}^+\rightsquigarrow\text{NADH} + \text{H}^+]{\text{Alcohol dehydrogenase}}$ Acetaldehyde $\xrightarrow[\text{NAD}^+\rightsquigarrow\text{NADH} + \text{H}^+]{\text{Acetaldehyde dehydrogenase}}$

Acetate $\xrightarrow{\text{Oxidation}}$ $CO_2 + H_2O + ATP$

Figure 11.1 Alcohol oxidation.

Increases in the NADH:NAD ratio inhibit the entrance of glycerol, lactic acid, and specific amino acids into the metabolic pathways that convert these metabolites to glucose, thus impairing gluconeogenesis. The high levels of NADH also block 2-carbon fragments from entry into the citric acid cycle, and as a result, these fragments become building blocks for fatty acids. Simultaneously, protein synthesis is depressed and protein carriers that normally carry fatty acids away from the liver are not manufactured, leading to the common alcoholic condition of fatty liver.

Alcohol metabolism leads to a shift toward lactate from pyruvate in the liver and to decreased use of lactic acid produced in muscles. Lactic acid interferes with the excretion of uric acid. This accumulation of uric acid may have symptoms similar to gout, but it is not "true" gout and clears up with abstinence from alcohol. Ketoacidosis may develop in addition to lactic acidosis because decreased oxidation of free fatty acids via the citric acid cycle leads to an increase in the formation of ketone bodies, β-hydroxybutyrate, and to a lesser degree, acetoacetate. With a virtually nonfat diet, alcohol does not induce ketonuria or hyperketonemia, which suggests that a combination of alcohol and dietary fat is necessary to produce these effects (10).

A moderate degree of hypertriglyceridemia is associated with alcohol intake. The enhanced NADH:NAD ratio causes an excess of hydrogen, some of which is shunted directly into the synthesis of α-glycerolphosphate, which leads to the trapping of fatty acids and the formation and accumulation of triglycerides.

MEOS and Catalase Pathways

In addition to the main pathway of oxidation by ADH in the cytosol, alcohol may also be metabolized by the microsomes that comprise the smooth endoplasmic reticulum (SER). The role of the MEOS is small, but it may play a predominant role at intoxicating levels of blood alcohol. The MEOS pathway requires reduced NAD phosphate (NADPH) rather than NAD^+ and may be a way of alleviating excess hydrogen equivalents in the liver. Because both the MEOS and the SER are involved in the metabolism of many drugs, this may also explain the unusual response of alcoholics to the action of many drugs (11). In the presence of an H_2O_2-generating system, catalase is also capable of oxidizing alcohol. However, only a small percentage of alcohol is oxidized via this pathway (11).

In people with no history of chronic exposure to alcohol, it is estimated that ~75% of alcohol is oxidized by the ADH pathway, whereas 25% probably involves the MEOS. At high concentrations and longer durations of intake, as much as 80% of alcohol metabolism could proceed via a non-ADH pathway. Therefore, steady and prolonged alcohol consumption allows drinkers to tolerate larger amounts of alcoholic beverages. In addition to the MEOS pathway, there are increases in the ability of the liver cells to synthesize ADH to help clear the blood of alcohol that may even double the amount of alcohol that an alcoholic can clear in 1 h (12).

EFFECTS OF ALCOHOL ON BLOOD GLUCOSE LEVELS

Alcohol can have both hypo- and hyperglycemic effects in people with diabetes. Alcohol can enhance glucose-stimulated insulin secretion (13) and reduce gluconeogenesis in the liver (14,15), and large amounts can cause peripheral insulin resistance by reducing glucose oxidation and storage (16). Thus, moderate (17) or severe hypoglycemia (18), no hypoglycemia at all (19,20), and hyperglycemia (21,22) have all been reported in people with diabetes after having alcoholic drinks.

Hypoglycemia can occur at blood alcohol levels that do not exceed the range of mild intoxication (23). Alcohol-induced hypoglycemia can develop within 6–36 h after moderate to heavy alcohol ingestion in individuals whose food intake has been markedly restricted. It may occur, however, even in occasional drinkers who have missed a meal or two (24). Two ounces of alcohol (20–25 g) may produce hypoglycemia in a fasting person, causing blood glucose levels of <40 mg/dl (2.2 mmol/l). The diagnosis of hypoglycemia may be obscured because its symptoms, especially alcoholic breath odor, are similar to those resulting from alcohol ingestion.

Ingestion of moderate amounts of alcohol also blunts the awareness of hypoglycemia. After nondiabetic subjects and subjects with type 1 diabetes drank either an alcoholic or a placebo beverage, their blood glucose levels were lowered to 45 mg/dl (2.2 mmol/l) for 40 min. During hypoglycemia, in both groups, moderate alcohol ingestion decreased awareness, blunted finger tremor, and increased reaction time and sweating without affecting the counterregulatory response. Despite being aware of facial flushing, blurred vision, palpitations, and sweating, only 2 of 15 subjects "felt hypoglycemia" after drinking alcohol, compared with 11 of 15 after the placebo beverage (25).

If alcohol inhibits gluconeogenesis, it might be speculated that alcohol could be a hypoglycemic agent, especially in people with type 2 diabetes. Puhakainen et al. (26) attempted to determine whether alcohol is hypoglycemic after an overnight fast in people with type 2 diabetes in whom gluconeogenesis is markedly increased. Total hepatic glucose output was measured after alcohol and saline ingestion. The inhibition of gluconeogenesis by alcohol was not sufficient to reduce total hepatic glucose output; therefore, alcohol would not be useful as a hypoglycemic agent. The ability of the liver to maintain hepatic glucose output in the presence of alcohol is probably due to accelerated glycogenolysis.

Alcohol can also augment the plasma insulin response to glucose. Moderate amounts of alcohol can enhance the glucose-lowering action of exogenous insulin and oral hypoglycemic agents. Although it does not affect the rate and degree of decline in plasma glucose, alcohol appears to alter the phase of glucose rebound. It interferes with hepatic gluconeogenesis and induces hypoglycemia whenever gluconeogenesis is required to maintain normal glucose levels (18). It also acutely interferes with the counterregulation of insulin-induced hypoglycemia that usually occurs when plasma insulin levels are low and glucagon levels are elevated. The hypoglycemia induced by alcohol is not ameliorated by glucagon because it is caused by the indirect impairment of gluconeogenesis and is not associated with excessive insulin secretion (18).

There are also adverse effects of chronic alcohol consumption. In people with type 2 diabetes, chronic alcohol intake can impair glycemic control; lead to increased lipolysis, ketogenesis, and hypertriglyceridemia; and become a risk factor for neuropathy (21). In addition, in some patients, alcohol abuse leads to overt diabetes (22). The effects induced by alcohol are reversed after abstinence from alcohol (21,22). Thus, patients with diabetes may need to be more cautious than the general public regarding chronic use of alcohol.

Table 11.1 summarizes the acute studies done using moderate amounts of alcohol in people with type 1 or type 2 diabetes. As can be seen, moderate amounts of alcohol have no acute impact on blood glucose levels in people with either type of diabetes. However, for individuals with type 1 diabetes, a risk of late-onset hypoglycemia may exist. In individuals with type 2 diabetes, the risk of alcohol-induced acute hypoglycemia is modest.

Alcohol and Insulin Sensitivity

Although large doses of ethanol have been shown to impair insulin-mediated glucose uptake (34,35), chronic effects of moderate intake may be quite the opposite. Lazarus et al. (36) examined the relationship between measures of insulin resistance and alcohol intake among 938 nondiabetic men from Boston, Massachusetts. After adjusting for

Table 11.1 Summary of Research Using Moderate Ingestion of Alcohol in Individuals with Type 1 and Type 2 Diabetes

Author (Reference)	Subjects	Study Design	Results	Study Conclusion
Walsh and O'Sullivan (27)	20 subjects with diabetes (7 on insulin, 10 on oral agents, 3 on diet alone)	2 1/2 h after their last meal at 1800, subjects slowly (over 90–120 min) drank either a drink containing 35 ml of alcohol mixed with orange juice, an isocaloric glucose drink, or no drink; BG tests done every 3–4 h for the next 24 h	Over 24 h there were no significant differences in BG for the three study periods; two subjects on insulin became hypoglycemic after alcohol.	Reasonable to permit moderate amounts of alcohol; food intake should not be reduced to compensate for extra calorie load from alcohol.
McMonagle and Felig (28)	5 nondiabetic subjects and 5 subjects with type 2 diabetes	1 h after lunch either 60 ml of alcohol diluted with water or a low-calorie beverage given in four equal hourly doses was ingested; at 1700 a glucose load was ingested	In both groups, BG levels after the glucose load were 30–80 mg/dl lower and the insulin response was 35 –40% higher after alcohol ingestion.	Alcohol enhances glucose-stimulated insulin secretion, which may contribute to a BG-lowering effect of alcohol in type 2 diabetes.
Avogaro et al. (29)	5 nondiabetic and 5 euglycemic subjects with type 1 diabetes (controlled by artificial pancreas)	Fed isocaloric meals with or without red wine (35% of caloric intake from alcohol) at lunch and dinner; followed for 15 h	BG levels were not significantly modified by alcohol, but metabolites that depend on an increase in liver NADH: NAD ratio were altered: increased lactate and 3-hydroxybutyrate levels, decreased pyruvate levels.	No impairment in glucose levels with moderate intake of alcohol with meals; alterations in other intermediate metabolites similar in both groups.

Reference	Subjects	Method	Results	Conclusions
Singh et al. (30)	10 subjects with type 2 diabetes (7 on oral agents, 3 on diet alone) and 14 nondiabetic subjects	OGTT conducted using 75-g glucose load and 1 week later repeated with addition of 43 g alcohol	Alcohol did not affect glucose tolerance, plasma insulin or C-peptide responses, or glucagon response.	Ingestion of moderate amounts of alcohol has no adverse effect on glucose tolerance in nondiabetic or type 2 diabetic individuals.
Lange et al. (17)	23 subjects with type 1 diabetes	Mineral water, diet beer, or whiskey (9.56 g alcohol/kg) were given after the evening snack to study effect of moderate amounts of alcohol on BG levels	After alcohol consumption, BG levels were significantly lower between 0700 and 1100; the number of hypoglycemic episodes the morning after alcohol ingestion was also greater.	Moderate amounts of alcohol ingested after dinner may increase the risk of hypoglycemia the next morning.
Spraul et al. (31)	8 male subjects with type 1 diabetes connected to a constant intravenous insulin infusion	~7 h after breakfast with steady-state glycemia, subjects ingested in randomized order on different days: 1) 500 ml carbohydrate depleted diet beer (3 g CHO, 20 g alcohol); 2) 500 ml ordinary German beer (18 g CHO, 20 g alcohol); 3) 500 ml dextrose solution (18 g CHO); 4) 500 ml dextrose plus alcohol solution (18 g CHO, 20 g alcohol); 5) control, no drink ingested	Glycemic responses to regular beer, dextrose solution, and dextrose with alcohol solution were similar (~80 mg/dl); after CHO-depleted beer, glycemic response decreased by ~18 mg/dl, significantly different than control.	CHO-containing beer has a glycemic index similar to other common CHO foods; CHO-depleted beer without food may decrease glucose levels.
Menzel et al. (32)	8 subjects with type 1 diabetes	1 g alcohol/kg ingested 2 h after usual supper	No signs of hypoglycemia following ingestion, but several episodes of hypoglycemia were seen 14 h after ingestion.	Subjects need to eat on schedule when consuming alcohol.

(Continued)

Table 11.1 Summary of Research Using Moderate Ingestion of Alcohol in Individuals with Type 1 and Type 2 Diabetes (*Continued*)

Author (Reference)	Subjects	Study Design	Results	Study Conclusion
Gin et al. (19)	5 men with type 1 diabetes connected to a Biostator and 10 men with type 2 diabetes treated with an oral agent	Ate the same lunch with the same volume of either water or red wine (2 glasses); glucose tolerance was evaluated over 4 h from the postprandial glycemic levels	Moderate intake of wine with meal had no effect on postprandial glucose response in either group and no significant difference in total insulin need in type 1 subjects.	Moderate intake of wine with a meal has no hypoglycemic effect and does not alter insulin need in type 1 diabetes.
Christiansen et al. (33)	12 subjects with type 2 diabetes (4 on oral agents, 8 on diet alone)	Consumed a light meal with 300 ml of water, 300 ml dry white wine, 300 ml sweet white wine, or 300 ml dry white wine with glucose added to determine the effects of dry or sweet wines	Similar glucose, insulin, and triglyceride responses were reported in all four situations.	People with well-controlled type 2 diabetes can drink moderate amounts of wine with meals; whether the wine is dry or sweet has no impact on glycemic control.
Koivisto et al. (20)	19 males with type 1 diabetes and 16 subjects with type 2 diabetes (14 on oral agents, 2 on diet alone)	Alcohol (1 g/kg, ~40 ml of vodka before, 400 ml of red wine during, and 40 ml of cognac after a meal) or an equal amount of water was given during a dinner; blood glucose and serum insulin levels were compared along with hypoglycemic episodes until 1000 the morning after the dinner	In type 1 diabetes, BG and serum insulin responses were identical after the dinner with or without alcohol; in type 2 diabetes, BG response was identical but alcohol slightly enhanced insulin response to meal; no hypoglycemic glucose levels in either group.	Social alcohol intake with a dinner does not alter postmeal or next-morning glucose homeostasis in either type 1 or type 2 diabetes.

BG, blood glucose; CHO, carbohydrate; OGTT, oral glucose tolerance test.

potential confounders, analysis revealed that subjects consuming moderate amounts of alcohol (10 g or more, but <30 g/day) had the lowest insulin and fasting insulin resistance index values. Fasting insulin resistance index and fasting insulin levels were higher in those subjects reporting no alcohol intake, low intake (<10 g/day), and high intake (30 g or more/day). Insulin resistance and associated hyperinsulinemia have been associated with the development of coronary heart disease. Thus, Lazarus et al. suggested the possibility that the coronary heart disease–protective effects of moderate alcohol use are at least partially mediated by the effects of alcohol on insulin. The biological mechanism by which moderate levels of intake lead to lower levels of insulin resistance is not known.

Light-to-moderate alcohol consumption in healthy men and women has been associated with enhanced insulin-mediated glucose uptake and lower plasma glucose and insulin concentrations. Facchini et al. (37) measured plasma glucose and insulin responses in light-to-moderate drinkers (10–30 g/day) and nondrinkers given an oral glucose challenge. Fasting plasma lipid and lipoprotein concentrations were also measured. The light-to-moderate drinkers had lower integrated plasma glucose and insulin responses to the glucose challenge and higher fasting HDL cholesterol levels compared with the nondrinkers. The researchers suggested that changes in glucose and insulin metabolism may contribute to the lower risk of coronary heart disease associated with light-to-moderate drinking. However, they also cautioned that the results should not be interpreted to mean that alcohol consumption should be encouraged to improve insulin-mediated glucose disposal, because the dangers of excessive alcohol intake are well appreciated.

In summary, in the absence of carbohydrate, insulin responses are not affected by alcohol; however, in people with type 2 diabetes, there may be a slightly greater insulin response when a moderate amount of alcohol is taken with carbohydrate. In people with type 1 diabetes, insulin needs are unchanged when alcohol is given with meals.

ALCOHOL AND LIPIDS

Chronic intake of alcohol in light-to-moderate amounts (approximately two to four drinks per day) is associated with a decrease in coronary heart disease, presumably due to the concomitant increase in HDL cholesterol (38–40). HDL is carried in roughly equivalent amounts of a less dense HDL_2 subfraction that is epidemiologically associated with reduced coronary heart disease and a more dense HDL_3 subfraction. Exercise has been found primarily to elevate HDL_2 and decrease HDL_3, whereas alcohol increases HDL_3 and has no significant effect on levels of HDL_2 (41,42). More recently, alcohol consumption has been shown to be associated with increased levels of both HDL_2 and HDL_3, and both subfractions are associated with decreased risk of heart disease (43). However, with alcohol, the difference between daily small-to-moderate amounts and large quantities may be the difference between preventing and causing disease. Heavy alcohol consumption is a leading avoidable cause of death in the U.S. Therefore, exercise rather than alcohol is usually recommended as the preferred means to increase HDL cholesterol levels. It should be noted that few of the studies relating to lipids and alcohol ingestion are performed in people with diabetes. Furthermore, it is not known whether information from short-term alcohol studies can be generalized to long-term moderate alcohol consumption.

Alcohol consumption and diabetes are also associated with hypertriglyceridemia. Alcohol ingestion increases the capacity for lipoprotein synthesis, especially very-low-density lipoprotein (VLDL), which is enhanced by a high-fat diet, particularly in people with diabetes and in those who have a genetic predisposition to lipid abnormalities. In people with severe hypertriglyceridemia, untreated diabetes was found to be the most common cause. Alcohol use was the second most common cause, and obesity was the third most common. The amount of alcohol consumed was in some cases equivalent to moderate social drinking (44). Israelsson (45) reported that >90% of the subjects with triglyceride levels >350 mg/dl (4.0 mmol/l) were obese, were glucose intolerant, or were suspected of consuming high levels of alcohol. Because alcohol has the potential to raise triglycerides, especially in susceptible individuals, ingestion of alcohol should be discouraged in people with hypertriglyceridemia, regardless of whether they do or do not have diabetes.

ALCOHOL AND CALORIES

Whether alcohol intake and body weight are correlated is controversial. The efficiency with which calories from alcohol are used depends on the quantity and frequency of its ingestion. Over long periods of time, excessive alcohol is metabolized predominantly by the MEOS, which leads to increased loss of energy from alcohol as heat. In contrast, when intake is light to moderate, alcohol is metabolized primarily by the ADH, with less waste of energy.

Suter et al. (46) measured the impact of alcohol consumption (25% of subject's caloric requirement) on energy expenditure, substrate oxidation rate, and substrate balance in men consuming normal diets. Carbohydrate and protein oxidation were essentially unaffected by the ingestion of alcohol or by its metabolism, whereas fat oxidation was reduced by ~50%. It appears that alcohol exerts a "lipid sparing" effect when consumed with normal amounts of food. Calories should be counted as if they were provided by dietary fat rather than carbohydrate (47).

In heavy drinkers, food intake is reduced to the point of inducing weight loss, emaciation, and sometimes malnutrition; whereas more moderate amounts of alcohol consumed with the normal diet raise the proportion of dietary energy consumed as fat, which may promote the development of obesity. Diets containing a substantial amount of fat facilitate fat accumulation because of the high caloric density of fatty foods and because one is driven to eat amounts sufficient to maintain stable glycogen levels (48). When increased alcohol intake leads to positive energy balance, accumulation of fat is the consequence. But even for people consuming a normal diet, each ounce of alcohol represents about 0.5 oz of fat (47).

GUIDELINES FOR THE OCCASIONAL USE OF ALCOHOLIC BEVERAGES

For the majority of people with diabetes, occasional ingestion of an alcoholic beverage will have minimal effects on blood glucose or insulin levels. Information regarding the contraindications for the ingestion of alcoholic beverages and guidelines for moderation in drinking should be presented to individuals so that they can make their own decisions (49,50).

People who should abstain from alcohol use include alcohol abusers; individuals with pancreatitis, hypertriglyceridemia, gastritis, frequent hypoglycemic reactions, and certain types of kidney and heart disease; and pregnant women. No one should drink alcohol before driving. In people treated with insulin, alcohol without food can predispose to hypoglycemia, and there is a danger that blood glucose levels can fall several hours after ingestion of alcoholic beverages.

Under normal circumstances and with food, blood glucose levels will not be affected by the moderate use of alcohol when diabetes is well controlled. Table 11.2 lists alcoholic beverages with the percentage and grams of alcohol in an average drink. Individuals should be prepared to follow the intake of alcohol with food or, better yet, to consume alcoholic beverages with or after a meal. For people using insulin, the alcoholic beverages should be considered an addition to the regular meal plan; no food should be omitted, because alcohol does not require insulin to be metabolized and because of the potential danger of hypoglycemia. For people with type 2 diabetes, alcohol calories are best substituted for fat calories or exchanges (1 drink = 2 fat exchanges). However, in reality, it is unusual for individuals to have two extra fat exchanges to substitute for alcohol, so alcohol in all individuals is usually consumed in addition to the regular meal plan.

Meals and snacks should be taken on time and selected with usual care. Alcohol can have a relaxing effect and may dull judgment. Hypoglycemia during the morning after consuming alcohol can be avoided by awakening at the usual time, testing blood glucose levels, and eating a usual breakfast.

Table 11.2 Percentage and Grams of Alcohol in Alcoholic Beverages

	Alcohol %	Average Serving Size (oz/ml)	Alcohol (g) in Average Serving
Distilled spirits (80 proof)	40	1.5/45	14
Beer	3.2–4.5	12/360	13
Wines	9–20 (11.5 ave)	4/112	12
Cocktails	33.4 (ave)	2–4/56–112	18 (ave)
Liqueurs	20–55	1.5/45	13

Ave, average.

The decision to use or not to use alcohol must be made by the individual with diabetes. Individuals should be educated about the effects of alcohol on metabolic parameters if they are to make the best decision for their health and well-being.

REFERENCES

1. Subar AF, Krebs-Smith SM, Cook A, Kahle LL: Dietary sources of nutrients among US adults, 1989 to 1991. *J Am Diet Assoc* 98:537–547, 1998

2. Block G, Dresser CM, Herman AM, Carroll MD: Nutrient sources in the American diet: quantitative data from the NHANES II survey. II. Macronutrients and fats. *Am J Epidemiol* 122:27–40, 1985

3. Braum-Baicker C: The health benefits of moderate alcohol consumption: a review of the literature. *Drug Alcohol Depend* 15:207–227, 1985

4. Lieber CS: Alcohol and the liver: 1994 update. *Gastroenterology* 106:1085–1105, 1994

5. The American Diabetes Association: Nutrition recommendations and principles for people with diabetes (Position Statement). *Diabetes Care* 21(Suppl. 1):S32–S35, 1998

6. U.S. Department of Agriculture, U.S. Department of Health and Human Services: *Nutrition and Your Health: Dietary Guidelines for Americans.* 4th ed. Hyattsville, MD, USDA's Human Nutrition Information Service, 1992

7. Lieber CS: Liver adaptation and injury in alcoholism. *N Engl J Med* 288:356–362, 1973

8. Padova C, Worner TM, Julkunen RJ, Lieber CS: Effects of fasting and chronic alcohol consumption on the first-pass metabolism of ethanol. *Gastroenterology* 92:1169–1173, 1987

9. Isselbacher KJ: Metabolic and hepatic effects of alcohol. *N Engl J Med* 296:612–616, 1977

10. Lefeuve A, Adler H, Lieber CS: Effect of ethanol on ketone metabolism. *J Clin Invest* 49:1775–1782, 1990

11. Lieber CS: Hepatic and metabolic effects of alcohol (1966–1973). *Gastroenterology* 65:821–846, 1973

12. Lieber CS: The metabolism of alcohol. *Sci Am* 234:25–33, 1976

13. Nikkila EA, Taskinen M-R: Ethanol-induced alterations of glucose tolerance, postglucose hypoglycemia and insulin secretion in normal, obese, and diabetic subjects. *Diabetes* 24:933–943, 1975

14. Madison L, Lochner A, Wulff J: Ethanol-induced hypoglycemia: mechanism of suppression of hepatic gluconeogenesis. *Diabetes* 16:252–258, 1967

15. Puhakainen I, Koivisto VA, Yki-Jarvinen H: No reduction in total hepatic glucose output by inhibition of gluconeogenesis with ethanol in NIDDM patients. *Diabetes* 40:1319–1327, 1991

16. Yki-Jarvinen H, Koivisto VA, Ylikahri R, Taskinen M-R: Acute effects of ethanol and acetate on glucose kinetics in normal subjects. *Am J Physiol* 254:E175–E180, 1988

17. Lange J, Arends J, Willms B: Alcohol-induced hypoglycemia in type 1 diabetics. *Med Klin* 86:551–554, 1991

18. Arky RA, Veverbrantd E, Abramson EA: Irreversible hypoglycemia: a complication of alcohol and insulin. *JAMA* 206:575–578, 1968

19. Gin H, Morlat P, Ragnaut JM, Aubertin J: Short-term effect of red wine (consumed during the meals) on insulin requirement and glucose tolerance in diabetic patients. *Diabetes Care* 15:546–548, 1992

20. Koivisto VA, Tulokas S, Toivonen M, Haapa E, Pelkonen R: Alcohol with a meal has no adverse effects on postprandial glucose homeostasis in diabetic patients. *Diabetes Care* 16:1612–1614, 1993

21. Ben G, Gnidi L, Maran A, Gigante A, Duner E, Iori E, Tiengo A, Avogaro A: Effects of chronic alcohol intake on carbohydrate and lipid metabolism in subjects with type II (non-insulin-dependent) diabetes. *Am J Med* 90:70–76, 1991

22. Feingold KR, Siperstein MD: Normalization of fasting blood glucose levels in insulin-requiring diabetes: the role of ethanol abstention. *Diabetes Care* 6:186–188, 1983

23. Freinkel N, Arky RA, Singer DL, Kohen A, Bleicher SJ, Anderson JD, Silbert CK, Foster A: Alcohol hypoglycemia. IV. Current concepts of its pathogenesis. *Diabetes* 14:350–361, 1965

24. Marks V: Alcohol and CHO metabolism. *Clin Endocrinol Metab* 7:333–349, 1978

25. Kerr D, Macdonald IA, Heller SR, Tattersall RB: Alcohol causes hypoglycaemic unawareness in healthy volunteers and patients with type 1 (insulin-dependent) diabetes. *Diabetologia* 33:216–221, 1990

26. Puhakainen I, Koivisto VA, Yki-Jarvinen H: No reduction in total hepatic glucose output by inhibition of gluconeogenesis with ethanol in NIDDM patients. *Diabetes* 40:1319–1327, 1991

27. Walsh CH, O'Sullivan DJ: Effect of moderate alcohol intake on control of diabetes. *Diabetes* 23:440–442, 1974

28. McMonagle J, Felig P: Effects of ethanol ingestion on glucose tolerance and insulin secretion in normal and diabetic subjects. *Metabolism* 24:625–632, 1975

29. Avogaro A, Duner E, Marescotti C, Ferrara D, Del Prato S, Nosadini R, Tiengo A: Metabolic effects of moderate alcohol intake with meals in insulin-dependent diabetics controlled by artificial endocrine pancreas (AEP) and in normal subjects. *Metabolism* 32:463–469, 1983

30. Singh SP, Kumar Y, Snyder AK, Ellyin FE, Gilden JL: Effect of alcohol on glucose tolerance in normal and noninsulin-dependent diabetic subjects. *Alcohol Clin Exp Res* 12:727–730, 1988

31. Spraul M, Chantelau E, Schonbach A-M, Berger M: Glycemic effects of beer in IDDM patients: studies with constant insulin delivery. *Diabetes Care* 11:659–661, 1988

32. Menzel R, Mentel DC, Brunstein U, Heinke P: Effect of moderate ethanol ingestion on overnight diabetes control and hormone secretion in type I diabetic patients (Abstract). *Diabetologia* 34:A188, 1991

33. Christiansen C, Thomsen C, Rasmussen O, Balle M, Hauerslev C, Hansen C, Hermansen K: Wine for type 2 diabetic patients? *Diabetic Med* 10:958–961, 1993

34. Shah J: Alcohol decreases insulin sensitivity in healthy subjects. *Alcohol* 23:103–109, 1988

35. Avogaro A, Fontana P, Valerio A, Trevisan R, Riccio A, Del Prato S, Nosadini R, Tiengo A, Crepaldi G: Alcohol impairs insulin sensitivity in normal subjects. *Diabetes Res* 5:23–27, 1987

36. Lazarus R, Sparrow D, Weiss ST: Alcohol intake and insulin levels. *Am J Epidemiol* 145:909–916, 1997

37. Facchini F, Ida Chen Y-D, Reaven GM: Light-to-moderate alcohol intake is associated with enhanced insulin sensitivity. *Diabetes Care* 17:115–119, 1994

38. Steinberg D, Pearson TA, Kuller LH: Alcohol and atherosclerosis. *Ann Intern Med* 114:967–976, 1991

39. Suh I, Shaten BJ, Cutler JA, Kuller LH: Alcohol use and mortality from coronary heart disease: the role of high-density lipoprotein cholesterol. *Ann Intern Med* 116:881–887, 1992

40. Burr ML, Fehily AM, Butland BK, Bolton CH, Eastham RD: Alcohol and high-density lipoprotein cholesterol: a randomized controlled trial. *Br J Nutr* 56:81–86, 1986

41. Haskell WL, Camargo C, Williams PT, Uranizam KM, Krauss RM, Lindgren FT, Wood PW: The effect of cessation and resumption of moderate alcohol intake on serum high-density-lipoprotein subfractions. *N Engl J Med* 310:805–810, 1984

42. Hartung GH, Foreyt JP, Mitchell RE, Mitchell JG, Revver RS, Grotto AM: Effects of alcohol intake on high-density lipoprotein cholesterol levels in runners and in active men. *JAMA* 249:747–750, 1983

43. Gaziano JM, Buring JE, Breslow JL, Goldhaber SZ, Rosner B, VanDenburgh M, Willett W, Hennekens CH: Moderate alcohol intake, increased levels of high-density lipoprotein and its subfractions, and decreased risk of myocardial infarction. *N Engl J Med* 329:1829–1834, 1993

44. Chait A, Brunzell JD: Severe triglyceridemia: role of familial and acquired disorder. *Metabolism* 32:209–213, 1983

45. Israelsson B: Role of alcohol, glucose intolerance and obesity in hypertriglyceridemia. *Atherosclerosis* 62:123–127, 1986

46. Suter PM, Schuta Y, Jequier E: The effect of ethanol on fat storage in healthy subjects. *N Engl J Med* 326:983–987, 1992

47. Flatt JP: Body weight, fat storage, and alcohol metabolism. *Nutrition Rev* 50:267–270, 1992

48. Flatt JP: Importance of nutrient balance in body weight regulation. *Diabetes Metab Rev* 49:33–45, 1991

49. Franz MJ: Alcohol and diabetes. I. Metabolism and guidelines. *Diabetes Spectrum* 3:136–144, 1990

50. Franz MJ: Alcohol and diabetes. II. Its metabolism and guidelines for occasional use. *Diabetes Spectrum* 3:210–216, 1990

Ms. Franz is Director of Nutrition and Professional Education at the International Diabetes Center, Institute for Research and Education, HealthSystem Minnesota, Minneapolis, MN.

Nutrition Issues
of Special Populations

12. Nutrition Therapy for Children and Adolescents with Diabetes

ANGELA R. SHARP, MPH, RD, CDE

Highlights

- A major goal is ensuring adequate calories for normal growth and development in children and adolescents with type 1 diabetes. Height and weight should be recorded on growth charts every 3–6 months, and the meal plan should be evaluated and adjusted to provide sufficient calories and nutrients for proper growth.
- A variety of meal planning approaches can be used for children and adolescents with diabetes.
- Nutrition self-management education must be provided to children, adolescents, and their families over a period of time and in a continual process. Initial education on meal planning for diabetes should take place within the first 1–2 weeks following diagnosis. In-depth education should provide more detailed information and flexibility for planning meals and snacks. Continued in-depth and ongoing education is essential because of the continual lifestyle changes that children and adolescents experience.

INTRODUCTION

Medical nutrition therapy (MNT) for children and adolescents with diabetes has been enhanced by a variety of factors that have guided practitioners toward a more flexible approach to helping patients manage diabetes. Important advances in pediatric diabetes nutrition management include development of nutrition recommendations (1,2) and of nutrition practice guidelines for type 1 diabetes (3), results of the Diabetes Control and Complications Trial (DCCT) (4), and pharmacological improvements.

The American Diabetes Association (ADA) nutrition recommendations for the treatment of type 1 diabetes provide practical guidance to diabetes nutrition practitioners and a solid framework of nutrition care for their pediatric patients. Most recently, the Diabetes Care and Education Practice Group of The American Dietetic Association has developed a set of nutrition practice guidelines for type 1 diabetes that help to formulate a logical and sequential plan of nutrition care to improve metabolic control in patients with diabetes. The much-anticipated results of the DCCT uncovered important information about the prevention of diabetes-related complications and the acute risks of intensive diabetes management that could be applied to pediatric patients in a clinical setting. The DCCT also offered new insights into the use of flexible meal planning strategies such as carbohydrate counting. Recent advances in the pharmacological treatment of diabetes, namely the development of lispro insulin (5,6), have opened a new chapter in diabetes management by offering a more physiological, rapid-acting insulin that can be combined with other insulins and matched to unconventional meal plans.

GOALS OF MEDICAL NUTRITION THERAPY IN CHILDREN AND ADOLESCENTS

The ADA goals for MNT are a standard reference for nutrition care and a primary component for use in developing a nutrition care plan for children and adolescents with type 1 diabetes (Table 12.1). While the nutrition goals are a reference point for care, the specific nutrition and health needs of individual pediatric patients should be considered when formulating the actual nutrition care plan. Nutrition care goals

---

Table 12.1 Goals of Medical Nutrition Therapy for Children and Adolescents with Diabetes

1. Maintenance of near-normal blood glucose levels by balancing food intake with insulin and activity levels.
2. Achievement of optimal lipid levels.
3. Provision of adequate calories for normal growth and development.
4. Prevention, delay, or treatment of nutrition-related risk factors and complications.
5. Improvement of overall health through optimal nutrition.

From Holzmeister LA: Medical nutrition therapy for children and adolescents with diabetes. *Diabetes Spectrum* 10:268–274, 1997.

developed for the pediatric population should be updated regularly to accommodate normal stages of growth and development in children and adolescents.

Maintaining normal blood glucose control is a primary treatment goal in children with diabetes. The DCCT documented a 47–76% reduction in the incidence of long-term complications in patients who were taught intensive management of their disease (4). While the DCCT study population comprised primarily adults, adolescents made up a percentage of the study cohort (~15%, ranging from 13 to 17 years of age at entry). Adolescents in the DCCT were found to have similar improvements in blood glucose control and a reduced risk of complications when compared with adult participants. Despite their improved glycemic control, however, the adolescents did prove more difficult to manage, gain more weight, have a higher incidence of hypoglycemia, and have higher blood glucose values overall as compared with the adult cohort (7). Along with the DCCT, other studies have documented a complication-reducing effect of intensive diabetes management in adolescents, including a reduction in microvascular complications (8). Barriers to the application of the DCCT in children have been identified, including the need for trained staff in a multidisciplinary practice setting and the existence of family-centered psychosocial difficulties that hinder the achievement of glycemic goals (9).

While blood glucose control is an important clinical goal in managing diabetes, care must be taken to prevent hypoglycemic events in young children, who are at risk of impaired brain development resulting from multiple hypoglycemic episodes (10,11). Glycemic goals for young children are generally less stringent than those for older children and adolescents, and intensive blood glucose management is not recommended for children under the age of 13 (12). Parents of very young children with diabetes should be cautioned about the potential effects of hypoglycemia on the growing brain, and glycemic goals should be reviewed regularly to reinforce compliance.

There is conflict in the literature regarding the protective effect of age against microvascular complications in diabetes. It has been suggested that children may be afforded some degree of protection from complications in diabetes (13); however, recent studies have shown that children and adolescents with diabetes demonstrate a rate of microvascular complications similar to that in an adult study population (13,14).

Diabetes is a major risk factor for the development of cardiovascular disease (CVD). Children and adolescents with diabetes appear to be at greater risk for developing CVD than are their matched nondiabetic counterparts (15). Maintaining normal blood lipid levels in children with diabetes is therefore an important and necessary goal in preventing cardiovascular complications.

Lipid management in children and adolescents with diabetes should begin with achievement of glycemic goals. Children and adolescents in groups at high risk for developing lipid abnormalities, including those with a family history of lipid abnormalities or CVD, should be screened and monitored according to guidelines issued by the National Cholesterol Education Program (NCEP) Report of the Expert Panel on Blood Cholesterol Levels in Children and Adolescents (16) and the American Academy of Pediatrics (17) (Table 12.2). A stepwise approach to the dietary management of lipid abnormalities suggested by the NCEP and the American Heart Association (18) recommends a reduction in total fat, saturated fat, and cholesterol for children over the age of 2 years.

Provision of adequate calories for normal growth and development in children and adolescents with diabetes is a key component of MNT. Children and adolescents with diabetes generally grow 5–10% below normal standards as a result of poor glycemic control or other factors (19). Therefore, it is important to monitor pediatric growth by measuring height and weight every 3–6 months and recording it on a National Center for Health Statistics growth chart (20).

Caloric requirements for children with diabetes can be calculated using a number of different formulas (Table 12.3). Children do, however, appear to have the inherent ability to select appropriate amounts and types of food to sustain normal growth. Often, the most accurate predictor of a child's calorie and nutrient need is based on a history of usual food intake, providing that growth and development are within normal limits (21). Population-based nutrition guidelines, such as the Recommended Dietary Allowances, tend to overestimate actual calorie needs in children and adolescents and may be less beneficial for determining specific calorie requirements (22). Nutrition assessment tools such as 24-h recall, 3-day food records, and food frequency questionnaires can be used in conjunction with a computer nutrient analysis program to determine usual nutrient intake.

Once calorie and nutrient needs are established, they can be adjusted to accommodate growth or prevent accelerated weight gain. At the time of

---

Table 12.2 Classification of Total and LDL Cholesterol Levels in Children and Adolescents from Families with Hypercholesterolemia or Premature Cardiovascular Disease

Category	Total Cholesterol (mg/dl)	LDL Cholesterol (mg/dl)
Acceptable	<170	<110
Borderline	170–199	110–129
High	>200	>130

From the National Cholesterol Education Program (16).

Table 12.3　Estimating Caloric Requirements for Youth

- Base calories on nutrition assessment
- Validate caloric needs
  - –Method 1: 1,000 kcal for 1st year
    Add 100 kcal/year up to age 11
    Girls 11–15 years, add 100 kcal or less/year
    Girls >15 years, calculate as an adult
    Boys 11–15 years, add 200 kcal/year
    Boys >15 years, 23 kcal/lb (50 kcal/kg) very active, 18 kcal/lb
    　(40 kcal/kg) usual, 15–16 kcal/lb (30–35 kcal/kg) sedentary
  - –Method 2: 1,000 kcal for 1st year
    Add 125 kcal × age for boys
    Add 100 kcal × age for girls
    Add up to 20% more kcal for activity
- For toddlers between 1 and 3 years, 40 kcal per inch length

From the American Diabetes Association (21).

diagnosis, children or adolescents with diabetes usually require additional calories to promote catch-up growth. Children with intensively managed diabetes generally gain more weight than do children on conventional insulin regimens, secondary to improved glycemic control and utilization of nutrients (4). Preventing weight gain in an intensively managed pediatric population is accomplished by carefully monitoring growth, especially rate of weight gain, with nutrition intervention as needed. Children and adolescents, along with their families, should be taught meal planning basics to prevent excess weight gain. Regular physical activity should be encouraged, and children should be taught the proper treatment of hypoglycemia to prevent excess calorie intake and weight gain.

Childhood obesity and parental history of diabetes appear to play a major role in the development of type 2 diabetes in children and adolescents (23). Type 2 diabetes is believed to account for 2–3% of diabetes cases in the pediatric population, with a greater prevalence seen in children belonging to high-risk ethnic groups. Similar mechanisms related to insulin resistance and the failure of the pancreas to produce adequate compensatory insulin seem to occur in children who develop type 2 diabetes.

Therapeutic options for the treatment of type 2 diabetes in children and adolescents include diet and exercise, oral hypoglycemic agents, and insulin. Unfortunately, weight control through diet and exercise is generally not a successful option in pediatric patients, and pharmacological treatment must be considered. There is little information on the use of oral hypoglycemic agents in the pediatric population, and insulin therapy is often the treatment of choice for managing blood glucose levels.

Preventing or delaying type 2 diabetes in children and adolescents may be accomplished by encouraging lifestyle modifications that promote weight management and regular physical activity. Screening children from high-risk ethnic populations or with a strong family history of diabetes has also been suggested.

Preventing acute and chronic diabetes complications with MNT in children and adolescents is an important diabetes management goal. Children and adolescents and their families should be taught the proper treatment of hypoglycemia. A general recommendation for the treatment of a hypoglycemic episode in children is the consumption of 15 g of carbohydrate, preferably in the form of a glucose tablet, although any readily available carbohydrate source will suffice in an emergency. There is no evidence to suggest that carbohydrate used to treat hypoglycemia should be combined with protein to enhance recovery (24). Blood glucose should be retested 15 min after treatment with carbohydrate, and an additional 15 g carbohydrate should be given as needed until blood glucose returns to the target range.

In the event that hypoglycemia does occur, it is important that children and their families be aware of the proper method of treatment. It is also important to teach concepts related to the prevention of future hypoglycemic episodes. Hypoglycemic episodes can be avoided by teaching children and families the proper management of diet, including consumption of regular, consistent meals and snacks with a balance of nutrients, including carbohydrate. Children and adolescents should be taught to carry a source of carbohydrate with them at all times, and this principle should be reinforced regularly. Principles of blood glucose management during acute illness, including use of well-tolerated carbohydrate sources in place of usual choices, should be taught at the time of diabetes diagnosis.

Basic nutrition principles can be taught to children and families using a variety of resources. The individual meal plan is an excellent starting point for teaching basic concepts of variety, portion control, and lower fat and moderate fiber content. Children should consume approximately their age plus 5 g of fiber per day, according to recent guidelines (25). Other resources that are helpful for teaching basic concepts of nutrition include the USDA Food Guide Pyramid, the guidelines for the National Cancer Institute Five a Day Program, and nutrition information from the National Dairy Council. The Internet is fast becoming a nutrition information channel for children and adolescents with diabetes and includes a variety of excellent interactive sites on topics related to nutrition and diabetes care.

INTERVENTION AND TREATMENT

Meal Planning Approaches

An individualized food plan is an excellent tool for implementing basic nutrition guidelines and meeting specific goals related to diabetes care in children and adolescents. The DCCT clearly indicated that the food plan was a necessary component of diabetes management to help patients achieve glycemic goals (26). It is important to teach children and adolescents the basic concepts and rationale for food planning early in diagnosis and to review and reinforce the concepts regularly to improve adherence. The basic concepts of a food plan should be taught to young children in a developmentally appropriate manner, with specific details given to parents, other family members, and caretakers. Older children and adolescents are often capable of understanding the basics of a meal plan, but require parental support and guidance for adherence.

A variety of approaches to meal planning exist and can be implemented successfully with children and adolescents. Widely used methods for meal planning include carbohydrate counting, the exchange system, and simplified meal planning guidelines. To promote adherence, the method chosen should be based on individual needs and level of understanding (27).

Carbohydrate counting. Carbohydrate counting is a meal planning method based on the principle that all types of carbohydrate (except fiber) are digested, the majority being absorbed into the bloodstream as molecules of glucose, and that the total amount of carbohydrate consumed has a greater effect on blood glucose elevations than does the specific type consumed. Children and families are taught that glucose requires insulin for entry into cells and that short-acting bolus doses of insulin are "matched" to the usual amount of carbohydrate consumed at meals. Principles of portion control and consistent intake of carbohydrate at meals and snacks are taught for blood glucose control. Children are taught to identify carbohydrate in foods by using exchange lists and by reading labels.

A carbohydrate-counting meal plan is developed according to the usual amount of carbohydrate children and adolescents consume at meals and snacks, which can vary according to age, level of activity, and usual eating patterns. Meal patterns are never predetermined, but are instead based on individual intake, which can vary widely among children and adolescents. Specific calorie levels are generally not recommended as long as growth is appropriate. General rather than specific guidelines for intake of foods that do not contain carbohydrate, including meats and meat substitutes, nonstarchy vegetables, and fats, are provided. Care should be taken to ensure that children and adolescents on carbohydrate-counting meal plans balance their intake with a variety of foods from all food groups to ensure a nutritionally adequate diet.

Carbohydrate counting is a relatively simple meal planning method that is easy to teach. It is generally well-accepted by children and adolescents with diabetes and their families. The concept that "all foods can fit" into a carbohydrate-counting meal plan should be taught and reinforced regularly. This is accomplished easily by teaching label reading and by providing resources on the carbohydrate content of favorite foods, including snacks and fast food.

Individual carbohydrate-counting meal plans are often age-dependent. Toddlers and young children often consume variable amounts of food because of rapid changes in growth that result in an unpredictable appetite. Toddlers and young children typically follow a "grazing" meal and snack schedule, consuming smaller amounts of food more frequently throughout the day. Older children and preadolescents tend to eat more consistent amounts at the same time each day because of school schedules and more predictable appetites. Older children typically eat three meals and at least two or three snacks each day. Adolescents often eat at inconsistent times, and the amount of carbohydrate they consume is often quite variable. They are more prone to skipping meals and snacks, especially the morning snack, because of school and work schedules.

Other meal planning methods. The *Exchange Lists for Meal Planning* (28), developed jointly by The American Dietetic Association and the ADA, is a standard meal planning reference for children and adolescents with diabetes. The exchange lists were recently expanded and updated to reflect the trend toward carbohydrate management for blood glucose control. Use of the exchange system allows for the development of a more specific meal plan based on calories and macronutrients and is especially helpful for use in formulating a meal plan based on specific nutrition needs in addition to glycemic control.

Carbohydrate-counting and exchange meal planning tools use a similar system to identify carbohydrate-containing foods and portion sizes and may be used interchangeably. As a result, children and adolescents who have been instructed on the exchange system usually have little difficulty converting to a carbohydrate-counting meal plan and often enjoy the resulting flexibility.

Simplified meal planning guidelines that provide basic information on the effect of carbohydrate on blood glucose levels and information on sources of carbohydrate can be used in place of more specific meal planning methods. Nutrition education materials that are specific to different cultures and languages are also helpful for teaching meal planning concepts.

Physical Activity

Physical activity generally reduces insulin requirements in children and adolescents with diabetes. Hypoglycemia that may occur in the presence of physical activity can be managed by an increase in carbohydrate consumption or a reduction in exogenous insulin. A general rule of thumb for the prevention of hypoglycemia caused by activity is the addition of 15 g of carbohydrate per hour of activity (29). Very young children may require only one-half of that amount. Additional carbohydrate can be added to the meal or snack that precedes activity, or it may be consumed during the activity itself. Additional carbohydrate may need to be added to postexercise meals and snacks to prevent delayed hypoglycemia (30).

For children and adolescents who require a reduction in insulin to prevent hypoglycemia during exercise, the general recommendation is to reduce the short- or rapid-acting insulin present during the time of activity by 1–2 U, depending on the initial insulin dose and type of activity. Long-lasting events usually require an adjustment in both the short and long-acting doses of insulin (31). It is generally suggested that children consume carbohydrate for activity rather than make an insulin adjustment because the additional calories enhance growth and because food adjustments afford greater predictability in blood glucose control.

Usual levels of physical activity in children and adolescents with diabetes should be taken into account when developing a meal plan, and food adjustments for additional activity should be taught at diagnosis and reviewed regularly. Physically active children and adolescents generally consume appropriate amounts of carbohydrate to fuel activity, and extra carbohydrate consumed for activity is usually reflected in the meal plan. Children who are sedentary or sporadically active may not consume adequate carbohydrate for additional physical activity and may require carbohydrate additions to their meal plan.

Hyperglycemia may occur with physical activity. Hyperglycemia in children and adolescents with diabetes is generally associated with an insulin deficiency, resulting from an improper insulin regimen or a missed injection. It may also be seen in very active children who experience increased levels of stress hormones, including adrenaline, which promote glycolysis. Hyperglycemia in exercise is often difficult to manage because of its unpredictability. Children and adolescents who experience stress-induced hyperglycemia before exercise may not require the addition of carbohydrate before exercise, but they may require additional postexercise carbohydrate, such as a larger supper or bedtime snack, to prevent delayed hypoglycemia.

Children and adolescents participate in a variety of activities that should be considered when developing the individual meal plan. Toddlers and young children are often intermittently active throughout the day, usually in the form of play. The meal plan for a toddler should support activity with small, frequent feedings to prevent hypoglycemia. As children grow, they are more likely to participate in organized sports. Young children often consume regularly planned meals and snacks during the day. Additional carbohydrate may be offered at the usual meal or snack preceding the planned activity. Older children and preadolescents are often active in organized activity and physical education class during the school day. Again, carbohydrate adjustments can be made to the usual meal plan to account for the additional activity.

Children and adolescents with diabetes should be encouraged to be active and participate in sports and other organized activities for health and social benefits. Children in the U.S. watch excessive amounts of television, which decreases the opportunity for vigorous exercise (32). Physical activity may have a lipid-lowering effect in adolescents with diabetes, which is beneficial for the prevention of CVD (33). Children and adolescents with diabetes should be encouraged to consume an adequate amount of fluid before, during, and after activity to prevent dehydration. A general guideline for the consumption of fluids is 4–8 oz before activity, at least 4 oz every 15 min during activity, and liberal fluid intake after activity to replace losses (34). Children with diabetes may consume carbohydrate-containing fluids, such as diluted fruit juices or commercial sport drinks, for fluid and carbohydrate replacement during activity.

Insulin Regimens

The variety of insulin regimens available for children and adolescents with diabetes can be as individual as the children themselves and is limited only by the creativity of the practitioner. Children and adolescents are often instructed on a conventional insulin regimen at the time of diagnosis, but they may be switched to more intensive therapy or multiple daily injections (MDIs), depending on blood glucose values.

An important development in insulin pharmacology was the creation of lispro insulin, a human insulin analog with physiological properties similar to endogenous insulin produced and secreted by the pancreas. Lispro is rapidly absorbed into the bloodstream and acts quickly to decrease postprandial blood glucose. Because of its rapid action, lispro must be injected at the time of meal consumption to prevent hypoglycemia.

Lispro is useful when developing insulin-to-carbohydrate ratios for increased flexibility in meal planning. Generally, a ratio of 1 U insulin per 15–20 g carbohydrate has been suggested; however, in children and adolescents, this ratio often varies with age and activity level as well as meal composition and timing (35). Young children often require a smaller dose of insulin in relation to carbohydrate consumed, while insulin-resistant adolescents may require more, often as much as 2 U insulin for every

15 g carbohydrate. A carbohydrate-to-insulin ratio is easily determined by measuring preprandial and 2-h postprandial blood glucose levels and comparing them. Lispro seems to exhibit greater efficacy when used in conjunction with a meal that contains a high percentage of carbohydrate in relation to other nutrients, such as fat (36).

The insulin pump (continuous subcutaneous insulin infusion [CSII]) provides another treatment option for intensive management of blood glucose in children and adolescents. However, there are a number of barriers that may limit blood glucose control, and the decision to institute pump use in this population must be carefully considered (37). Children and adolescents interested in diabetes management with CSII should be reminded that insulin pump technology is based on a single-loop feed-back mechanism. An insulin pump cannot detect blood glucose fluc-tuations throughout the day or in response to a meal. Children and adolescents on the pump must take responsibility for the additional blood glucose testing and carbohydrate counting that is required to achieve optimal blood glucose control. Families interested in blood glucose man-agement with an insulin pump must weigh the costs and benefits of CSII with those of MDI because it appears that there may be no additional benefit in terms of overall blood glucose control (38).

NUTRITION EDUCATION TOPICS

MNT for children and adolescents with diabetes encompasses a variety of education topics that can be discussed at the time of diagnosis or as part of the continuing education process. It is helpful to categorize the edu-cation process into a logical sequence to ensure that all pertinent areas are covered and to avoid overwhelming families with an abundance of infor-mation (39). Initial nutrition education strategies, such as the formulation of a meal plan, can focus on basic survival skills necessary for diabetes management. Ongoing nutrition education strategies can offer greater detail and specific information on pertinent nutrition topics.

Initial Education

Nutrition education topics addressed at diabetes diagnosis should focus on food components that influence blood glucose levels, and a meal plan should be established. Emphasis should be placed on the identifica-tion of carbohydrate-containing foods using exchange lists and food labels, and the concept of meal timing and consistent carbohydrate intake for insulin synchronization should be discussed. Special dietary needs such as food allergies, lactose intolerance, and gluten sensitivity should be incorporated into the meal plan, and vegetarian diets or cultural diet con-cerns can be addressed. Prevention and treatment of hypoglycemia with carbohydrate and sources of carbohydrate for use during illness should also be discussed. Physical activity and diabetes management should be addressed.

In-Depth Nutrition Education

Diabetes nutrition topics that can be addressed as part of the in-depth education process include monitoring and discussion of growth and weight gain, including poor growth or excess weight gain. The meal plan should be reviewed and modified based on schedule or appetite changes resulting from increased growth. The current insulin regimen should be noted in relation to the present meal plan and activity level, and appropriate changes should be made to the insulin regimen as required. Use of results of blood glucose monitoring to develop carbohydrate-to-insulin ratios can be addressed. Special occasions, such as birthday parties, holidays, and dining out, can be taken into account for increased flexibility in meal planning. Guidelines for travel should be addressed. Basic guidelines for making healthy food choices can be offered using a variety of general health resources. Topics such as the use of sugar and fat replacers, nutrition supplements, and alcohol are additional points for discussion (21).

Continuing Nutrition Education Topics

Continuing diabetes education should be an ongoing process that provides an opportunity for monitoring growth and weight gain, making meal plan adjustments, and problem solving in areas of concern related to nutrition and diabetes management. Discussion of special events, holidays, and schedule changes provides children and adolescents a sense of confidence for making decisions. Encouraging independence in making food choices and insulin adjustments is important for developing mastery of self-management principles. Troubleshooting issues related to sports and physical activity and continuing to encourage a healthy, active lifestyle are important.

Age Components of Nutrition Education

The challenges of nutrition education for children and adolescents with diabetes are often age-related and require consideration of the specific nutrition and development needs of different age-groups. The defining characteristics of different age-groups must be considered when providing nutrition care to children and adolescents.

Toddlers. Managing the daily variation in eating patterns of toddlers with diabetes is often a challenge to both parents and health care providers.

Inconsistency in meal timing and amount of food consumed is common as independence gains momentum and the rapid growth of infancy declines. Typical patterns of intake are uncommon in toddlers with diabetes, making blood glucose control difficult. Toddlers usually prefer to graze, eating small, frequent meals throughout the day. They are more prone to food jags and selective eating, often resulting in battles with parents. Meal plans for toddlers should be based on usual intake and age-appropriate portions of food. A schedule of regular meals and snacks containing carbohydrate should be offered throughout the day to fuel sporadic activity and prevent hypoglycemia. Suggestions should be given for alternate sources of carbohydrate in the event that food refusal does occur. Daycare providers and others involved in the care of toddlers with diabetes should be instructed on the basics of meal planning and prevention and treatment of hypoglycemia. Parents of toddlers with diabetes must be instructed to avoid withholding food in cases of hyperglycemia.

Preschool and school-aged children. Preschool and school-aged children usually follow a more consistent meal plan. Growth is also more consistent, resulting in greater appetite and intake predictability. Older children usually enjoy taking an active role in food preparation and meal planning and should be encouraged to do so.

Preschool and school-aged children generally eat consistent amounts of carbohydrate at the same time each day. They usually prefer to eat three meals and snacks between meals. A morning snack is common during the school day, and afternoon snacks are also favored. Older children may begin to consume more meals and snacks away from home, with birthday or overnight parties becoming more common. Parents of older children should be instructed on the management of diabetes during special occasions, with guidelines given for insulin or food adjustments to prevent hypoglycemia.

Older children often begin to participate in organized sports and activities, and participation in physical education class at school is common. The meal plan should be reviewed on a regular basis to ensure that meals and snacks correspond to the usual activity patterns, and recommendations for increasing food for activity should be reinforced regularly.

Adolescents. Adolescents with diabetes often have variable meal schedules because of work, school, and other activities and responsibilities. They are responsible for their food choices and usually have decided whether or not to follow a meal plan, with mismanagement of the meal plan a common occurrence (40). Peer influence regarding food choices is common and can have an impact on meal plan adherence.

Common concerns related to meal planning in adolescence include general inconsistency relative to meal timing, meal frequency, and amount of carbohydrate consumed. Issues of growth and variable appetite and intake related to growth spurts in early adolescence are common, only to be replaced with slowed growth and concerns with weight gain in late adolescence. Conventional insulin regimens often are not practical for adolescents; however, it is often difficult to convince them of the need for MDIs to better manage blood glucose levels.

Sports and other physical activities often play a central role in the lives of adolescents, and an assessment of involvement in activity should be conducted on a regular basis, with appropriate adjustments in insulin regimen and meal plan suggested. Suggestions for snacks and foods to use to supplement activity should be made. Sports-minded adolescents may inquire about sports nutrition supplements to promote weight gain and can be instructed on alternative choices. Adolescents who are very active are usually on smaller doses of insulin or can be instructed on insulin adjustments for activities of long duration.

Body image and weight management concerns in adolescent females with diabetes are of particular concern. Disordered eating habits and weight control behaviors are common in adolescent girls with type 1 diabetes (41) and occur more frequently than in matched nondiabetic control subjects (42). Adolescents with diabetes should be screened regularly for insulin omission and eating disorders to prevent the serious medical consequences of very poor glycemic control. Warning signs that may be indicative of an eating disorder in adolescents include lack of adequate weight gain or growth, significant weight loss without illness, and erratic blood glucose levels with suboptimal overall glycemic control (43).

Other issues of concern in adolescents with diabetes include the potential use of alcohol. Adolescents must be instructed on the potential hypoglycemic effects of alcohol and on responsible drinking should they choose to use alcohol. Adolescents who drive should be instructed on blood glucose monitoring before driving and carrying a source of carbohydrate with them at all times in case hypoglycemia should occur. Finally, adolescents with diabetes may experiment with alternative eating patterns, such as a vegetarian diet, or they may choose to use nutritional supplements. Practical information on these topics will enable adolescents to make wise choices for their health.

SUMMARY

Children and adolescents with diabetes often present diabetes management challenges not commonly seen in the adult population. Optimal blood glucose management in the pediatric population should rely on the use of basic diabetes care guidelines that have been individualized to meet age- or development-specific needs. Basic diabetes and nutrition care guidelines offer a framework of care, but they must be individualized to meet the constantly changing needs of children and adolescents. Dietitians must take a big-picture approach to diabetes management when working with children and adolescents. The constantly changing growth, developmental, and social needs of children and adolescents with diabetes require a dynamic, flexible plan of care that provides optimal blood glucose control but does not restrict the joy of childhood.

REFERENCES

1. Franz MJ, Horton ES, Bantle JP, Beebe CA, Brunzell JD, Coulston AM, Henry RR, Hoogwerf BJ, Stacpool PW: Nutrition principles for the management of diabetes and related complications. *Diabetes Care* 17:490–518, 1994

2. American Diabetes Association: Nutrition recommendations and principles for people with diabetes (Position Statement). *Diabetes Care* 21 (Suppl. 1):S32–S35, 1998

3. Kulkarni KD, Castle G, Gregory R, Holmes A, Leontos C, Powers MA, Snetselaar L, Splett PL, Wylie-Rosett J: Nutrition practice guidelines for type 1 diabetes: an overview of the content and application. *Diabetes Spectrum* 10:248–256, 1997

4. The DCCT Research Group: The effect of intensive treatment of diabetes on the development and progression of long-term complications in insulin-dependent diabetes mellitus. *N Engl J Med* 329:977–986, 1993

5. Pamponelli S, Torlone E, Ialli C, DelSindaco P, Ciofetta M, Lepore M, Bartocci L, Brunetti P, Bolli CB: Improved postprandial metabolic control after subcutaneous insulin injection of a short-acting insulin analog in IDDM of short duration with residual β-cell function. *Diabetes Care* 18:1452–1459, 1995

6. Heinemann L, Heise T, Wohl L, Trentmann ME, Ampudin J, Starke AAR, Berger M: Prandial glycemia after a carbohydrate-rich meal in type 1 diabetic patients using the rapid acting insulin analogue [Lys (B28), Pro(B29)] human insulin. *Diabetic Med* 13: 625–629, 1996

7. Drash J: The child, adolescent and the Diabetes Control and Complications Trial (Editorial). *Diabetes Care* 16:1515–1516 , 1993

8. Danne T, Weber B, Reinhard H, Enders I, Burger W, Hovener G: Long-term glycemic control has a nonlinear association to the frequency of background retinopathy in adolescents with diabetes: follow-up of the Berlin retinopathy study. *Diabetes Care* 17:1390–1396, 1994

9. Brink SJ, Moltz K: The message of the DCCT for children and adolescents. *Diabetes Spectrum* 10:259–267, 1997

10. Ryan C, Vega A, Drash A: Cognitive deficits in adolescents who developed diabetes early in life. *Pediatrics* 75:921–927, 1985

11. Rovet JF, Ehrlich RM, Hoppe M: Intellectual deficits associated with early onset of insulin-dependent diabetes mellitus in children. *Diabetes Care* 10:510–515, 1987

12. Malone JI: Lessons for pediatricians from the Diabetes Control and Complications Trial. *Pediatr Ann* 23:295–299, 1994

13. Kostraba JN, Dorman JS, Orchard TJ, Becker DJ, Ohki Y, Ellis D, Dott BH, Lobes LA, LaPorte RE, Drash AL: Contribution of diabetes duration before puberty of development of microvascular complications in IDDM subjects. *Diabetes Care* 12:686–692, 1989

14. Donaghue KC, Fung ATW, Hing S, Fairchild J, King J, Chan A, Howard NJ, Silink M: The effect of prepubertal diabetes duration on diabetes. *Diabetes Care* 20:77–80, 1997

15. Brink SJ: Pediatric and adolescent nutrition issues. In *Pediatric and Adolescent Diabetes Mellitus*. Brink SJ, Ed. Chicago, Year Book, 1987, pp. 284–291

16. National Cholesterol Education Program: *Report of the Expert Panel on Blood Cholesterol Levels in Children and Adolescents*. Bethesda, MD, U.S. Department of Health and Human Services, 1991 (National Heart, Lung and Blood Institute publ. no. 91-2732)

17. American Academy of Pediatrics. Statement on cholesterol. *Pediatrics* 90:469–473, 1992

18. American Heart Association Nutrition Committee: Rationale of the diet-heart statement of the American Heart Association: report of the Nutrition Committee. *Circulation* 88:3008–3029, 1993

19. Wise JE, Kolb EL, Sauder SE: Effect of glycemic control on growth velocity in children with insulin-dependent diabetes mellitus. *Diabetes Care* 15:826–830, 1992

20. Hamill PVV, Drizd RA, Johnson CL, Reed RB, Roche AF, Moore WM: Physical growth: National Center for Health Statistics percentiles. *Am J Clin Nutr* 32:607–629, 1979

21. American Diabetes Association: *Maximizing the Role of Nutrition in Diabetes Management*. Alexandria, VA, American Diabetes Association, 1995

22. World Health Organization: *Energy and Protein Requirements*. Geneva, World Health Org., 1985 (Tech. Rep. Ser., no. 724)

23. Glaser NS: Non-insulin dependent diabetes mellitus in childhood and adolescence. *Ped Clin N Am* 44:307–337, 1997

24. Gray RO, Butler PC, Beers TR, Kryshak RJ, Rizza RA: Comparison of the ability of bread versus bread plus meat to treat and prevent subsequent hypoglycemia in patients with insulin-dependent diabetes mellitus. *J Clin Endocrinol Metab* 81:1508–1511, 1996

25. Williams CL, Bollella M, Wynder EL: A new recommendation for dietary fiber in childhood. *Pediatrics* 96:S985–S988, 1995

26. Delahanty LM, Halfor BN: The role of diet behavior in achieving improved glycemic control in intensively treated patients in the Diabetes Control and Complications Trial. *Diabetes Care* 16:1453–1458, 1993

27. Weissbert-Benchell J, Glasgow AM, Tynan WD, Wirtz P, Turek J, Ward J: Adolescent diabetes management and mismanagement. *Diabetes Care* 18:77–82, 1995

28. American Diabetes Association, The American Dietetic Association: *Exchange Lists for Meal Planning*. Alexandria, VA, American Diabetes Association, 1995

29. Wasserman DH, Zinman B: Exercise in individuals with IDDM (Technical Review). *Diabetes Care* 17:924–947, 1990

30. MacDonald MJ: Postexercise late-onset hypoglycemia in insulin-dependent diabetic patients. *Diabetes Care* 10:584–588, 1987

31. Franz MJ, Barry B: *Diabetes and Exercise, Guidelines for Safe and Enjoyable Activity*. Minneapolis, MN, International Diabetes Center, 1993

32. Andersen RE, Cresp CJ, Bartlett SJ, Cheskin JL, Pratt M: Relationship of physical activity and television watching with body weight and level of fatness among children: results from the third National Health and Nutrition Examination Survey. *JAMA* 279:938–960, 1998

33. Austin A, Warty J, Janosky J, Arslanian S: The relationship of physical fitness to lipid and lipoprotein(a) levels in adolescents with IDDM. *Diabetes Care* 16:421–425, 1993

34. Bar-Or O, Barr S, Bergeron M, Carey R, Clarkson P, Houtkooper L, Rivera-Brown A, Rowland T, Steen S, Barrington: Youth in sport: nutritional needs. *Gatorade Sports Science Exchange Roundtable* 8, 1997

35. Boland E, Savoye M: Nutrition strategies for adolescents with insulin-dependent diabetes mellitus. *Lippincott's Primary Care Practice* 1:270–284, 1997

36. Strachan MWJ, Frier B: Optimal time of administration of insulin lispro: importance of meal consumption. *Diabetes Care* 21:26–31, 1998

37. Boland E, Ahern J, Grey M: A primer on the use of insulin pumps in adolescents. *Diabetes Educ* 24:78–86, 1998

38. Diabetes Control and Complications Trial Research Group: Implementation of treatment protocols in the Diabetes Control and Complications Trial. *Diabetes Care* 18:361–376, 1995

39. American Diabetes Association: *Diabetes Education Goals.* Alexandria, VA, American Diabetes Association, 1995

40. Lorenz RA, Christensen MN, Pichert JW: Diet-related knowledge, skills and adherence among children with insulin-dependent diabetes mellitus. *Pediatrics* 75:872–876, 1985

41. Peveler RC, Fairburn CG, Boller I, Dunger D: Eating disorders in adolescents with IDDM. *Diabetes Care* 15:1356–1360, 1992

42. Neumark-Sztainer D, Story M, Toporoff E, Cassuto N, Resnick MD, Blum RW: Psychosocial predictors of binge eating and purging behaviors among adolescents with and without diabetes mellitus. *J Adolescent Health* 19:289–296, 1996

43. Rodin GM, Daneman D: Eating disorders and IDDM. *Diabetes Care* 15:1402–1412, 1992

Ms. Sharp is a pediatric diabetes nutrition specialist at the International Diabetes Center, Institute for Research and Education, HealthSystem Minnesota, Minneapolis, MN.

13. Nutrition Therapy for Pregnancy and Lactation

CATHY FAGEN, MA, RD, CDE

Highlights

- Pregnancy nutrition therapy for women with prior-onset type 1 or type 2 diabetes starts with a prenatal meal plan before attempting conception to assist in achieving glycemic control and optimal body weight.
- To avoid hypoglycemia during pregnancy, regularity of meals and snacks is extremely important.
- Breastfeeding is recommended. A postpartum meal plan must take into account the energy demands of breastfeeding as well as its blood glucose–lowering effect.
- Nutrition therapy is the cornerstone of treatment for gestational diabetes mellitus (GDM). Intensive nutrition therapy along with daily blood glucose monitoring and an exercise program may be a viable alternative to insulin therapy in women with GDM.

INTRODUCTION

Studies on the effects of undernutrition as a consequence of World War II showed that the nutritional status of the pregnant woman affects the outcome of her pregnancy (1). Currently, research is being conducted on the fetal-origins hypothesis, which says that proper prenatal nutrition is important not only for a healthy pregnancy outcome, but also for the lifelong health of the infant. Infant birth weight is being related to risk of long-term adverse health outcomes such as hypertension, obesity, glucose intolerance, and cardiovascular disease (2).

During pregnancy, women with and without diabetes have similar nutritional needs. Nutrition-related concerns during pregnancy include weight gain and caloric requirements, adequate nutrients, and possible need for vitamin and mineral supplements. In women with prior-onset type 1 and type 2 diabetes and women with gestational diabetes mellitus (GDM), nutrition also has an impact on glycemic control.

NUTRITION-RELATED CONCERNS OF PREGNANCY

Weight Gain

Infant birth weight is consistently related to maternal size and the amount of weight gained during pregnancy. Larger mothers tend to have bigger babies, whereas underweight women have a greater incidence of low–birth weight (LBW) infants and premature deliveries (3). Short women are also are risk (4). In overweight and obese women, failure to gain at least 15–25 lb during pregnancy has been associated with increased risk of intrauterine growth retardation (IUGR) (5). By reaching a higher prepregnancy weight if underweight or by gaining adequate weight during pregnancy, women in these high-risk categories can improve their pregnancy outcomes (6).

The past decade has brought forth many publications with guidelines for improving nutritional status in pregnancy. The 1990 report by the Institute of Medicine (IOM), *Nutrition During Pregnancy* (7), recommends desirable weight gain during pregnancy based on evaluation of the scientific evidence on nutritional status and weight gain. The recommended weight gain ranges are based on the pregravid weight category or pregravid BMI (Table 13.1).

Just as important as the total weight gain is the rate of weight gain. A normal-weight woman typically gains 3–5 lb/month in her first trimester and 1–2 lb/week during the rest of her pregnancy. Overweight women should gain at less than half this rate. Women who gain <2 lb or >6. 5 lb in 1 month and women who have not gained at least 10 lb by mid-pregnancy should be seen by a registered dietitian for medical nutrition therapy.

Calories

Calorie requirements increase minimally in the first trimester and are estimated to be an additional 100 calories per day. In the second and third trimester, an additional 300 calories per day are theoretically required for increases in maternal blood volume, breast tissue, and uterus and adipose tissue; placental growth; fetal growth; and amniotic fluids. The distribution of this weight gain is given in Table 13.2. More than half of the total weight gain is attributed to maternal reproductive tissues, fluid, blood, and maternal stores. The maternal stores are composed largely of body fat, which serves as an energy reserve for pregnancy and lactation. Obese women (≥135% ideal body weight) do not need to gain this mater-

Table 13.1 Recommended Total Weight Gain Ranges for Pregnant Women, by Prepregnancy BMI

Weight-for-Height Category	Recommended Total Gain	
	kg	lb
Low (BMI <19.8)	12.5–18	28–40
Normal (BMI 19.8–26.0)	11.5–16	25–35
High (BMI >26.0–29.0)	7–11.5	15–25

Young adolescents and black women should strive for gains at the upper end of the recommended range. Short women (<157 cm, or 62 in) should strive for gains at the lower end of the range. The recommended target weight gain for obese women (BMI >29.0) is at least 6.0 kg (15 lb). From the National Academy of Sciences, Institute of Medicine, Food and Nutrition Board, Committee on Nutritional Status During Pregnancy and Lactation, Subcommittee on Dietary Intake and Nutrient Supplements During Pregnancy, Subcommittee on Nutritional Status and Weight Gain During Pregnancy (7).

nal body fat, but should be counseled on gaining at least 15 lb to account for the weight of the fetus and the maternal support tissues.

Nutrients

Not only maternal size and weight gain but also specific nutrients have been linked with pregnancy outcome. So in addition to eating extra calories, pregnant women need to eat a balanced diet. The food guide pyramid can serve as a checklist and educational tool in counseling the pregnant woman on nutritional needs during pregnancy. Also, the daily food guide demonstrates how a woman can meet her nutritional require-

Table 13.2 Distribution of Weight Gain During Pregnancy

	Weight (lb)
Fetus	7.5–8.5
Stores of fat and protein	7.5
Blood	4.0
Tissue fluids	2.7
Uterus	2.0
Amniotic fluid	1.8
Placenta and umbilical cord	1.5
Breasts	1.0
Total	28–29

ments by choosing an adequate number of servings from each of the food groups (Table 13.3).

Protein is needed for synthesis of new tissue in maternal organs and the fetus. The 1989 Recommended Dietary Allowance (RDA) for protein in pregnancy is 60 g/day (8). In the U.S., most women consume adequate protein, but their intake of fruits, vegetables, and dairy products is often inadequate. Vegetarians can meet the nutritional requirements of pregnancy if their diet is well planned (9). Food guidelines for vegetarians are outlined in Table 13.4.

Vitamin and Mineral Supplements

Iron needs are greatly increased during pregnancy to support tissue growth and increased blood supply. The IOM recommends a low-dose iron supplement of 30 mg/day during the second and third trimesters. Infants of women diagnosed with iron-deficiency anemia (hemoglobin <11.0 g/l, serum ferritin <12 µg/l) at 16 weeks' gestation had significantly higher risks of both LBW and prematurity (10). If iron-deficiency anemia is present, a higher dose of 60–120 mg/day ferrous iron supplement is required. However, research suggests that excess iron may lead to zinc depletion, which is associated with IUGR (11). Excessive doses of

Table 13.3 Daily Food Guide for Women

| Food Group | Minimum Number of Servings | | |
	Nonpregnant 11–24 years	Nonpregnant 25–50 years	Pregnant/Lactating 11–50 years
Protein foods	5*	5*	7†
Milk products	3	2	3
Breads, cereals, grains	7	6	7
Whole	4	4	4
Enriched	3	2	3
Fruits and vegetables			
Vitamin C–rich	1	1	1
Vitamin A–rich	1	1	1
Other	3	3	3
Unsaturated fats	3	3	3

*Equivalent to 5 oz of animal protein; at least 3 servings/week should be from the vegetable protein list. †Equivalent to 7 oz of animal protein; at least 1 serving/day should be from the vegetable protein list. From the California Department of Health Services, Maternal and Child Health Branch, Women, Infants, and Children Supplemental Food Branch (60).

Table 13.4 Food Guidelines for Pregnant Vegetarians

Food Group	Serving Size	Number of Servings	Comments
Grains	1 slice bread, 1/2 cup cooked cereal or pasta, 3/4 to 1 cup ready-to-eat cereal	7 or more	Choose whole or enriched grains
Legumes, nuts, seeds, milk	1/2 cup cooked beans; 1/2 cup tofu, tempeh, TVP; 3 oz meat analog; 2 Tbsp fortified soy or rice milk; 1 cup cow's milk; 1 cup yogurt	5 or more	Choose these calcium-rich foods often: chickpeas, black beans, vegetarian baked beans, calcium-set tofu, tempeh, TVP, almonds, almond butter, tahini, fortified soy milk, cow's milk, yogurt
Vegetables	1/2 cup cooked vegetables; 1 cup raw vegetables	4 or more	Choose these calcium-rich foods often: dark green leafy vegetables (kale, collard and mustard greens), broccoli, bok choy
Fruits	1/2 cup canned fruit or juice; 1 medium piece of fruit	4 or more	Choose these calcium-rich foods often: figs, fortified orange juice

These guidelines describe minimum servings for pregnant women. Women who do not meet calorie needs to support adequate weight gain should choose additional servings from the food groups and can also use added fats, such as oil and salad dressing, to increase calorie intake. TVP, textured vegetable protein. From the Vegetarian Nutrition Practice Group of The American Dietetic Association (9).

iron supplements (i.e., 300 mg t.i.d.) interfere with copper and zinc absorption and can cause havoc for the woman's gastrointestinal tract. The pregnant woman should be counseled on dietary sources of iron and ways to enhance its absorption, such as consuming a source of vitamin C with the iron-rich food. Good sources of iron are meat, poultry, organ meats, clams, oysters, shrimp, whole grains, enriched grains, leafy green vegetables, dried fruit, prune juice, dried legumes, soybeans, tofu, and blackstrap molasses.

Folic acid is necessary for cell replication and plays a crucial role in pregnancy. The most important finding in recent years has been the relationship between maternal folic acid status and neural tube defects (NTDs). In 1991, the Medical Research Council Vitamin Study Group reported the results of a well-designed, prospective, randomized study of folic acid supplementation for the prevention of NTDs in high-risk pregnancies (12). The data conclusively demonstrated that daily 0.4-mg doses of folic acid before and during early pregnancy resulted in a 71% reduction of recurrence of NTDs. In 1992, the Public Health Service recommended that all women of childbearing age who are capable of becoming pregnant should take 0.4 mg of folic acid daily (13). Other researchers are reporting that periconceptional folic acid supplementation also reduces the rate of other major nongenetic syndromatic congenital abnormalities (14) and orofacial clefts (15). The Food and Drug Administration (FDA) ruled that effective January 1998, products made with enriched flour or grain products, such as bread, rice, and pasta, will contain additional folic acid in the same way they contain additional iron, niacin, and other vitamins. Food sources of folic acid are spinach, leafy green vegetables, liver, lentils, black-eyed peas, red kidney beans, broccoli, Brussels sprouts, beets, okra, green peas, asparagus, legumes, orange and grapefruit juice, and fortified cereals. Even when eating fortified foods and a folate-rich diet, many women will not consume enough folic acid to prevent birth defects, thus the recommendation of a daily folic acid supplement for women of child-bearing age.

Zinc is needed for the function of tissues and is essential for growth. Animal studies have provided strong support for a relationship between zinc status and pregnancy outcome. Women with low pregravid weight and low plasma zinc levels benefit from zinc supplementation, which leads to higher–birth weight infants (16). The average zinc intake of pregnant women is 11.1 mg/day, while the RDA is 15 mg/day (17). Zinc absorption is inhibited with high intakes of phytates, iron, and calcium. Pregnant women should be counseled on consuming adequate sources of zinc, such as shellfish (oysters), meat, poultry, whole grains, dried beans, and nuts.

Calcium is needed for the formation of bones and teeth and has essential roles in muscle contraction, nerve functioning, blood clotting, blood pressure, and immune defense. Successful pregnancies occur with widely varying intakes of calcium. The Dietary Reference Intakes established an Adequate Intake for calcium of 1,000 mg/day for women >19 years of age to replace the 1989 RDA of 1,200 mg/day for pregnancy and lactation (18). The reason for this lowered recommendation is that maternal hormones increase calcium absorption and utilization. The pregnant and lactating woman can meet her calcium needs by consuming three or more servings a day from the milk group. Other dietary sources of calcium are broccoli, greens, legumes, blackstrap molasses, tofu with calcium added during processing, and some seaweed and sea vegetables.

A balanced diet that results in appropriate weight gain during pregnancy generally supplies the vitamins and minerals needed for pregnancy. However, many physicians prescribe a prenatal vitamin-mineral supplement because of the uncertainty of their patient's nutritional status and intake. The IOM did not find sufficient evidence to recommend routine use of prenatal vitamins except in high-risk pregnancies (i.e., short-interval pregnancy, history of LBW infant, multiple gestation, substance abuse, adolescent mother, etc.) (7).

The clinical recommendation is routine assessment of the pregnant woman's dietary pattern using a food history or food-frequency questionnaire, augmented by questions about special problems or conditions that might affect her nutritional adequacy or needs. Food is considered the optimal vehicle for delivering nutrients, and the recommendation to supplement the diet with vitamins or minerals should be based on evidence of a benefit as well as a lack of harmful effects (7).

Other Substances

The use of alcohol is discouraged during pregnancy because of its potential adverse effects on the fetus (19). Caffeine use should be limited for the same reason (7). Artificial sweeteners are considered safe for consumption; however, there have been no adequate long-term studies in humans during pregnancy. Moderation in their consumption during pregnancy seems appropriate (20).

SPECIAL CONCERNS OF PREGNANCY
AND PRIOR-ONSET TYPE 1 AND TYPE 2 DIABETES

Women with diabetes need to achieve and sustain optimal glycemic control before and during pregnancy. The specific level of glycemia that is needed to avoid the complications associated with diabetes and pregnancy is not known (21). The major focus of diabetes and pregnancy programs is prevention of diabetes-associated complications through preconception counseling and intensive diabetes management with a multidisciplinary team.

Glycemic Control

The problems associated with a pregnancy accompanied by diabetes are outlined in Figure 13.1. The most disconcerting problem for the woman is the increased risk for fetal birth defects. Clinical trials in humans indicate that the risk for congenital anomalies is related to hyperglycemia

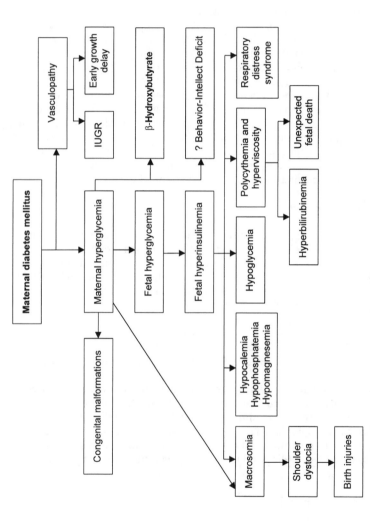

Figure 13.1 Potential problems when diabetes is a factor.

during the organogenesis stage, which is the first 6 weeks of pregnancy (22,23). First trimester glycosylated hemoglobin levels are used as an indicator of glycemic control during organogenesis. An elevated level indicates an increased risk for congenital malformations, but is not a reliable predictor of outcome in every woman. Other factors that have been implicated in diabetes-associated birth defects are ketone bodies, hypoglycemia, somatomedin-inhibiting factors, and free oxygen radicals (24–26). Routine screening of pregnant women with diabetes should include maternal alpha-fetoprotein and an ultrasonic evaluation that includes a general anatomic survey and fetal echocardiogram (27).

Adhering to stringent regimens before and after conception has been shown to lower the incidence of birth defects from 10% (28) to 2% (29), which is equal to that of the general population. Also, women with excellent diabetes control have a lower spontaneous abortion rate than the general population (30), whereas poor glycemic control during the periconceptional and early phase of pregnancy results in increased spontaneous abortion rates (31).

Tight metabolic control and improved management protocols have also dramatically reduced the incidence of the problems shown in Figure 13.1. Women who have complications associated with diabetes have vascular alterations that contribute to higher maternal morbidity and mortality rates. These women need a complete physical examination and laboratory workup to assess the presence of any pathological condition in the eyes, kidneys, and cardiovascular system. Pregnancy is not absolutely contraindicated in these conditions, but the woman would be counseled on her increased risk of complications. Some complications that are already present need to be treated before planning a pregnancy. These are discussed in a technical review by Kitzmiller et al. (32).

Ideally, women with type 1 or type 2 diabetes should achieve optimal glycemic control before attempting conception. Women with type 2 diabetes need to be changed from oral agents to insulin therapy during the preconception period because of the hypoglycemic effects of oral agents on the fetus. Attempts to achieve normoglycemia with intensive insulin therapy increase the risk of hypoglycemia (33). Women on insulin need to be counseled on the risk of hypoglycemic episodes in pregnancy (27,34). It is imperative to include family members and significant others in the education and management of hypoglycemia. Guidelines to achieve normoglycemia in prepregnant women are available in the literature (32,35–37) as well as in diabetes and pregnancy programs (27,38).

Medical Nutrition Therapy

Nutrition therapy guidelines include achieving optimal body weight and starting a prenatal meal plan before attempting conception. This is to stabilize blood glucose levels and avoid fluctuations from diet changes in early pregnancy. Calorie recommendations are based on prepregnancy weight and weight-gain goals. It is important to individualize this recommendation because individuals' metabolisms differ. A suggested guideline is 30 kcal/kg/day for women at desirable body weight (DBW), 24 kcal/kg/day for women >120% DBW, and 36–40 kcal/kg/day for women <90% DBW (35).

The American Diabetes Association (ADA) nutrition recommendations stress the importance of individualizing diet recommendations (39). Medical nutrition therapy includes a nutrition assessment and patient interview to take into consideration medical history, clinical data, blood glucose records, food history, exercise pattern, and psychosocial and economic living conditions when developing an individualized meal plan. The distribution of calories and carbohydrates in the meal plan will be based on the woman's food habits, her blood glucose records, and the physiological effects of pregnancy on her body.

The goal of medical nutrition therapy in a pregnancy with diabetes is to maintain normal blood glucose levels while meeting the nutritional needs of pregnancy. Regularity of meals and snacks is extremely important to avoid hypoglycemia secondary to the continuous fetal draw of glucose from the mother. Because blood glucose goals are lower in pregnancy and because the hormones of pregnancy make insulin less effective, the woman may have to eliminate certain foods that trigger a glycemic response for her (27). This places tremendous value on her dedication and motivation for self-monitoring of blood glucose (SMBG) and for keeping accurate records of her daily food intake. The support of a diabetes care team has been shown to have a positive effect on achieving blood glucose control with intensive management (29,33,40).

Lactation

The nutritional quality of a woman's diet is just as important in the postpartum period as it is in pregnancy. Not only is the woman recovering from the physiological stresses of pregnancy and delivery, but she is also now dealing with the additional demands of her new baby.

A meal plan for weight loss should be developed with the woman in her last trimester or at her postpartum visit. A gradual weight loss of 1–2 lb/month should be emphasized, especially if the woman is breastfeeding.

Breastfeeding is recommended for women with diabetes. Energy requirements during lactation may be partially met by maternal fat stores. During the first 6 months of lactation, the woman needs to consume an additional ~200 kcal above her pregnancy meal plan.

Murtaugh et al. (41) described the effects of lactation on glycemia and energy intake in women with type 1 diabetes. Achieving desired glucose control goals during lactation was reported to be difficult. They suggest that 35 kcal/kg should be prescribed to achieve moderate (4.5 lb) weight loss per month during lactation. Frequent contact and changes in intervention are necessary to maintain glycemic control.

Since breastfeeding lowers blood glucose levels, women need to eat a snack containing carbohydrate and protein either before or during breastfeeding. It is important to encourage the woman to nap after meals or snacks and not before, because she may sleep through her eating time, which may result in hypoglycemia. For this same reason, nighttime snacks are very important. Adding a source of protein to the snack can provide additional bulk with minimal effects on blood glucose level. Fluid intake is important for adequate milk production, but drinking beyond thirst has no beneficial effect.

Women who elect to bottle-feed can continue the same pregnancy meal plan after delivery to provide adequate nutrients for recovery. A moderate hypocaloric diet and exercise program for loss of weight gained during pregnancy can be started after the recovery period and approval of her physician.

NUTRITION-RELATED CONCERNS OF GESTATIONAL DIABETES

Normal pregnancy is accompanied by changes in the intermediary metabolism of all fuels, especially carbohydrate (42). Fasting blood glucose levels decrease to 55–65 mg/dl, and diurnal blood glucose levels rarely exceed 100 mg/dl except after meals (43).

Women who develop GDM, 3–5% of the pregnant population, are not able to meet the demands for increased production of insulin, have delayed secretion, or are strongly insulin resistant (44). Risk factors associated with these conditions are first-degree relative with diabetes, previous history of GDM, overweight (>120% DBW), age >25 years, and high-risk ethnic group (45). Diagnostic testing procedures have been challenged, and the 4th International Workshop on GDM reviewed the research on this topic in March of 1997. A summary of the panel's recommendations was published in a supplement to the journal *Diabetes Care* (46).

Medical Nutrition Therapy

The goal of medical nutrition therapy for GDM is the same as for women with type 1 or type 2 diabetes: optimal blood glucose control with adequate nutrition for both mother and fetus. Nutrition recommendations to be incorporated into the individualized meal plan are listed in Table 13.5.

Table 13.5 Nutrition Recommendations for Women with GDM

Factor	Recommendation
Energy	Consume energy necessary to maintain desirable weight gain during pregnancy.
Carbohydrate	Percentage depends on individual eating habits and effect on blood glucose goals.
Sucrose and caloric sweeteners	Use depends on effect on blood glucose levels.
Fiber	Consume 20–35 g dietary fiber a day from a wide variety of food sources.
Protein	Consume 10 g/day above the RDA (i.e., a total of 60 g/day).
Fat	Percentage is based on nutrition assessment and treatment goals; less than 10% of energy should be from saturated fat.
Alternative sweeteners	Restrict use of saccharin. Use of aspartame and acesulfame K in moderation is acceptable.
Sodium	Sodium restriction has not been found to be beneficial in alleviating gestational hypertension.
Alcohol	Consumption is not advisable during pregnancy.
Caffeine	Moderate use is acceptable.
Vitamins and minerals	IOM does not recommend routine use of multivitamin/mineral supplementation. Instead, it recommends that the nutritional adequacy of individual dietary habits be assessed to determine need for supplementation. Ferrous iron supplement (30 mg) is recommended to provide for the increased iron needs of pregnancy.

From Fagen et al. (52).

The recommendation for energy intake is to consume energy necessary to maintain desirable weight gain during pregnancy. This may be no more than an additional ~50–100 kcal/day for the first 34–36 weeks and an additional ~200–300 kcal/day for the final few weeks (47). The use of hypocaloric diets (1,200 kcal/day) in the management of obese women with GDM may reduce hyperglycemia and fetal birth weight, but it also increases free fatty acids and ketone levels in maternal blood. Studies by Knopp et al. (48) conclude that modest caloric reduction (1,600–1,800 kcal/day) results in reduced mean glucose without elevations in free fatty acids or ketones in the urine. A study by Snyder et al. (49) concluded that euglycemia and appropriate weight gain and birthweights were achieved with 23–25 kcal/kg for obese women with GDM and 30–34 kcal/kg for normal-weight women (49). This is consistent with the recommended daily caloric intake for pregnancy. Women who are underweight need 36–40 kcal/kg (35). Daily food records, weekly weight checks, and urine ketone testing will help determine the individual woman's caloric needs.

Intensive Nutrition Management

A meal plan limiting total carbohydrate intake and distributing it throughout the day into three meals and two to four snacks can be used to achieve normal blood glucose levels in GDM (50). A summary of intensive nutritional therapy for GDM is outlined in Table 13.6. It has been suggested that carbohydrate intake at breakfast be limited to 30 g because of the morning release of cortisol, a contra-insulin hormone (51,52). Different types of carbohydrate produce variable postprandial blood glucose responses. A 30- to 35-g carbohydrate breakfast consisting of bran flakes and milk caused significantly higher 1-h postprandial blood glucose levels than did a 30- to 35-g carbohydrate breakfast of whole-wheat bread and fruit or whole-wheat bread alone (53). Breakfast seems to produce more variability in postprandial blood glucose levels

---

Table 13.6 Summary of Intensive Nutritional Therapy for GDM

- Meal pattern
  - Three meals plus three or more snacks (2- to 3-h intervals; breakfast meal with low carbohydrate content)
  - ADA exchange pattern individualized

- Composition (nutrition therapy and exercise only, no insulin)
  - 38–45% carbohydrate (minimum of 150 g/day; 38% carbohydrate used as long as no ketonuria present)
  - 20–25% protein (1.3 g/kg)
  - 30–40% fat (mono- or polyunsaturated emphasized)

- Energy levels
  - Second trimester, 25–30 kcal/kg IBW prepregnant
  - Third trimester, 30–35 kcal/kg IBW prepregnant

- Weight gain
  - Kilocalorie level adjusted to achieve appropriate weight gain for prepregnancy BMI category

---

IBW, ideal body weight. Adapted from Gunderson (51).

than do the midday and evening meals (54). Frequent SMBG enables women to identify their individual glycemic responses to different sources of carbohydrate at different times of the day. Some clinicians find that during pregnancy, the more processed a food is the greater the glycemic response and the higher the elevation in postprandial blood glucose. Unrefined whole-grain breads, noninstant oatmeal, legumes, and lentils are recommended because of their lower glycemic responses (27,51). SMBG in conjunction with daily food records will help determine individual glycemic responses to meals and food products (e.g., breakfast, pizza, fast-food hamburgers, and lactose-containing foods) (55–58). With intense management, women with GDM learn to control their blood glucose levels by modifying food choices and portion sizes (51). Use of intensive nutrition therapy with daily SMBG (52) and an exercise program (59,60) may be a viable alternative to insulin therapy for a large population of women with GDM. A study by Jovanovic et al. (59) concluded that diet plus cardiovascular conditioning lowered blood glucose levels more than diet alone. Some women, despite their efforts at dietary manipulation of carbohydrate intake, will require the assistance of exogenous insulin to achieve normoglycemia. These are usually women with elevated fasting blood glucose levels.

Lactation

Breastfeeding is encouraged, and women should not follow a hypocaloric diet until lactation is terminated. A minimum intake of 1,800 kcal/day meets the nutritional requirements of lactation and should induce a slow weight loss of 1–2 lb/month (61). Overweight women can lose up to 4. 5 lb/month without affecting milk volume.

Cost-Effectiveness of Medical Nutrition Therapy

Assessment of the costs and benefits of managing GDM with programs that use intensive nutrition therapy has been studied by Kitzmiller et al. (62). Program input costs per case and outcome costs per case were higher for the women requiring insulin treatment than for those on nutrition therapy alone. One program used a randomized controlled trial to study the outcomes of using postprandial SMBG-based adjustments of medical nutrition therapy and insulin therapy versus premeal SMBG (63). Input costs were somewhat higher for postprandial blood glucose monitoring, but outcome costs were lower because of fewer cesarean sections and neonatal admissions to intensive care units as compared with the premeal testing group. The use of postprandial blood glucose values as the basis for adjustments in nutrition and insulin therapy proved more cost-effective and indicates that about $3 would be saved in outcome costs for every $1 expended for the greater input cost (62). Unfortunately, this study looked only at women already on insulin therapy. Research is needed to identify the characteristics of women who may achieve optimal perinatal outcomes by following intensive nutrition therapy without the use of insulin (51).

Another area of study that is difficult but could demonstrate cost-effectiveness of medical nutrition therapy is outcome evaluation of the woman's food and eating habits and general indicators of health for the subsequent years after delivery. Women with GDM are at high risk of developing GDM in subsequent pregnancies and type 2 diabetes later in life. Maintaining a reasonable body weight and active lifestyle helps reduce the risk of future glucose intolerance.

For an extensive coverage of medical nutrition therapy for GDM, refer to the *Nutrition Practice Guidelines for Gestational Diabetes Mellitus* published by The American Dietetic Association (50).

REFERENCES

1. Susser M, Smith Z: Timing in prenatal nutrition: a reprise of the Dutch Famine Study. *Nutr Rev* 52:84, 1994

2. Barker DJP: Fetal origins of coronary heart disease. *BMJ* 311:171–174, 1995

3. Rosso P, Salas SP: Mechanism of fetal growth retardation in the underweight mother. In *Nutrient Regulation During Pregnancy, Lactation, and Infant Growth*. Allen L, King J, Lonnerdal B, Eds. New York, Plenum, 1994

4. Luke B, Jonaitis MA, Petrie RH: A consideration of height as a function of prepregnancy nutritional background and its potential influence on birth weight. *J Am Diet Assoc* 84:176, 1984

5. Edwards LE, Hellerstedt WL, Alton IR, Story M, Himes JH: Pregnancy complications and birth outcomes in obese and normal weight women: effects of gestational weight change. *Obstet Gynecol* 87:389–394, 1996

6. Luke B: Nutritional influences on fetal growth. *Clin Obstet Gynecol* 37:538–549, 1994

7. Institute of Medicine, Food and Nutrition Board, Committee on Nutritional Status During Pregnancy and Lactation, Subcommittee on Dietary Intake and Nutrient Supplements During Pregnancy, Subcommittee on Nutritional Status and Weight Gain During Pregnancy: *Nutrition During Pregnancy*. Washington, DC, National Academy Press, 1990, pp. 1–23

8. Food and Nutrition Board, National Research Council, National Academy of Sciences: *Recommended Dietary Allowances.* 10th ed. Washington, DC, National Academy Press, 1989

9. Vegetarian Nutrition, a Dietetic Practice Group of The American Dietetic Association: Vegetarian diets in pregnancy. In *Issues in Vegetarian Dietetics.* Chicago, IL, The American Dietetic Association, 1996

10. Scholl TO, Hedler ML, Fischer RL, Shearer JW: Anemia vs. iron deficiency: increased risk of preterm delivery in a prospective study. *Am J Clin Nutr* 55:985–988, 1992

11. Hemminki E, Merilainen J: Long-term follow-up of mothers and their infants in a randomized trial on iron prophylaxis during pregnancy. *Am J Obstet Gynecol* 173:205–209, 1995

12. Medical Research Council Vitamin Study Group: Prevention of neural tube defects: results of the Medical Research Council Vitamin Study. *Lancet* 338:131–137, 1991

13. PHS (Department of Health and Human Services, Public Health Service): Recommendation for the use of folic acid to reduce the number of cases of spina bifida and other neural tube defects. *MMWP* 41/RR-14:1–7, 1992

14. Czeizel AE: Prevention of congenital abnormalities by periconceptional multivitamin supplementation. *BMJ* 306:1645–1648, 1993

15. Shaw GM, Lammer EJ, Wasserman CR, O'Malley CD, Tolarova MM: Risks of orofacial clefts in children born to women using multivitamins containing folic acid periconceptually. *Lancet* 346:393–397, 1995

16. Goldenberg RL, Tamura T, Neggers Y, Copper RL, Johnston KE, Du Bard MB, Hauth JC: The effect of zinc supplementation on pregnancy outcome. *JAMA* 274:463–468, 1995

17. Murtaugh MA, Weingart J: Individual nutrient effects on length of gestation and pregnancy outcome. *Sem Perinatol* 19:197–210, 1995

18. Institute of Medicine, Food and Nutrition Board: *Dietary Reference Intakes for Calcium, Phosphorus, Magnesium, Vitamin D, and Fluoride.* Washington, DC, National Academy Press, 1997

19. Hanson JW, Streissguth AP, Smith DW: The effects of moderate alcohol consumption during pregnancy on fetal growth and morphogenesis. *J Pediatr* 92:457, 1978

20. Stone Neuhouser ML: Nutrition during pregnancy and lactation. In *Krause's Food, Nutrition and Diet Therapy*. 9th ed. Mahan LK, Escott-Stump S, Eds. Philadelphia, WB Saunders, 1996, pp. 181–212

21. Langer O: Is normoglycemia the correct threshold to prevent complications in the pregnant diabetic patient? *Diabetes Rev* 4:2–10, 1996

22. Goldman JA, Dickerd D, Feldberg D: Pregnancy outcome in patients with insulin-dependent diabetes mellitus with preconceptual diabetic control: a comparative study. *Am J Obstet Gynecol* 155:193–197, 1986

23. Kitzmiller JL, Gavin LA, Gin GD, Jovanovic-Peterson L, Main EK, Zigrang WD: Preconception care of diabetes: glycemic control prevents congenital anomalies. *JAMA* 265:731–736, 1991

24. Horton WE Jr, Sadler TW: Effects of maternal diabetes on early embryogenesis: alterations in morphogenesis produced by the ketone body, β-hydroxybutyrate. *Diabetes* 32:610–616, 1983

25. Freinkel N: Diabetic embryopathy and fuel-mediated organ teratogenesis: lessons from animal models. *Horm Metab Res* 20:473, 1988

26. Miodovnik M, Mimouni F, Dignan PS, Berk MA, Ballard JL, Siddiqi TA, Khoury J, Tsang RC: Major malformations in infants of IDDM women: vasculopathy and early first-trimester pool glycemic control. *Diabetes Care* 11:713–718, 1988

27. *Sweet Success California Diabetes and Pregnancy Program Guidelines for Care*. Revised edition. Sacramento, CA, State of California Department of Health Services, Maternal and Child Health, 1998

28. Mills JL: Malformations in infants of diabetic mothers. *Teratology* 25:385, 1982

29. Cousins L: The California Diabetes and Pregnancy Program: a statewide collaborative program for the preconception and prenatal care of diabetic women. *Clin Obstet Gynecol* 5:443–460, 1991

30. Mills JL, Simpson JL, Driscoll SG, Jovanovik-Peterson L, Van Allen M, Aarons JH, Metzger B, Bieber FR, Knopp RH, Holmes LB, et al.: The National Institute of Child Health and Human Development Diabetes in Early Pregnancy Study: incidence of spontaneous abortion among normal women and insulin-dependent diabetic women whose pregnancies were identified within 21 days of conception. *N Engl J Med* 319:1617–1623, 1988

31. Miodovnik M, Skillman C, Holroyde JC, Butler JB, Wendel JS, Siddiqi TA: Elevated maternal glycohemoglobin in early pregnancy

and spontaneous abortion among insulin-dependent diabetic women. *Am J Obstet Gynecol* 153:439–442, 1985

32. Kitzmiller JL, Buchanan TA, Kjos S, Combs CA, Ratner RE: Preconception care of diabetes, congenital malformations, and spontaneous abortions. *Diabetes Care* 19:514–541, 1996

33. The Diabetes Control and Complications Trial Research Group: The effect of intensive treatment of diabetes on the development and progression of long-term complications in insulin-dependent diabetes mellitus. *N Engl J Med* 329:977–986, 1993

34. Reece EA, Honko CJ, Jagaay Z: When the pregnancy is complicated by diabetes. *Contemporary OB/GYN* 42–61, 1995

35. Jovanovic-Peterson L, Abrams RS, Coustan DR, Cowett RM, Jornsay D, Miller EH, Papatheodorou NH, Patterson AM: Prepregnancy counseling and management of women with pre-existing diabetes or previous gestational diabetes. In *Medical Management of Pregnancy Complicated by Diabetes*. Jovanovic-Peterson L, Ed. Alexandria, VA, American Diabetes Association, 1993

36. Jovanovic-Peterson L, Peterson CM: The art and science of maintenance of normoglycemia in pregnancies complicated by insulin-dependent diabetes mellitus. *Endocrine Pract* 2:130–143, 1996

37. American Diabetes Association: Preconception care of women with diabetes (Position Statement). *Diabetes Care* 21 (Suppl. 1):S56–S59, 1998

38. Willhoite B, Bennert H: The impact of preconception counseling on pregnancy outcomes: the experience of the Maine Diabetes in Pregnancy Program. Poster 22 presented at a satellite symposium to the 14th International Diabetes Foundation Congress, Newport, Rhode Island, June 1991

39. American Diabetes Association: Nutrition recommendations and principles for people with diabetes mellitus (Position Statement). *Diabetes Care* 21 (Suppl. 1):S32–S35, 1998

40. Kitzmiller JL: Sweet Success with diabetes. *Diabetes Care* 16 (Suppl. 3):107–121, 1993

41. Murtaugh MA, Ferris AM, Capacchione CM, Reese EA: Energy intake and glycemia in lactating women with type 1 diabetes. *J Am Diet Assoc* 98:642–648, 1998

42. Freinkel N: Intermediary metabolism in pregnancy. In *Williams Textbook of Endocrinology*. 7th ed. Foster DW, Wilson JD, Eds. Philadelphia, WB Saunders, 1985, pp. 438–451

43. Gillmer MDG, Beard RW, Brooke FM, Oakley NW: Carbohydrate metabolism in pregnancy: diurnal plasma glucose profile in normal and diabetic women. *Br Med J* 3:399–404, 1975

44. Hollingsworth DR: Alterations of maternal metabolism in normal and diabetic pregnancies: differences in insulin-dependent, non-insulin dependent, and gestational diabetes. *Am J Obstet Gynecol* 146:417–429, 1983

45. Expert Committee on Diagnosis and Classification of Diabetes Mellitus: Report of the Expert Committee on Diagnosis and Classification of Diabetes Mellitus. *Diabetes Care* 20:1183–1197, 1997

46. Metzger BE, Coustan DR, The Organizing Committee: Summary and recommendations of the Fourth International Workshop-Conference on Gestational Diabetes Mellitus. *Diabetes Care* 21 (Suppl. 2):B161–B167, 1998

47. Durnin JV, McKillop FM, Grant S, Fitzgerald G: Is nutritional status endangered by virtually no extra intake during pregnancy? *Lancet* ii:823–825, 1985

48. Knopp RH, Mages MS, Rassys V, Benedetti T, Bonet B: Hypocaloric diets and ketogenesis in the management of obese gestational diabetic women. *J Am Coll Nutr* 10:649–667, 1991

49. Snyder J, Gray-Donald K, Koski KG: Predictors of infant birth weight in gestational diabetes. *Am J Clin Nutr* 59:1409–1414, 1994

50. The American Dietetic Association: *Nutrition Practice Guidelines for Gestational Diabetes Mellitus.* Chicago, IL, The American Dietetic Association. In press

51. Gunderson EP: Intensive nutrition therapy for gestational diabetes: rationale and current issues. *Diabetes Care* 20:221–226, 1997

52. Fagen C, King J, Erick M: Nutrition management in women with gestational diabetes mellitus: a review by ADA's Diabetes Care and Education Dietetic Practice Group. *J Am Diet Assoc* 95:460–467, 1995

53. Regenstein A, Flanagan G, Coulstan A, Durzin M: Metabolic response to carbohydrate variation in gestational diabetes (Abstract). *Diabetes* 45 (Suppl. 2):336A, 1996

54. Peterson CM, Jovanovic-Peterson L: Percentage of carbohydrate and glycemic response to breakfast, lunch, and dinner in women with gestational diabetes. *Diabetes* 40 (Suppl. 2):172–174, 1991

55. Lenner RA: Studies of glycemia and glucosuria in diabetics after breakfast meals of different composition. *Am J Clin Nutr* 29:716–725, 1976

56. Ahern JA, Gatcomb PM, Held NA, Pettit WA, Tamboralane WV: Exaggerated hyperglycemia after a pizza meal in well-controlled diabetes. *Diabetes Care* 16:578–580, 1993

57. Viachokosta FV, Piper CM, Gleason R, Kinzel L, Kahn CR: Dietary carbohydrate, a Big Mac, and insulin requirements in type 1 diabetes. *Diabetes Care* 11:330–336, 1988

58. Mahaffey PJ, Podell SK: Euglycemic control of gestational diabetes mellitus by specific dietary manipulation, a case study presentation. *Diabetes Educ* 17:460–465, 1991

59. Jovanovic-Peterson L, Durak EP, Peterson CM: Randomized trial of diet versus diet plus cardiovascular conditioning on glucose levels in gestational diabetes. *Am J Obstet Gynecol* 161:415–419, 1989

60. Mulford MI, Jovanovic-Peterson L, Peterson CM: Alternative therapies for the management of gestational diabetes. *Clin Perinatol* 20:611–634, 1993

61. *Nutrition During Pregnancy and the Postpartum Period: A Manual for Health Professionals.* Sacramento, CA, California Department of Health Services, Maternal Child Health Branch, Women, Infants, and Children Supplemental Food Branch, 1990

62. Kitzmiller JL, Elixhauser A, Carr S, Major CA, de Veciana M, Dang-Kilduff L, Weschler JM: Assessment of costs and benefits of management of gestational diabetes. *Diabetes Care* 21 (Suppl. 2): B123–B130, 1998

63. de Veciana M, Major CA, Morgan MA, Asrat T, Toohey JS, Lien JM, Evans AT: Postprandial versus preprandial blood glucose monitoring in women with gestational diabetes mellitus requiring insulin therapy. *N Engl J Med* 333:1237–1241, 1995

Ms. Fagen is a perinatal nutrition consultant at Long Beach Memorial Medical Center and regional coordinator for the California Diabetes and Pregnancy Program, Sweet Success.

14. Nutrition Therapy for the Older Adult with Diabetes

SUE MCLAUGHLIN, BS, RD, CDE, LMNT, LD

Highlights

- Approximately 19% of adults over age 60 have either diagnosed or undiagnosed diabetes, with 90% having type 2 diabetes. This percentage is greater in many ethnic groups.
- The first step toward effective diabetes management in the older adult is an individualized intervention program that begins with medical nutrition therapy and increased physical activity. Medications may also be needed to achieve adequate metabolic control.
- Malnutrition (both overnutrition and undernutrition) is a potentially serious health problem for the older person with diabetes. The need for weight loss in the obese older adult should be evaluated carefully. Nutrition screening programs of elderly populations living in institutions and community settings have reported malnutrition risk rates ranging from 25 to 85%.
- If poorly controlled, diabetes exacerbates the risk for malnutrition, and conversely, the reasons for the presence of malnutrition make diabetes management more difficult. Both conditions contribute to a decreased quality of life and a social and economic burden for our country. A thorough nutrition assessment and provision of adequate nutrition is essential if these problems are to be reduced in the elderly.
- Residents of long-term care facilities are at increased risk for malnutrition and dehydration. These conditions may be present at admission to the facility or may develop over time. Inappropriate food restrictions; lack of choice, variety, and appreciation for ethnic, cultural, and social preferences; and suboptimal diabetes care will contribute to poor health outcomes

if unrecognized and undertreated. By serving as resident advocates, nutrition care providers can have a significant impact on improving the care and quality of life for the older adult with diabetes.

INTRODUCTION

It is often difficult to define the age of the "older adult." Chronological age is not necessarily a good measure of vitality. An individual can be seemingly "old" at 30 with regard to mental outlook and lifestyle habits, whereas a 90-year-old can appear to be "forever young." This chapter focuses on individuals who are over the age of 65 years. Adults 65–74 years of age are often referred to as the "young old." Likewise, 75- to 84-year-olds are often referred to as "old," with the "oldest old" being 85 years or older.

Older adults comprise an increasingly greater percentage of the U.S. population. In 1994, 33.2 million Americans were over the age of 65 (12.7% of the population, or 1 in 8), compared with a projected 53.3 million (1 in every 6 Americans) by the year 2020 (1). This latter group is the fastest growing segment of our population.

Increasing age is known to be a major risk factor in the development of diabetes. Based on information from the Third National Health and Nutrition Examination Survey, 1988–1994 (NHANES III), the combination of diagnosed and undiagnosed diabetes in adults >60 years of age is reaching rates of 18.8% (2). Over 90% of older adults with diabetes have type 2 (3). Older adults from many ethnic groups are at even greater risk of developing diabetes. As Figure 14.1 illustrates, the problem of diabetes escalates as each ethnic group ages (4).

Diabetes is a leading cause of mortality in the U.S. (ranking seventh in 1994), and the highest rates have been noted in older Americans and in minority populations. Between 1980 and 1994, the greatest increase in diabetes death rates occurred in black males >65 years of age (5).

Beyond the personal hardship caused by diabetes, there are tremendous implications for the health care industry. In 1997, direct medical expenditures attributable to diabetes inpatient care (62%), outpatient services (25%), and nursing home care (13%) totaled $44 billion. Two-thirds of these costs were related to the care of the older person with diabetes. Outrageous as these statistics are, they do not include health care costs attributable to undiagnosed diabetes, individuals treated through the Department of Veterans Affairs, potential omissions of diabetes diagnosis due to improper ICD-9-CM coding, and overall nursing home costs (expected to be substantial), which most likely would cause the economic burden to be even higher than the above figures indicate (6).

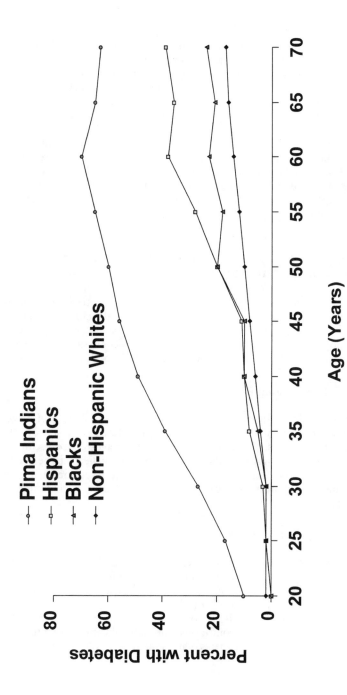

Figure 14.1 Diabetes and ethnicity. From King et al. (4).

Much of the research conducted to date on adults with diabetes is not specific to those over age 65. Furthermore, there are limited data regarding nutritional status and nutritional needs specific to the older adult with diabetes. Therefore, much of the clinical practice information available for medical nutrition therapy (MNT) has been extrapolated from studies done with younger adults with diabetes or older individuals who had not been diagnosed with diabetes.

In this chapter, risk factors associated with the development of diabetes and overall diabetes management for the older adult are reviewed first. Calories related to over- and undernutrition and other nutrient concerns are discussed as well as implementing MNT in the older adult. Finally, the important topic of diabetes care and nutrition therapy in long-term care facilities is discussed.

RISK FACTORS ASSOCIATED WITH DIABETES IN THE OLDER PERSON

What is the cause for the increased incidence of diabetes in individuals over age 65? While more research is needed, several factors are believed responsible: an age-related increase in insulin resistance, causing a deterioration in glucose metabolism; the presence of coexisting chronic disease conditions; physical inactivity; and changes in body composition.

Age-Related Insulin Resistance

Fasting blood glucose levels are known to increase slightly with age, at a rate of 1–2 mg/dl (0.06–0.11 mmol/l) per decade over age 30–40. Studies have suggested that this may be due to an age-related decline in β-cell function (7); however, the major alteration is believed to be due to peripheral changes in insulin metabolism and action, specifically insulin resistance caused by a postreceptor defect (8) or a decreased number of glucose transporters (9).

Coexisting Chronic Health Problems

Nearly 40% of individuals over age 65 report having at least one chronic condition that they find limiting. Most older adults with diabetes have at least one additional condition or disease. The most common chronic conditions include arthritis, hypertension, hearing impairments, cataracts, chronic sinusitis, ischemic heart disease, and orthopedic impairments (10). These conditions and the medications used to treat them may interfere with diabetes management.

Physical Inactivity

Physical inactivity has been suggested by some to be among the top three leading actual causes of death in the U.S. (11). According to estimates by the Centers for Disease Control, at least 60% of the U.S. adult population does not meet even the recommended minimum levels of physical activity (12). Physical inactivity is known to be higher in those over the age of 45, in non–college graduates, and in minorities (13–15). Physical activity is linked to increased insulin sensitivity; therefore, the age-related decline in insulin sensitivity is believed to be caused in part by a reduction in physical activity in this age-group (16).

Body Composition

Aging brings with it a decline in muscle mass (i.e., sarcopenia), which is accompanied by a decline in basal metabolic rate, muscle strength, activity, and caloric requirements (17). In sedentary individuals, the main determinant of energy expenditure is fat-free mass. This is known to decline by ~15% between the third and eighth decades of life. If older adults do not lower their caloric intake to compensate, weight gain and increased adipose tissue deposition will occur. In the elderly, excessive adipose accumulation occurs in the trunkal portion of the body. This upper-body, or abdominal, obesity, measured as waist-to-hip ratio, increases the risk of type 2 diabetes.

OVERALL DIABETES MANAGEMENT FOR THE OLDER ADULT

One of the primary goals of diabetes management is to assist in maintaining blood glucose levels within a target range, as determined by the older adult, family and/or caregivers, and other members of the diabetes team. The detrimental effects of both hyperglycemia and hypoglycemia for this population group have been acknowledged. However, fear of hypoglycemia, in and of itself, should not preclude efforts to lower blood glucose levels to within a desirable range. The consequences of prolonged, uncontrolled hyperglycemia in the elderly include urinary incontinence, sleep interference, dehydration, increased risk of falls and resultant immobility, increased platelet adhesiveness with increased risk of diabetes complications and related vascular compromise, visual impairment, decreased pain tolerance and increased use of analgesics, cognitive changes that may impact ability to carry out components of the diabetes management plan, and immune system impairment leading to increased infections, resulting in an overall diminished quality of life (18).

A number of factors, including chronological age, frailty, cognitive function, coexisting disease, level of social support, and potential consequences of both hyper- and hypoglycemia must be considered when determining goals for blood glucose in the older adult. Once goals have been established, intervention based on an individualized program that addresses these issues and begins with MNT and increased physical activity is the first step toward effective diabetes management and may prove to prevent, delay, or lessen the severity of diabetes complications in the older adult. Monitoring blood glucose and tracking HbA_{1c} results are key to interpreting the success of diabetes management.

MNT for the Older Adult with Diabetes

Nutrition recommendations for the general population with diabetes have been discussed previously in this book. Suggested goals of diabetes MNT for the older adult (Table 14.1) resemble those recommended for all people with diabetes, as identified in the American Diabetes Association (ADA) nutrition recommendations (19). As is true for younger individuals, diabetes nutrition recommendations must be individualized, accommodating personal lifestyle habits. For many older adults with diabetes, balancing food intake with endogenous insulin may achieve target blood glucose levels. If not, many options for the use of medication are available, but all still require attention to food choices.

Providing effective MNT to the older adult will occur only if attention is given to several other factors as discussed here.

Physiological changes of aging. The physiological changes of aging affect the overall nutritional status of older adults. These changes include altered thirst, dentition, swallowing, and gastrointestinal function; sensory losses; decreased metabolic rate; anorexia; and early satiety. Pain, discomfort, or loss of appetite related to these changes may result in altered food choices, with a resultant impact on glycemic control.

Table 14.1 Goals of Medical Nutrition Therapy for the Older Adult with Diabetes

- Maintain blood glucose levels within target range
- Provide appropriate calories and nutrients
- Assist with management of coexisting medical diseases
- Prevent, delay, or treat nutrition-related complications
- Promote safety, quality of life, and overall health.

From the American Diabetes Association Clinical Education Program Diabetes Care for the Older Adult, 1996.

Table 14.2 Psychosocial Factors That Impact Diabetes Management in Older Adults

■ Depression	■ Safety
■ Stress and anxiety disorders	■ Cultural practices
■ Alcohol and drug abuse	■ Housing/living conditions
■ Comorbid illnesses and polypharmacy	■ Health beliefs
■ Presence of diabetes complications	■ Transportation difficulties
■ Social support mechanisms	■ Financial concerns
■ Abuse	■ Cognitive changes and
■ Sexuality	dementia

Adapted from the American Diabetes Association Clinical Education Program Diabetes Care for the Older Adult, 1996.

Psychosocial factors. Psychosocial factors have a significant impact on the ability of an older adult to manage diabetes and on how one's quality of life is perceived. Table 14.2 lists some of these factors. Several are discussed at length.

Depression is the most common emotional disorder of later life. It often goes unrecognized or undertreated, but it is believed to be present in 5–10% of community residents over age 65 and in 15–25% of long-term care residents (20). Factors that may contribute to depression in the older adult include physiological changes of aging, diagnosis of diabetes complications or other medical conditions, use of prescription medications or substance abuse, and perhaps most significantly, losses— economic losses, social losses, and losses in living conditions, level of independence, and functional ability. Regardless of the cause, once depression is present, it will interact negatively with diabetes and the components of diabetes management. It has been associated with poor glycemic control, diabetes complications, and factors related to glucose dysregulation: obesity, physical inactivity, and an inability to follow through with lifestyle intervention programs (21). A depression scale, such as the Geriatric Depression Scale (22), Beck Inventory (23), and others, should be administered to alert the health care team to potential difficulties in following through with components of diabetes management so that appropriate therapy may be initiated.

Loss of independence and functional ability is one of the greatest challenges to the older adult (24). The functional assessment is used to evaluate how well one performs the activities of daily living (25), or personal care activities, such as the ability to feed oneself, and the instrumental activities of daily living (26), or home management activities, which include more complex and demanding activities, such as the ability to shop, prepare meals, manage money, administer medications, etc.

These assessments become increasingly valuable as an individual ages, as cognitive changes occur, and as social support systems for the older adult diminish. They assist the health care professional in focusing on the older adult's capabilities and when deficits are noted, are helpful in identifying and activating community resources such as Meals on Wheels, home health care services, and agencies for the visually impaired, which can address identified needs and facilitate diabetes management.

Social isolation also places older adults at high risk for malnutrition, depression, and other problems. Loneliness has been related to dietary inadequacies as well (27). In 1994, 30% of all noninstitutionalized older adults lived alone (40% of older women, 16% of older men) (28). Social factors are known to influence rates of compliance to any medical regimen, including diabetes management.

Financial limitations affect all aspects of the older person's life. Specific to diabetes management is the ability to purchase adequate and appropriate food choices and access to medical care. While the economic status of older Americans has increased overall in the past two decades, almost 19% of this population group were poor ($8,967/year for a couple, or $7,108/year for one living alone) or nearly poor in 1994. This figure does not include homeless elders. Those at greatest risk include Hispanics, African Americans, those with less than 8 years of education, inner-city dwellers, and black women living alone (28).

Cultural factors and changes in cognition also affect the food choices that older adults make.

Physical Activity

The merits of physical activity and exercise as critical components of a diabetes management program and healthy lifestyle are discussed elsewhere in this book. As noted earlier in this chapter, declining physical activity, a reduction in lean muscle mass, and an increase in adipose tissue are believed to contribute to the development of type 2 diabetes in the older adult.

In recent years, an increasingly greater number of studies have shown that healthy older people can exercise safely and that exercising regularly may result in increased aerobic potential, strength, balance, and flexibility (29–32). In addition, both experimental and observational studies have demonstrated that older people who participate in an exercise program find improvements in risk factors (lipids, bone density, insulin resistance) for several of the major chronic diseases, including diabetes (33–36). Furthermore, high levels of physical activity have been associated with a lower incidence of physical disability, falls, hip fractures, and mortality (37–42).

When determining an appropriate exercise regimen for the older person with diabetes, it is best to examine the potential risks (e.g., fluctuations in blood glucose levels) and benefits (e.g., increased insulin sensitivity and glucose tolerance) of implementing such a program. Because of an increased incidence of diabetes complications in this older age-group (e.g., neuropathy, visual problems, cardiovascular damage) and an increased risk for injury and prolonged rate of recovery, it is critical that guidelines/precautions be followed closely to promote a safe and positive exercise experience.

Medications

Whether oral medication, insulin, or combination therapy is prescribed, the medication must be matched to food patterns, rather than the reverse. Because of cognitive changes, depression, financial problems, and other factors, older adults may forget to eat or choose not to eat meals or snacks. A thorough nutrition history and education regarding the importance of a consistent pattern of meals and snacks, as well as discussion regarding signs, symptoms, prevention, and treatment of hypoglycemia will aid in preventing problems with extreme variances in blood glucose control and potentially dangerous situations.

Blood Glucose Monitoring

Blood glucose monitoring is a critical part of diabetes management at any age. Many older adults are accustomed to checking only fasting blood glucose levels—if they have been testing at all. When determining the frequency of blood glucose testing and the most informative times to test, several things should be considered: the intensity of glycemic control desired, type of diabetes medication prescribed, activity patterns, and knowledge level regarding the impact of food choices on blood glucose levels. Testing blood glucose 2 h postprandially is often a valuable teaching tool when evaluating the effect of various food choices on glycemic control.

A common misconception is that older adults are less capable of blood glucose monitoring than their younger counterparts. Yet in a study published in 1994 by Bernbaum et al. (43), individuals ages 65–79 were found to be as capable as those ages 28–54 in carrying out blood glucose monitoring. Frequency of error was not increased in the older group.

A plethora of blood glucose monitors are available, but the challenge is to match the monitor to the needs of the individual. Considerations for meter selection include visual acuity and manual dexterity of the patient, complexity of operation, blood sample size required, portability, ease of calibration, degree of cleaning required, extent of memory, and type of data storage desired.

Medicare now covers the cost of diabetes supplies, including blood glucose monitors, test strips, lancets, etc., when prescribed by the physician, whether the older adult has type 1 or type 2 diabetes. It is hoped that this will help to increase the frequency of blood glucose testing and, with education, will assist the older person in improving diabetes management.

CALORIE AND NUTRIENT CONCERNS FOR THE OLDER ADULT

Calories

A major goal of MNT is to provide adequate calories and nutrients. Caloric requirements have been shown to decrease by 20–30% between the ages of 20 and 60 years (44). The needs of each individual will depend on age, sex, BMI, physical activity patterns, and presence of disease and/or disability. While caloric requirements decrease, the need for specific nutrients may increase with age (45). This may present a challenge to the nutrition educator, as an attempt is made to provide a meal plan that incorporates individual food preferences, promotes attainment and maintenance of a reasonable body weight, and also prevents nutrient deficiencies.

Malnutrition (both overnutrition, or obesity, and undernutrition, or protein-calorie malnutrition) presents potentially serious health problems for the older person with diabetes. It is often assumed that the older adult with diabetes is obese; however, the prevalence of obesity in older adults with type 2 diabetes is only 20%. Data from NHANES II indicate that while obesity is quite common in middle age, it is less prevalent after age 65.

To date, there has been little agreement on appropriate weight standards for defining obesity in older adults. A desirable range for BMI of 24–29 for those over 66 years of age has been suggested by the National Institute on Aging (46). The Recommended Dietary Allowances (RDAs) and newly revised U.S. Dietary Guidelines suggest lower weight-height standards. Regardless, there is little disagreement that a BMI of >30 presents a major health risk. A study by Galanos et al. (47) found BMI to be related to functional capability in community-dwelling elderly individuals. Extremes in BMI (either high or low) were found to place older adults at risk for functional disability.

The need for weight loss in the obese older adult should be evaluated carefully. Mild calorie restriction (i.e., 150–300 fewer calories per day) for gradual weight loss, coupled with an exercise prescription that focuses on non–weight-bearing activity, such as water aerobics, or low-intensity activity, such as walking, may result in improved glycemic control and is preferable to calorie restriction, which may result in nutrient deficiencies, lower metabolic rate, and decreased perception of quality of life.

Calorie requirements should be determined based on the nutrition history. However, because of changes in cognition, literacy problems, and a variety of other reasons, incomplete and/or inaccurate data may be collected. Including family members or friends when gathering information, as well as using scientific formulas such as the Harris-Benedict equation (48), may be useful in estimating needs.

Statistical data specific to malnutrition in the elderly person with diabetes is limited. However, nutrition screening programs in a wide variety of institutional and community settings have reported malnutrition risk rates ranging from 25 to 85% in the elderly population as a whole (49). An evaluation of the Elderly Nutrition Program of the Older Americans Act (i.e., community-based nutrition programs) indicates that 67–88% of participants are at moderate to high nutritional risk (50). Low body weight has been associated with increased morbidity and mortality in the elderly.

In a collaborative multidisciplinary effort by the American Academy of Family Physicians, The American Dietetic Association, and the National Council on Aging, the Nutrition Screening Initiative developed tools to assist in screening and assessment of nutritional risk: the DETERMINE Your Nutritional Health checklist and Level I and II screens. These tools identify risk factors for malnutrition among older adults (51). As the cumulative number of risk factors increases, so does the likelihood for malnutrition (Table 14.3).

High rates of malnutrition often lead to more frequent physician visits, lengthier and costlier hospitalizations, more readmissions, riskier surgeries, and premature admissions to long-term care facilities. If poorly controlled, diabetes exacerbates the risk for malnutrition, and conversely, the reasons for malnutrition in the older person with diabetes (e.g., food insecurities, etc.) will only make diabetes management more difficult.

Table 14.3 Risk Factors for Malnutrition in the Older Adult

- Inadequate food intake and food insecurity
- Social isolation
- Depression
- Dementia
- Dependency and functional ability, or the degree of dependency required by an older adult to complete the activities of daily living
- Poor oral health, including chewing and swallowing problems
- Presence of acute or chronic diseases or conditions
- Polypharmacy
- Advanced age
- Chronic hyperglycemia

The combination of these two conditions contributes to a decreased quality of life for the elderly and a social and economic burden for our country as a whole. A thorough nutritional assessment and identification of treatment alternatives is essential if these problems are to be reduced in this population.

Nutrient Concerns

The new Dietary Reference Intakes will provide RDAs or Adequate Intakes based on life-stage group. Separate recommendations for nutrients for men and women ages 51–70 years and >70 years will be reported. Two reports have been issued for nutrients and food components (52,53), with at least four additional groups of nutrients and food components planned for review over the next 3–4 years.

Protein. Individual recommendations for protein intake in the older adult should consider status of current body stores (prealbumin, serum albumin, etc.); potential for increased needs during wound healing, infection, and other stressors; and status of renal function. Research by Campbell et al. (54) suggests that protein requirements for older adults may exceed the RDA of 0.8 g/kg body wt and that 1.0–1.25 g/kg body wt may be more appropriate. Protein needs have been estimated using a factor from 1 g/kg/day during periods of low stress to 2 g/kg/day during severe stress. However, because of decreased appetite and intake, the latter value is often difficult to achieve orally in older adults. A controlled protein intake (0.8 g/kg ideal body wt) has been suggested with the onset of nephropathy for those with diabetes (55); however, the risk-to-benefit ratio must be carefully evaluated in the older adult because of the risk of malnutrition.

Fat. Cardiovascular disease (CVD) is well-recognized as one of the most prevalent chronic illnesses in the older adult. In 1994, ~33% of all diabetes-related hospital discharges had CVD as the primary discharge diagnosis. Age-specific rates of hospital discharge with CVD, ischemic heart disease, and stroke increased with age; in 1994, individuals over 75 years of age were almost 10 times as likely as those under 45 years of age to be hospitalized for CVD (5).

Given the relationship between a decreased intake of saturated fat and a reduction in serum cholesterol in younger adults, it might appear reasonable to predict similar results in older adults. However, the relationship between atherosclerosis and dyslipidemia in the older adult is complex because of multiple etiologies contributing to the atherosclerosis: genetics, hypertension, smoking, obesity, hyperinsulinemia, dyslipidemia, lack of physical activity, and renal disease.

As for younger adults, the ADA nutrition recommendations suggest that the fat content of the meal plan be based on the nutrition assessment and individualized treatment goals. For example, in a young-old adult (age 65–74) who is obese, a reduced intake of total and saturated fat and cholesterol may assist in lowering elevated blood lipids, reducing body weight and adipose tissue, and improving blood glucose control via decreased insulin resistance; however, the same recommendations for an old (age 75–84) or oldest-old (age ≥85) adult may predispose to deficiencies of various nutrients. For the majority of older adults, dietary restrictions should be limited to National Cholesterol Education Program Step 1 guidelines (56).

Carbohydrate. Research specific to carbohydrate intake for the older adult is lacking. Recommendations do not differ from those for younger adults. Because of the age-related decline in carbohydrate tolerance, particular attention to carbohydrate load at meals and distribution throughout the day seems prudent. As with other aspects of meal planning, individualization is the key. Older adults who have not received diabetes education in recent years will require updates regarding the use of sucrose and sucrose-containing foods and the recognition of the impact of total carbohydrate on glycemic control.

Fiber. A large number of older adults complain of constipation. The average and notably low fiber intake in the U.S. is 8–10 g/day. Increased fiber intake accompanied by adequate fluid intake seems prudent for this age-group; however, the recommended intake of 20–35 g/day for the general healthy adult population may be too high for many.

Health care professionals should be alert for a condition known as terminal reservoir syndrome, which is caused by poor motility in the last segment of the sigmoid colon, causing constipation along with accumulation of fecal material. Increased fiber intake along with inadequate fluid intake often aggravates the condition, worsening the constipation and possibly causing fecal impaction (57).

Alcohol. Alcohol abuse is a serious problem in the older population. It reportedly affects up to 10% of community dwellers and as many as 40% of long-term care residents (58). Decreased appetite, omission of nutrient-dense foods, dehydration, and increased risk of either hyper- or hypoglycemia (related to food intake) are all potential detrimental effects of alcohol abuse. A prudent recommendation for alcohol use would be to suggest that if they drink at all, women and men should consume no more than one or two drinks per day, respectively.

Sodium. A high sodium intake has been shown to increase the risk of hypertension in sodium-sensitive individuals. Of adults aged 65 and over (with and without diabetes), 44–76% are reportedly hypertensive (59).

Incidence is particularly high in the black population. The ADA nutrition recommendations suggest that the general population limit intake of sodium to 3,000 mg/day and to <2,400 mg/day for those with mild to moderate hypertension or congestive heart failure. Because of the relatively high rates of hypertension in the elderly, a sodium-restricted diet and weight loss may be helpful. However, before advising sodium restriction, recognize that older adults are known to have a diminished taste perception (60). Combined with severe sodium restriction, this may result in inadequate food intake and malnutrition over time. If a 3-month trial of sodium restriction does not produce changes in condition, it may be in the patient's best interest to relax sodium recommendations and make adjustments in medication.

Micronutrients. Aging and diabetes have been independently associated with altered micronutrient status. Chronic hyperglycemia has been found to cause altered micronutrient status (not limited to the older population), specifically an excess loss of water-soluble vitamins and minerals (61). Reed and Mooradian (62) have reviewed the vitamin and mineral status of older adults with diabetes. Vitamins B_6, B_{12}, C, and D and the trace element zinc were found to be decreased in many individuals. Thiamin (vitamin B_1), folate, and the trace minerals chromium, selenium, and magnesium were decreased in some. Levels of vitamins A and E and iron were usually normal. Manganese may be increased or show no change. Copper is often increased.

Unfortunately, the older population is often vulnerable to non–research-based recommendations regarding use of nutritional supplements. Older adults should be advised first of the need to look carefully at the nutritional content of their meal plans for overall variety and compare them to the guidelines of the USDA Food Guide Pyramid and second of the need for a clinical laboratory evaluation to determine whether a true deficiency exists before supplementation is initiated.

Basic multivitamin/mineral supplements are among the most highly used nonprescription medications in the U.S. Data from NHANES II suggests that nearly 39% of the U.S. population aged 51–74 regularly takes this type of supplement. It also found that those older adults most likely to take them were also most likely to have an adequate nutritional intake (63).

IMPLEMENTING DIABETES MNT FOR THE OLDER ADULT

The four-step model of diabetes MNT (assessment, goal setting, intervention, and evaluation) provides a framework for providing continuous care for people of any age (64). Individualized treatment, in which the unique experiences and characteristics of the older adult are noted, and involvement by the family or caregiver in every step of the model (as appropriate) often increase the reliability of the information gathered and the chances for successful implementation.

As is true for younger individuals, diabetes medication should be matched to food intake and activity patterns, not vice versa. Older adults are not likely to make significant changes in eating patterns that have been established over a lifetime (e.g., a large meal at noon or two meals per day). The nutrition educator's time will be much better spent if the focus is on consistent intake of amounts and on the times meals and snacks are eaten. Education regarding pattern management, including guidelines for carbohydrate distribution throughout the day, and hypo-glycemia prevention and treatment can help to reinforce the importance of consistency and blood glucose monitoring in diabetes management.

Teaching older adults is rewarding, yet it often presents unique challenges to the educator that are specific to this age-group. It is important to recognize that just as diabetes treatment changes over time, so do a person's educational needs. Diabetes education must be seen as a lifelong continuum with emphasis on individualization and ongoing assessment. Suggested strategies for teaching effectively are summarized in Table 14.4.

Because diabetes often goes unrecognized or undertreated, many older patients may not receive adequate diabetes education. Jenny (65) found that older adults are frequently overlooked. In a study of four age-

---

Table 14.4 Strategies for Teaching Older Adults Effectively

- Teach in a setting free of background noise and other distractions
- Assess vision, hearing, and cognitive losses
- Assess educational needs and readiness to learn
- Recognize the influence of cultural, ethnic, and religious practices on behavior
- Screen for depression and anxiety, which interfere with learning
- Offer both one-on-one and group classes to provide socialization and support
- Include family and/or caregivers in teaching sessions
- Listen; utilize principles of adult learning: address client concerns first
- Individualize teaching and beware of ageism
- Actively involve client in decision making, from goal setting through evaluation
- Adapt teaching materials/style to meet client needs
- Present material in a variety of teaching formats
- Focus messages and limit teaching sessions to 45 min each
- Provide written information on key points for later reference
- Discuss or role-play real-life scenarios
- Demonstrate needed skills and observe return demonstration
- Allow time for questions

groups with diabetes, older adults were found to have the highest level of motivation but the second lowest level of instruction. Those with a mean age of 72 years received the least amount of diabetes education of any of the groups. Reasons for this inadequacy may include lack of understanding regarding the seriousness of the disease by both patients and health care professionals, ageism (i.e., prejudice against the elderly) among family members and health care providers, perception that providing diabetes education is too difficult or not worthwhile, financial constraints, transportation difficulties, social stigmas, functional dependence, and others. It is ironic that the population group with the greatest accumulation of knowledge and life experiences should be the least educated regarding how to manage this serious disease.

SPECIAL CONSIDERATIONS FOR RESIDENTS OF LONG-TERM CARE FACILITIES

According to a 1996 U.S. Census Bureau report, ~1% of young-old (age 65–74) adults were residing in long-term care facilities, compared with ~24% of the oldest old (age ≥85) (1). The older adult residing in a long-term care facility has the same needs as his community-dwelling counterpart, with several significant differences. For example, individuals in the long-term facility typically have reduced functional ability, thereby requiring more assistance in the activities of daily living; a greater number of comorbid conditions and thus an increased risk for drug-nutrient interactions; an increased rate of malnutrition and dehydration; and a greater rate of depression.

Malnutrition has been reported at rates of 10–85% in long-term care facilities (66). This is due in part to the admission of malnourished elders (previously community dwellers) whose nutritional status has declined secondary to illness or prolonged hospitalization. Nonetheless, if unrecognized, the visible signs and symptoms of nutrition deficiency may be mistaken for normal aging processes. Nutrition department staff are responsible for providing flavorful food of high quality that includes variety, choice, and consideration for the ethnic, cultural, and social preferences of the resident. Food that lacks these characteristics, as well as inappropriate restrictions, may serve to prolong or promote malnutrition. Nutrition providers must pay special attention to these and other psychosocial factors if they are to have a positive impact on the nutritional status of and level of care provided to all residents, including those with diabetes.

Nutrition intervention to reverse malnutrition typically includes *1)* modification in nutrient density and content, e.g., liberalized fat intake, larger portions of meat, etc.; *2)* modification in consistency and use of nutritional supplements; *3)* enteral nutrition support; and *4)* parenteral nutrition support.

Long-term care facilities have typically provided food to residents with diabetes by following a calorie-controlled menu (i.e., a 1,500-, 1,800-, or 2,000-calorie diet). In a study conducted by Coulston et al. (67), the glycemic control of residents of two long-term care facilities was evaluated after provision of a standard diabetic diet versus a regular diet. Acknowledging that this was a small study and that the subjects' glycemic control was good at the onset, the results indicated that short-term substitution of a regular diet versus a standard diabetic diet did not result in a deterioration of glycemic control for residents of these facilities.

The ADA suggests that as an alternative, long-term care facilities consider a newer approach in menu provision, i.e., the regular menu with a consistent carbohydrate content at meals (68,69). Basic principles of the diabetic diet are incorporated (controlled fat, protein at 10–20% of total calories, balance, and variety) with carbohydrate distribution throughout the day. A basic premise is that carbohydrate be provided in consistent amounts at meals and snacks from one day to the next (i.e., x amount of carbohydrate at the morning meal 7 days a week, y amount at the midday or evening meal 7 days a week, and so on). Calorie-restricted diets would not be used; however, the calorie content of an individual's diet could easily be adjusted to meet needs by altering meat portions, adjusting added fats, or changing snack composition. This system is suggested as a means to control glycemia while providing residents with a greater variety of carbohydrate-containing foods, including small portions of desserts. Research in this area is needed to give guidance regarding the optimal methods of meeting the nutritional needs of older adults with diabetes who reside in these facilities.

Weight loss is an indicator of poor nutritional status and is known to be a predictor of mortality in the elderly (70). Both undiagnosed and undertreated diabetes may contribute to weight loss in the older adult. As Table 14.5 illustrates, underweight may be more of a problem than obesity in long-term care residents. In subjects with diabetes, as in subjects without diabetes, slightly over 20% in each group were below average body weight, while only 8.5% were obese or overweight (71). Diagnosis and provision of appropriate treatment of hyperglycemia are critical. Both monitoring blood glucose and tracking weight trends in the long-term care resident will help to identify where adjustments in the diabetes management plan and further nutrition intervention are warranted.

Dehydration is a major problem in the older adult population, with the risk being highest in the oldest old (age ≥85), African Americans, and men. There are several reasons for the increased risk: reduced thirst sensation, decline in renal function with decreased ability to concentrate urine and conserve free water, changes in functional status, cognitive changes, medication side effects, and mobility disorders (72). In addition, fear of either incontinence or falls en route to the toilet may cause elders to decrease their intake of fluids. The risk of dehydration is height-

Table 14.5 Body Weight among Nursing Home Residents

	Subjects with Diabetes	Subjects without Diabetes
Age (years)	81 ± 1.6	78 ± 0.9
>20% ABW	4 (8.5%)	8 (9.0%)
<20% ABW	10 (21%)	20 (23%)

ABW, average body weight. From Mooradian et al. (71).

ened for those who are comparatively more frail and reside in long-term care. For the older adult with diabetes, dehydration poses a serious concern because inadequate fluid intake and hyperglycemia may result in a potentially deadly condition known as hyperglycemic hyperosmolar nonketotic syndrome (HHNS).

HHNS is characterized by very high blood glucose, without the presence of ketones. Glucose levels range from 400 to 2,800 mg/dl (22.2 to 155.5 mmol/l), with an average of just over 1,000 mg/dl (55.6 mmol/l). On initial exam, most patients have had polyuria and polydipsia for days or weeks. They are markedly dehydrated, with dry mucous membranes and doughy skin. Those who are mentally alert usually complain of extreme thirst, weakness, and fatigue. Mental status may range from mild confusion to hallucinations to coma. Treatment of HHNS includes hospitalization with insulin administration and fluid replacement, including electrolytes (73).

Prevention of HHNS includes provision of adequate fluids and documentation that they are taken by the older adult, as well as control of blood glucose. Daily fluid requirements have been calculated based on 30 ml water/kg body wt, with additional fluids recommended if any of the following conditions are present: infection, mild vomiting (≥500 ml/day), diarrhea (≥1,000 ml/day), elevated environmental temperature, diuretic or multiple medication use, high-protein feedings, history of dehydration, or out-of-control diabetes (74).

While critical, providing appropriate MNT to the long-term care resident with diabetes is just one component of a much larger concern: ensuring that these individuals receive high-quality, comprehensive diabetes care. Because of a variety of factors (e.g., lack of knowledge regarding current diabetes management practices, financial constraints, limited direct care staff), there may be a reluctance or lack of appreciation for intensifying diabetes management in this population group. Nutrition professionals with expertise in diabetes care must act as resident advocates. By sharing standards of care and "best practices" information with the staff and administration of the long-term care facility, significant progress in improving the care and quality of life for these older adults can be realized.

SUMMARY

Older adults comprise an increasingly greater percentage of the U.S. population. By the year 2000 it has been projected that there will be over 53 million people over age 65 (20% of the population). Older populations are disproportionately affected by diabetes. The impact is even more striking in older minority populations. Risk factors associated with diabetes in the older person include age-related changes in insulin resistance, coexisting chronic health conditions, physical inactivity, and body composition.

Diabetes management for the older person may be challenging for a number of reasons. Biological changes occur with the aging process that affect the nutrition prescription recommended for diabetes management, and psychosocial factors have a significant impact on older adults' abilities to successfully manage their diabetes and on the quality of life they are able to realize. Many older Americans are at risk for nutrition deficiencies, and protein-calorie deficiency often goes unrecognized. Most older adults with diabetes are not obese. Undernutrition is a much greater problem in the older population, especially among long-term care residents. Older adults with diabetes who reside in long-term care facilities are at greater risk for malnutrition than for obesity and are at greater risk than those living at home.

Eating habits and physical activity patterns have a significant role in the management and prevention of type 2 diabetes. If trends continue, an increasing number of overweight and/or physically inactive individuals can be expected to have an impact on the health care system like never before. How we tackle diabetes today will surely return to applaud or haunt us in the years to come. As nutrition professionals concerned about diabetes care, our role will be pivotal in deciding what the next 30–40 years will bring.

REFERENCES

1. U.S. Census Bureau: Sixty-five plus in the United States, Statistical Brief. http://www.census.gov/ftp/pub/socdemo/www/agebrief.html, June 6, 1996

2. Harris MI, Flegal KM, Cowie CC, Eberhardt MS, Goldstein DE, Little RR, Wiedmeyer HM, Byrd-Holt DD: Prevalence of diabetes, impaired fasting glucose, and impaired glucose tolerance in U.S. adults: the Third National Health and Nutrition Examination Survey, 1988–1994. *Diabetes Care* 21:518–524, 1998

3. Madshad S: Classification of diabetes in older adults. *Diabetes Care* 13:93–96, 1990

4. King H, Rewers M, WHO Ad Hoc Diabetes Reporting Group: Global estimates for prevalence of diabetes mellitus and impaired glucose tolerance in adults. *Diabetes Care* 16:157–177, 1993

5. Centers for Disease Control and Prevention: *Diabetes Surveillance, 1997*. Atlanta, GA, U.S. Department of Health and Human Services, Centers for Disease Control and Prevention, 1997

6. American Diabetes Association: Economic consequences of diabetes mellitus in the U.S. in 1997. *Diabetes Care* 21:296–309, 1998

7. Chen M, Bergman RN, Porte D Jr: Insulin resistance and β-cell dysfunction in aging: the importance of dietary carbohydrate. *J Clin Endocrinol Metab* 67:951–957, 1988

8. Fink RI, Kolterman OG, Griffin J, Olefsky JM: Mechanism of insulin resistance in aging. *J Clin Invest* 71:1523–1535, 1983

9. Jackson RA: Mechanisms of age-related glucose intolerance. *Diabetes Care* 13 (Suppl. 2):9–19, 1990

10. National Center for Health Statistics: *Current Estimates from the National Health Interview Survey, 1992*. Hyattsville, MD, Public Health Service, 1994 (ser. 10, no. 189, PHS 94-1517)

11. McGinnis JM, Foege WH: Actual causes of death in the United States. *JAMA* 270:2207–2212, 1993

12. U.S. Department of Health and Human Services: *Physical Activity and Health: A Report of the Surgeon General*. Atlanta, GA, U.S. Department of Health and Human Services, Centers for Disease Control and Prevention, National Center for Chronic Disease Prevention and Health Promotion, 1996

13. Clark DO: Racial and educational differences in physical activity among older adults. *Gerontologist* 35:472–480, 1995

14. Galuska DA, Serdula M, Pamuk E, Siegel PZ, Byers T: Trends in overweight among U.S. adults from 1987 to 1993: a multistate telephone survey. *Am J Public Health* 86:1729–1735, 1996

15. Pate RR, Pratt M, Blair SN, Haskell WL, Macera CA, Bouchard C, Buchner DM, Ettinger W, Heath GW, King AC, Kriska A, Leon AS, Marcus BH, Morris J, Paffenbarger RS, Patrick K, Pollock ML, Rippe JM, Sallis J, Wilmore JH: Physical activity and public health: a recommendation from the Centers for Disease Control and Prevention and the American College of Sports Medicine. *JAMA* 273:402–407, 1995

16. Goldberg AP, Coon PJ: Non-insulin dependent diabetes mellitus in the elderly: influence of obesity and physical inactivity. *Endocrinol Metab Clin* 16:843–865, 1987

17. Evans WJ, Cyr-Campbell D: Nutrition, exercise, and healthy aging. *J Am Diet Assoc* 97:632–637, 1997

18. Morley JE: Diabetes and its complications in older people. In *Endocrinology and Metabolism in the Elderly.* Morley JE, Korenman SG, Eds. Boston, Blackwell Scientific Publications, 1992, pp. 373–387

19. American Diabetes Association: Nutrition recommendations and principles for people with diabetes mellitus (Position Statement). *Diabetes Care* 21 (Suppl. 1):S32–S35, 1998

20. National Institutes of Health Consensus Conference: Diagnosis and treatment of depression in late life. *JAMA* 268:1018–1024, 1992

21. Lustman PJ: Depression in adults with diabetes. *Diabetes Spectrum* 7:187–189, 1994

22. Yesavage JA, Brink TL, Rose TL, Lum O, Huang V, Adey M, Leirer VO: Development and validation of a geriatric depression screening scale: a preliminary report. *J Psychiatr Res* 17:37–49, 1983

23. Beck AT, Ward CH, Mendelson M, Mock J, Erbaugh J: An inventory for measuring depression. *Arch Gen Psychiatry* 4:561–571, 1961

24. Krall LP, Beaser RS: Diabetes and aging. In *Joslin's Diabetes Manual.* 12th ed. Philadelphia, Lea & Febinger, 1989, pp. 240–245

25. Katz S, Ford AB, Moskowitz RW, Jackson BA, Jaffe MW: Studies of illness in the aged: the index of ADL. *JAMA* 185:914–919, 1963

26. *The OARS Methodology: Multidimensional Functional Assessment Questionnaire.* 2nd ed. Durham, NC, Duke University Center for the Study of Aging and Human Development, 1978, pp. 169–170

27. Walker D, Beauchene RE: The relationship of loneliness, social isolation and physical health to dietary adequacy of independently living elderly. *J Am Diet Assoc* 91:300–304, 1991

28. Fowles DG: *A Profile of Older Americans: 1995.* Washington, DC, American Association of Retired Persons and USDHHS Administration on Aging, 1995

29. Hunter GR, Treuth MS, Weinsier RL, Kekes-Szabo T, Kell SH, Roth DL, Nicholson C: The effects of strength conditioning on older women's ability to perform daily tasks. *J Am Geriatr Soc* 43:756–760, 1995

30. Green JS, Crouse SF: The effects of endurance training on functional capability in the elderly: a meta-analysis. *Med Sci Sports Exercise* 27:920–926, 1995

31. Skelton DA, Young A, Greig CA, Malbut KE: Effects of resistance training on strength, power, and selected functional abilities of women aged 75 and older. *J Am Geriatr Soc* 43: 1081–1087, 1995

32. Morganti CM, Nelson ME, Fiatarone MA, Dallal GE, Economos CD, Crawford BM, Evans WJ: Strength improvements with 1 year of progressive resistance training in older women. *Med Sci Sports Exercise* 27:906–912, 1995

33. Dengel DR, Hagberg JM, Coon PJ, Drinkwater DT, Goldberg AP: Effects of weight loss by diet alone or combined with aerobic exercise on body composition in older obese men. *Metabolism* 43:867–871, 1994

34. King AC, Haskell WL, Young DR, Oka RK, Stefanick ML: Long-term effects of varying intensities and formats of physical activity on participation rates, fitness, and lipoproteins in men and women aged 50 to 65 years. *Circulation* 91:2596–2604, 1995

35. Shaw JM, Snow-Harter C: Osteoporosis and physical activity. *Phys Activity Fitness Res Dig* 2:1–6, 1995

36. Casperson CJ, Kriska AM, Dearwater SR: Physical activity epidemiology as applied to elderly populations. *Bailliere's Clinic Rheumatol* 8:7–27, 1994

37. Simonsick EM, Lafferty ME, Phillips CL, Mendes de Leon CF, Kasl SV, Seeman TE, Fillenbaum G, Hebert P, Lemke JH: Risk due to inactivity in physically capable older adults. *Am J Public Health* 83:1443–1450, 1993

38. Rakowski W, Mor V: The association of physical activity with mortality among older adults in the longitudinal study of aging (1984–1988). *J Gerontol* 47:M122–M129, 1992

39. Fries JF, Singh G, Morfeld D, Hubert HB, Lane NE, Brown BW Jr: Running and the development of disability with age. *Ann Intern Med* 121:502–509, 1994

40. Blair SN, Kohl HW, Barlow CE, Paffenbarger RS, Gibbons LW, Macera CA: Changes in physical fitness and all-cause mortality. *JAMA* 273:1093–1098, 1995

41. Cummings SR, Nevitt MC, Browner WS, Stone K, Fox KM, Ensrud KE, Cauley J, Black D, Vogt TM: Risk factors for hip fracture in white women: Study of Osteoporotic Fractures Research Group. *N Engl J Med* 332:767–773, 1995

42. Province MA, Hadley EC, Hornbrook MC, Lipsitz LA, Miller JP, Mulrow CD, Ory MG, Sattin RW, Tinetti ME, Wolf SL: The

effects of exercise on falls in elderly patients: a preplanned meta-analysis of the FICSIT Trials: Frailty and Injuries: Cooperative Studies of Intervention Techniques. *JAMA* 273:1341–1347, 1995

43. Bernbaum MB, Albert SG, McGinnis J, Brusca S, Mooradian AD: The reliability of self blood glucose monitoring in elderly diabetic patients. *J Am Geriatr Soc* 42:779–781, 1994

44. McGandy RB, Barrows CH, Spanias A, Meredith A, Stone JL, Norris AH: Nutrient intakes and energy expenditure in men of different ages. *J Gerontol* 21:581–587, 1966

45. Russel RM: New views on the RDAs for older adults. *J Am Diet Assoc* 97:515–518, 1997

46. Dwyer JT: *Screening Older Americans' Nutritional Health: Current Practices and Future Possibilities.* Washington, DC, Nutrition Screening Initiative, 1991

47. Galanos AN, Pieper CF, Cornoni-Huntley JC, Bales CW, Fillenbaum GC: Nutrition and function: is there a relationship between body mass index and the functional capabilities of community-dwelling elderly? *J Am Geriatr Soc* 42:368–373, 1994

48. Frankenfield DC, Nuth ER, Rowe WA: The Harris-Benedict studies of human basal metabolism: history and limitations. *J Am Diet Assoc* 98:439–445, 1998

49. Peter D: *National Survey on Nutrition Screening and Treatment for the Elderly.* Washington, DC, Hart Research Associates, 1993

50. Ponza M, Ohls JC, Millen BE: *Serving Elders at Risk: The Older Americans Act Nutrition Programs, National Evaluation of the Elderly Nutrition Program, 1993–1995.* Washington, DC, Mathematical Policy Research, 1996

51. Nutrition Screening Initiative: *Nutrition Screening Manual for Professionals Caring for Older Americans.* Washington, DC, Nutrition Screening Initiative, 1991

52. Institute of Medicine, Food and Nutrition Board: *Dietary Reference Intakes for Calcium, Phosphorus, Magnesium, Vitamin D, and Fluoride.* Washington, DC, National Academy Press, 1997

53. Institute of Medicine, Food and Nutrition Board: *Dietary Reference Intakes for Thiamin, Riboflavin, Niacin, Vitamin B-6, Folate, Vitamin B-12, Pantothenic Acid, Biotin, and Choline.* Washington, DC, National Academy Press, 1998

54. Campbell WW, Crim MC, Dallal GE, Young VR, Evans WJ: Increased protein requirements in elderly people: new data and retrospective reassessments. *Am J Clin Nutr* 60:501–509, 1994

55. Brodsky IG, Robbins DC, Hiser E, Fuller SP, Fillyaw M, Devlin JT: Effects of low-protein diets on protein metabolism in insulin-dependent diabetes mellitus patients with early nephropathy. *J Clin Endocrinol Metab* 75:351–357, 1992

56. Expert Panel on Detection, Evaluation, and Treatment of High Blood Cholesterol in Adults: Summary of the second report of the National Cholesterol Education Program (NCEP) expert panel on detection, evaluation, and treatment of high blood cholesterol in adults (Adults Treatment Panel II). *JAMA* 269:3015–3023, 1993

57. Read NW, Abouzekry L, Read MG, Howell P, Ottewell D, Donnelly TC: Anorectal function in patients with fecal impaction. *Gastroenterology* 89:959–966, 1988

58. Egbert AM: The older alcoholic: recognizing the subtle clinical clues. *Geriatrics* 48:63–69, 1993

59. Sytkowski PA, Kannel WB, D'Agostino RB: Changes in risk factors and the decline in mortality from cardiovascular disease: the Framingham Heart Study. *N Engl J Med* 322:1635–1640, 1990

60. Kamath SV: Taste acuity and aging. *Am J Clin Nutr* 36:766–801, 1982

61. Mooradian AD, Failla M, Hoogwerf B, Maryniuk M, Wylie-Rosett J: Selected vitamins and minerals in diabetes (Technical Review). *Diabetes Care* 17:464–479, 1994

62. Reed RL, Mooradian AD: Nutritional status and dietary management of elderly diabetic patients. *Clin Geriatr Med* 6:883–901, 1990

63. Koplan JP, Annest JL, Layde PM, Rubin GL: Nutrient intake and supplementation in the United States (NHANES II). *Am J Public Health* 76:287–289, 1986

64. Tinker LF, Heins JM, Holler HJ: Commentary and translation: 1994 nutrition recommendations for diabetes. *J Am Diet Assoc* 94:507–511, 1994

65. Jenny JL: A comparison of four age-groups' adaptation to diabetes. *Can J Public Health* 75:237–244, 1984

66. Kerstetter JE, Holthausen BA, Fitz PA: Malnutrition in the institutionalized older adult. *J Am Diet Assoc* 92:1109–1116, 1992

67. Coulston AM, Mandelbaum D, Reaven GM: Dietary management of nursing home residents with non-insulin-dependent diabetes mellitus. *Am J Clin Nutr* 51:67–71, 1990

68. Schafer R, Bohannon B, Franz MJ, Freeman J, Holmes A, McLaughlin S, Haas L, Kruger D, Lorenz R, McMahon M: Trans-

lation of the diabetes nutrition recommendations for health care institutions (Technical Review). *Diabetes Care* 20:96–105, 1997

69. American Diabetes Association: Translation of the diabetes nutrition recommendations for health care facilities (Position Statement). *Diabetes Care* 21 (Suppl. 1):S66–S68, 1998

70. Henderson C: Nutrition and malnutrition in the elderly nursing home patient. *Clin Geriatr Med* 4:527–547, 1988

71. Mooradian AD, Osterweil D, Petrasek D, Morley JE: Diabetes mellitus in elderly nursing home patients. *J Am Geriatr Soc* 36:391–396, 1988

72. Weinberg AD, Menaker KL: Dehydration: evaluation and management in older adults: Council on Scientific Affairs, American Medical Association. *JAMA* 274:1552–1556, 1995

73. McCurdy DK: Hyperosmolar hyperglycemic nonketotic diabetic coma. *Med Clin North Am* 54:683–699, 1970

74. Campbell SM: Maintaining hydration status in elderly persons: problems and solutions. In *DNS Support Line*. Vol. XIV (3). Chicago, IL, American Dietetic Association, Dietitians in Nutrition Support Practice Group, 1992, pp. 7–10

Ms. McLaughlin is a diabetes and nutrition consultant in Omaha, NE.

15. Nutrition Therapy for Ethnic Populations

LEA ANN HOLZMEISTER, RD, CDE

Highlights

- The prevalence of type 2 diabetes is much higher among Native Americans, Asian Americans, Hispanic Americans, and African Americans. Complications also occur more often in minority populations.
- Successful diabetes prevention and treatment in diverse ethnic populations requires sensitivity to cultural differences in health beliefs and food habits.
- Food and food habits must be understood within the context of culture. Eating is a personal matter carrying with it great cultural significance.
- Cross-cultural counseling can be improved by health professionals using a four-step process involving self-evaluation, pre-interview research, in-depth interview, and unbiased analysis of the data.

INTRODUCTION

America is becoming increasingly multicultural. Hispanic Americans now comprise 8.6% of the U.S. population, and by the year 2050, they are expected to comprise 21% (1). Between 1970 and 1990, the number of people of Asian and Pacific Islander origin living in the U.S. increased almost fivefold (2).

Diabetes takes a toll on minority populations in the U.S. The prevalence of type 2 diabetes is much higher in Native Americans, Asian Americans, Hispanic Americans, and African Americans than in Americans of European descent (3). In people 45–74 years of age, the prevalence of diagnosed diabetes is 5.9% in non-Hispanic whites and Cuban Americans, 10.1% in non-Hispanic African Americans, and 14.3% in Mexican and Puerto Rican Americans. Although the prevalence of type 2 diabetes is variable in the more than 500 existing Native American tribes, the overall prevalence in Native Americans 19 years of age or older is 12.2%. In Pima Indians in Arizona, about half of the population between the ages of 30 and 64 has type 2 diabetes.

Diabetes complications occur more often in minority populations. In African Americans, the prevalence of blindness due to diabetic retinopathy (27–29%) is twice as high as that in whites (7–16%), but the prevalence is highest in Mexican Americans (32–40%). The incidence of end-stage renal disease in Native Americans compared with whites (6 times higher) is even greater than that reported in Mexican Americans compared with whites (4.5–6.6 times higher). Peripheral vascular disease is 84% more common in Mexican Americans than in whites.

Obesity and central-body obesity are risk factors for diabetes in African Americans, Hispanic Americans, Asian Americans, Pacific Islanders, and Native Americans. These risk factors are related to physical inactivity and a diet high in total and saturated fat. In those individuals with a genetic predisposition to diabetes, a westernized lifestyle leads to insulin resistance and diabetes. The incidence of type 2 diabetes could be reduced by almost 50% with obesity prevention.

CULTURAL INFLUENCES ON HEALTH AND NUTRITION

Successful diabetes prevention and treatment in diverse ethnic populations requires sensitivity to cultural differences in health beliefs and food habits. Each culture has a set of beliefs, assumptions, and values that shape the behavior of its members. A value system (widely held beliefs about what is worthwhile, desirable, or important for well-being) is a standard that people use to assess themselves and others. Developing knowledge, awareness, and respect for cultural differences and values influences the overall impact of intervention.

Cultures vary in their beliefs about the cause, prevention, and treatment of disease. These beliefs dictate the practices used to maintain health. Health practices can be folk practices, spiritual or psychic healing practices, or conventional medical practices (4). The value and perception of "good health" varies from one culture to another. Some cultures value duration of life more than quality of life. Thinness is considered to be a desirable health goal in some cultures, whereas in others it is perceived as poor health.

Diseases and illnesses are categorized differently among various cultures (5). A condition considered normal in one culture may be defined as a disease in another. Also, when no acute symptoms are present, clients may be unwilling to seek health care. Preventative health care, such as physical or eye examinations, may be avoided or considered unnecessary because no symptoms are present. For example, prenatal care may be delayed or avoided because childbirth is considered to be a natural and personal process.

The method by which health care is accessed is also influenced by cultural factors. Cultural healers or medicine men may be used instead of conventional medical care. Highly respected community or family members may provide physical and emotional support to believers. Unconventional beliefs and practices must be acknowledged and respected. Building on individual beliefs and involving support systems when developing an acceptable plan of care will ensure positive outcomes.

The foods and food habits of Americans reflect the diversity of the U.S. population. Each ethnic group has its own culturally based foods and food habits, and these must be understood within their own context. Eating is a personal matter, carrying with it great cultural significance. Food habits within a culture are influenced by numerous lifestyle factors such as income, availability of foods, societal level, religious beliefs, ethnic identity, household structure and composition, occupation, education, and nutrition knowledge (6). Understanding culturally based food and food habits is important when determining nutritional status and implementing dietary change. Because in the U.S. traditions have been influenced and modified through contact with other cultures, this understanding requires that the interactions between cultures be considered as well.

CROSS-CULTURAL COUNSELING

Cross-cultural nutrition counseling involves a health care professional working with a client from a different culture (7). The differences in ethnic heritages pose special challenges that require culturally sensitive communication strategies (5). The most common challenge facing the physician treating Mexican-American and Asian-American children and adolescents with type 2 diabetes has been reported to be communication (8). Knowledge about general ethnic, regional, and religious food habits and awareness of individual practices and preferences is essential to successful nutrition counseling (6). A four-step process involving self-evaluation, pre-interview research, in-depth interview, and unbiased data analysis has been developed to improve cross-cultural counseling (Table 15.1) (9).

Self-Evaluation

Self-evaluation is the first step to understanding another culture. Each individual has a specific ethnic, regional, and/or religious heritage unique

---

Table 15.1 Four Steps Toward Successful Cross-Cultural Counseling

Self-Evaluation
1. Identify cultural assumptions.
2. Evaluate culturally based categories of food use:
   - Is a food edible or inedible?
   - When is a food eaten?
   - What are considered meals and when are they eaten?
   - How are foods used symbolically?

Pre-Interview Research
1. Become familiar with the conventional worldview of client's culture.
2. Investigate immigration patterns to the U.S.
3. Learn about client's culturally based food habits:
   - What are traditional foods and ingredients?
   - What preparation methods are common?
   - What adaptations are often made in the U.S.?

In-Depth Interview
1. Ask questions about factors that influence food habits:
   - What is the client's ethnic identity?
   - How long has the client lived in the U.S.?
   - Where does the client live?
   - What are the client's religious beliefs?
   - What is the client's socioeconomic status?
   - What is the structure of the client's family?
   - What is the client's health status?
2. Determine the client's personal preferences regarding foods and food habits.

Unbiased Data Analysis
1. Evaluate the nutritional impact of the client's food habits:
   - Do they have positive health consequences?
   - Are they neutral?
   - Can their effect be determined?
   - Do they have demonstrably detrimental consequences?
2. Avoid ethnocentric or culturally biased approaches.

---

to him- or herself. Many assume that their culturally based values and attitudes are shared by all people and/or are superior to others. Ethnocentric assumptions may interfere with cross-cultural communication. For example, a health professional should not assume that a client follows the same meal pattern; meal patterns will vary from one culture to another. A typical American pattern is to eat three meals per day; however, eating two meals a day is the traditional pattern of many Native Americans and some Hispanic Americans.

Pre-Interview Research

The health professional must do pre-interview research to become familiar with the client's cultural background. Pre-interview research should uncover information on the client's country or region of origin, conventional worldview, immigration patterns to the U.S., traditional food habits, and common adaptations made in the U.S. (6). The world-view is a culture's outlook on life and includes factors such as religious values, role of the family, control over life, importance of human inter-actions versus importance of time, and family welfare versus individual welfare. Worldview can encompass food habits, health beliefs, and com-munication methods. A professional and client may experience value conflicts due to differences in cultural worldview (5).

Culturally based food habits are one of the most obvious expressions of ethnic, regional, or religious heritage of interest to health care profes-sionals involved in cross-cultural diet modifications (9). It is necessary to obtain knowledge about traditional food habits and adaptations made after immigration into the U.S. before counseling begins. Identifying the common ingredients consumed by a cultural group is fundamental. Conventional preparation methods and flavoring styles must be consid-ered as well. Health care professionals should also determine the way a specific culture defines a meal, when those meals are eaten, and the sym-bolic values attached to food. Developing this familiarity with traditional food habits serves as a basis for understanding individual adaptations.

In-Depth Interview

After the pre-interview research, an in-depth interview is used to establish the client's cultural background, adaptations made in the U.S., and personal preferences (9). Factors that influence individual food habits are ethnic identity, sex, age, length of time in the U.S., location of current residence, religious beliefs, socioeconomic status, family structure, and health status (10). In addition to exploring these factors, the in-depth interview should determine the client's personal preferences and establish exactly what the client is willing to modify in his or her diet. The pro-fessional should be aware that the client may consult with nontraditional health caregivers for metaphysical and spiritual health, which may affect recommended diet modifications.

Unbiased Data Analysis

The final step in successful cross-cultural counseling and culturally sensitive diet modification is unbiased analysis of the dietary data (9). The client's diet should be evaluated carefully within the context of the client's cultural and personal preferences, without ethnocentric approaches. The nutritional impact of food habits can be classified as having positive health consequences, neutral health consequences, unknown health consequences because of inadequate culturally specific data, and demonstrable detrimental health consequences (11).

Verbal and nonverbal communication are both important elements of cross-cultural counseling. The counselor's style of communication will reveal attitude and concern for the client. Messages are communicated by facial expressions and body movements that are specific to each culture (5). Awareness of eye contact, emotional expression, distance, body language, and other variations in nonverbal communications will avoid misunderstandings or inappropriate movements that may unintentionally offend clients. The health care professional should avoid verbal communication that is condescending or is done in an unpleasant tone. Articulation of each word and a positive tone are important, especially when working with a client whose native language is not English.

Fluency in spoken or written English does not correlate with intelligence. Some clients may not be able to read their native language. Some clients will be able to speak English well but not read it well, or vice versa. Therefore, do not assume that the level of fluency reflects the appropriate reading level when choosing written materials, whether they are in English or translated.

An interpreter must be included when counseling a non–English-speaking client. When working with an interpreter, instruct the interpreter on the goals of the program and the purpose of the counseling. Address the client directly instead of directing statements to the interpreter. Use language and examples the interpreter can understand and translate. Instruct the interpreter to use the client's own words instead of paraphrasing, and avoid complex ideas, difficult abstractions, or lengthy speeches without pauses.

In cross-cultural counseling, it may be difficult to get accurate information from clients. Establishing rapport and showing concern for the client will build a level of trust that encourages more accurate responses (5). To cross-check information, ask questions in several different ways. Using open-ended questions in counseling may increase the amount of information and accuracy of the information you obtain.

NUTRITION IMPLICATIONS OF FOOD HABITS

Specific differences between cultures in health beliefs, food practices, customs, and holidays and the nutrition implications of these differences are beyond the scope of this chapter. Information on selected ethnic groups has been published by The American Dietetic Association and the American Diabetes Association (12–21); see Table 15.2 for a sample table of contents. These publications have been developed for use by health

15.2 Sample Table of Contents of Ethnic and Regional Food Practice Series: Chinese American

- Diabetes in Chinese Americans
- Traditional Food and Health Beliefs
- Traditional Food Practices and Customs
- The Influence of American Food Habits
- Nutrition Implications of Current Dietary Practices
- Holiday Food Customs
- Culturally Appropriate Nutrition Counseling
- Current Nutrition Recommendations for Clients with Diabetes and Implications for Diet
- Meal Pattern for Traditional Chinese American Clients with Type 2 Diabetes
- Examples of Yin, Neutral, and Yang Foods
- Supplementary Exchange Lists for Chinese American Foods
- Nutrient Evaluation Database for Chinese Food Practices, Customs, and Holidays
- Glossary of Food Items
- Popular and Traditional Recipes–Modification with Nutrient Evaluations
- Additional Resources

professional who provide nutrition intervention and counseling to individuals with diabetes and their families. Each series is being revised to include a two-page client education sheet on diabetes meal planning. The current nutrition recommendations for clients with diabetes and implications for diet in selected groups have been compiled in Table 15.3.

REFERENCES

1. Stern MP, Mitchell BD: Diabetes in Hispanic Americans. In *Diabetes in America*. 2nd ed. Harris MI, Cowie CC, Stern MP, Boyko EJ, Reiber GE, Bennett PH, Eds. Bethesda, MD, National Institutes of Health, National Institute of Diabetes and Digestive and Kidney Diseases, 1995 (NIH publ. no. 95-1468), pp. 631–660

2. Fujimoto WY: Diabetes in Asian and Pacific Islander Americans. In *Diabetes in America*. 2nd ed. Harris MI, Cowie CC, Stern MP, Boyko EJ, Reiber GE, Bennett PH, Eds. Bethesda, MD, National Institutes of Health, National Institute of Diabetes and Digestive and Kidney Diseases, 1995 (NIH publ. no. 95-1468), pp. 661–682

3. American Diabetes Association: *Diabetes 1996: Vital Statistics*. Alexandria, VA, American Diabetes Association, 1996

4. Watkins EL, Johnson AE (Eds.): *Removing Cultural and Ethnic Barriers to Health Care, Proceedings of a National Conference.* Chapel Hill, NC, Univ. of North Carolina, 1979

5. U.S. Department of Agriculture, U.S. Department of Health and Human Services: *Cross-Cultural Counseling: A Guide for Nutrition and Health Counselors.* Washington, DC, U.S. Govt. Printing Office, 1987

6. Kittler PG, Sucher K: *Food and Culture in America: A Nutrition Handbook.* New York, Van Norstrand Reinhold, 1989

7. Magnus MH: What's your IQ on cross-cultural nutrition counseling? *Diabetes Educ* 22:57–62, 1996

8. Jones KL: Non-insulin dependent diabetes in children and adolescents: the therapeutic challenge. *Clin Pediatr* 37:103–110, 1998

9. Kittler PG, Sucher KP: Diet counseling in a multicultural society. *Diabetes Educ* 16:127–131, 1990

10. Pelto GH: Anthropological contributions to nutrition education research. *J Nutr Educ* 13:S2–S8, 1981

11. Jelliffe DB, Bennett FJ: Cultural and anthropological factors in infant and maternal nutrition. *Fed Proc* 20:185–188, 1961

12. Diabetes Care and Education Practice Group of The American Dietetic Association: *Ethnic and Regional Food Practices: Chinese American.* Chicago, IL and Alexandria, VA, The American Dietetic Association and the American Diabetes Association, 1998

13. Diabetes Care and Education Practice Group of The American Dietetic Association: *Ethnic and Regional Food Practices: Mexican American.* Chicago, IL and Alexandria, VA, The American Dietetic Association and the American Diabetes Association, 1998

14. Diabetes Care and Education Practice Group of The American Dietetic Association: *Ethnic and Regional Food Practices: Indian and Pakistani.* Chicago, IL and Alexandria, VA, The American Dietetic Association and the American Diabetes Association, 1996

15. Diabetes Care and Education Practice Group of The American Dietetic Association: *Ethnic and Regional Food Practices: Cajun and Creole.* Chicago, IL and Alexandria, VA, The American Dietetic Association and the American Diabetes Association, 1996

16. Diabetes Care and Education Practice Group of The American Dietetic Association: *Ethnic and Regional Food Practices: Filipino American.* Chicago, IL and Alexandria, VA, The American Dietetic Association and the American Diabetes Association, 1994

(References Continued on Page 292)

Table 15.3 Nutrition Implications for Selected Populations

	Calories	Protein	Total Fat and Cholesterol
Alaska Native	Encourage consumption of traditional foods. Discuss portion size. Decrease intake of low-nutrient-density American foods.	Moderate consumption of traditional fish, lean game meat, and sea animals. Low-fat cooking methods. Decrease intake of luncheon meat, bologna, wieners, sausage, and bacon. Encourage use of wild birds and dried fish.	Encourage consumption of omega-3–containing fish (salmon, herring, trout, and whitefish). Use small amounts of fish oil, seal oil, or margarine instead of butter or shortening. Limit organ meats to once a month.
Cajun and Creole	If overweight, reduce calories to achieve weight loss and to improve control of lipids, glucose, and blood pressure.	Encourage use of smaller portions of lean meat and substitutes. Cooked vegetables, beans, rice, and fruit can replace larger meat portions.	Use nonstick spray for well-seasoned cast-iron cookware; use oven-browned roux; replace bacon fat or lard with vegetable oil or margarine. Use low-fat cooking methods for meats. Skim fat off gumbo, gravy, stew, soup, fricassee after chilling. Use cocktail sauce instead of tartar sauce. Limit use of debris, tongue, sausage, chitterlings, boudin. Use lean ham or tasso in red beans instead of sausage. Use lean home-cooked meats instead of luncheon meats.
Chinese American	If overweight, reduce calories to achieve weight loss toward an appropriate weight for height. Encourage activities such as walking and tai chi.	Since the recommended level of milk and dairy consumption is relatively high for the Chinese population, additional protein from other food groups may be necessary. Encourage use of beans, tofu, or grains; meats are not customarily used in large quantities.	Reduce oil in cooking, especially in stir-frying; avoid lard or chicken fat in cooking; use peanut or polyunsaturated oils instead. Choose steaming over deep-fat frying. Skim fat off broths and soups. Avoid fatty meats such as pig feet, Chinese sausage, and marbled meat. Limit use of duckling and organ meats. Make noodle soups instead of fried noodles and boiled rice instead of fried rice. Use low-fat milk.

with Diabetes

Carbohydrate	Alternative Sweeteners	Sodium	Alcohol
Encourage consumption of vegetables (i.e., wild greens) and gardening. Encourage berry picking and use of fresh fruits, canned fruit in juice or water, and whole fruit in place of juice. Encourage use of whole-wheat flour in bread making, whole-grain cereals, and other whole-grain products.	Choose water or diet soda instead of regular soda, sugar-sweetened fruit drinks, or fruit punches. If needed, use alternative sweeteners in coffee, tea, and on cereal. Make clients aware of sugar-free products available.	Use less salt in cooking; taste food before adding salt; decrease intake of salty snack foods; use low-sodium soy sauce; rinse vegetables and cook in fresh water. Encourage plain dried fish and home-prepared foods instead of processed dinners.	Abstinence is best choice. Avoid binge drinking. Offer referrals to those with indications of abuse.
Use rice, French bread, or corn bread, dried beans and peas, starchy vegetables without added fat. On special occasions, use small portions of sweets, e.g., massepain, petites gateaux secs, plain King cake, or cane syrup.	Substitute diet soda for regular soft drinks. Use artificial sweeteners in beverages.	Substitute lean home-cooked meats for luncheon or canned meats. Avoid adding salt at mealtime. Cook rice in unsalted water.	Average consumption in this culture is more than advised limit. Select nonalcoholic beer; dilute wine and distilled liquor with ice cubes. Reduce frequency and quantity.
Continue to use allowable amounts of rice, rice congee, egg/rice/mung bean noodles, steamed buns. Sweeten broths with artificial sweeteners. Vegetables, fruits, brown rice, whole-wheat noodles, soybeans, and soybean products are good sources of fiber.	Substitute diet sodas for regular sodas and sweetened fruit drinks. Use nonnutritive sweeteners in beverages and sweet broths.	Use low-sodium seasonings, such as ginger, scallions, garlic, and coriander. Discourage use of monosodium glutamate, oyster sauce, shrimp paste, soy sauce, and other high-sodium seasonings for flavoring. Limit use of salted, canned, and preserved meat.	Beer is the alcoholic beverage of choice. Select light beer for fewer calories. Mix hard liquor with water, soda, or lots of ice cubes.

(Continued)

Table 15.3 Nutrition Implications for Selected Populations

	Calories	Protein	Total Fat and Cholesterol
Filipino American	Encourage overweight clients to select lower-calorie foods, especially snack foods. Portion control should be emphasized.	Be aware that most clients' protein intakes are probably adequate, if not high. Encourage continued use of fish, lean meats, and seafood and less use of glandular organs. Reduce frequency and quantity of intake of fatty meats; teach clients to trim visible fats and avoid chicken and pork skins. Use fortified milk containing added vitamins A and D. Substitute yogurt for non-milk drinkers.	Encourage clients to eat more fish, such as salmon, herring, trout, and whitefish, instead of fatty meats. Avoid butter, lard, and shortening. Encourage use of low-fat cooking methods. Use evaporated fat-free milk, fresh milk, or low-fat milk instead of whole milk. Substitute enriched cereal or bread for bacon, eggs, and sausage for breakfast. Avoid glandular organs or reduce consumption to once per month. Use oils low in saturated fats but high in polyunsaturates for cooking and salad dressings.
Hmong American	Encourage consumption of traditional foods and discourage high intake of low-nutrient-density American foods. Portion control should be emphasized.	Protein intake, especially of animal sources, probably has increased since immigration. Demonstrate portion sizes and encourage consumption of standard portion sizes of meat. Emphasize that there is no need to have meat at every meal.	Encourage replacement of pork lard with vegetable oil. Reinforce stir-frying with a small amount of oil. Discourage use of fatty cuts of meat, and encourage limited intake of organ meats. Encourage trimming fat from meat and removing skin from poultry.

with Diabetes (*Continued*)

Carbohydrate	Alternative Sweeteners	Sodium	Alcohol
Encourage a variety of carbohydrate foods, such as legumes and beans, which are high in fiber and can be used as meat substitutes. Because sweets and desserts play an important role in the social life of Filipinos, traditional sweet items can be substituted for food items of equal carbohydrate content on occasion. Use alternative sweeteners to sweeten foods. Encourage use of whole fruits instead of juice. Encourage continued use of traditional vegetable choices when available.	Use alternative sweeteners in desserts and sweets to reduce calories.	The typical Filipino uses salt and salt-rich condiments generously during cooking or on the table. Suggest that clients cut down on salt and salty condiments like toyo (soy sauce), patis (fish sauce), bagoong alamang (shrimp sauce), and vetsin (monosodium glutamate). Avoid or decrease salty main dishes such as daint (dried fish), tinapa (salted, smoked fish), tucino (pork, bacon-style), tapa (similar to beef jerky), and itlog maalat (salted eggs). Avoid salty snacks, such as salted nuts, chips, and cracklings.	For habitual alcohol use, especially beer and local wines, clients should be cautioned against adverse effects of alcohol on diabetes. Teach importance of eating food with drinks and sipping slowly.
Encourage continued consumption of wide variety of vegetables and fruits. Introduce clients to whole-grain bread and cereal products using the actual food item (Hmong clients often buy items on visual recognition). Encourage brown rice as a replacement for white rice. High-sugar foods may need to be divided into three groups: everyday foods, "some day" foods, and "not too many day" foods.	Explain the differences between alternative sweeteners and sugar. Describe how diet soft drinks differ from regular soft drinks. Discourage overconsumption of all sweeteners.	Encourage use of low-sodium seasonings (lemon grass, garlic, dill, coriander, lemon juice, lime juice, green onions, Thai chili peppers, and fresh herbs from the garden). Suggest limiting use of monosodium glutamate, fish sauce, and salt. Suggest occasional use of low-sodium soy sauce and pickled mustard greens.	Encourage limiting alcohol consumption at social gatherings.

(*Continued*)

Table 15.3 Nutrition Implications for Selected Populations

	Calories	Protein	Total Fat and Cholesterol
Indian and Pakistani	Attainment and maintenance of a reasonable body weight is encouraged. Yoga or other acceptable exercises can be encouraged as a first step.	The strict vegetarian's diet may provide around 10% protein, but nonvegetarians, lacto-vegetarians, and lacto-ovo-vegetarians have higher protein intakes. Encourage clients to use cereal-lentil dishes as source of vegetable protein more often, instead of omitting them in the acculturation process. Encourage use of lean meats, fish, and poultry. Educate about portion control.	Encourage use of monounsaturated fats, such as olive oil, instead of coconut oil or shortening, as well as fat-free milk, yogurt, and low-fat cheese instead of whole milk and heavy sour cream. Increase awareness of fat in gravies and curries. Explain that homemade paneer cheese can be made from low-fat milk and baked instead of deep-fried. Encourage low-fat cooking methods. Emphasize legume and vegetable dishes with low-fat preparation methods. Varied spices and condiments can bring out flavor while reducing ghee and oil.
Jewish	Teach portion control by practice of weighing and measuring foods to achieve prescribed calorie level.	Recommend use of smaller portions of lean protein sources. Encourage use of fresh, smoked, or water-packed canned fish (e.g., gelfite fish or sardines) instead of corned beef, pastrami, tongue, and salami. Suggest vegetarian main dishes, such as pea and bean soups, vegetarian burgers, and chili. Many wheat gluten and soy products are now Kosher.	Recommend use of reduced-fat or fat-free cheeses. Use nonstick pans with fat-free vegetable spray or portioned amount of oil instead of butter, stick margarine, or chicken fat (schmaltz). Pareve (neutral) nondairy creamers are often used as a dairy substitute at meat meals. Instead use light or fat-free versions. Use reduced-fat or low-fat chicken and turkey franks, bologna, and pastrami in place of beef hot dogs, knockwurst, and cold cuts. Use low-fat ingredients in food preparation.

with Diabetes (*Continued*)

Carbohydrate	Alternative Sweeteners	Sodium	Alcohol
Suggest methods of cooking breads and rice with no fat or use of vegetable spray, as well as modifying the total fat content. Encourage switching to brown rice. For the vegetarian client, low-fat tofu, low-fat dairy cheeses, or egg white may be suggested to supply protein. Emphasize portion control and consider carbohydrate content of legumes.	Try to reduce calories in concentrated desserts through use of alternative sweeteners.	Limit intake of salted pickles, chutneys, pappads, and high-sodium snacks. Encourage use of spices and lemon juice to replace salt and enhance taste.	Dilute wine or hard liquor with large amounts of ice. Select light beer instead of regular. Advise reduction or abstinence.
Emphasize use of complex carbohydrates (potatoes, whole-wheat noodles, brown rice, kasha, beans, peas, legumes, and whole-grain breads, crackers, and cereals) to increase fiber intake. Use fresh fruits and vegetables instead of juices and sweetened canned fruit and fruit compotes. Traditional desserts, such as mandlebrot, sponge cake, honey cake, poppy seed cake, and plain cookies, can be used on occasion. Use lower-fat preparation methods for foods such as knishes, kishka, kugels, potato pancakes, and cookies.	Sugar-free candies, gums, syrups, no-sugar-added cookies, cakes, yogurt, pudding, and jam are acceptable and should be incorporated into the meal plan.	Limit use of high-sodium foods, such has herring, lox, pickles, canned chicken broth or soups, delicatessen meats (corned beef, pickled tongue, hot dogs, pastrami), and cheese. Encourage use of reduced-sodium soups, herbs, and spices to season food. Recommend use of center cuts of meat from kosher butcher because salt from koshering process does not penetrate as much.	Traditional sweet kosher wine has 15 g carbohydrate in 4 oz (1/2 cup) and should be consumed in moderate amounts. Dry kosher wines are available and may be used for sacramental purposes.

(*Continued*)

Table 15.3 Nutrition Implications for Selected Populations

	Calories	Protein	Total Fat and Cholesterol
Mexican American	Teach portion control to achieve prescribed calorie intake.	For those who do not drink milk regularly, daily protein intake for the average 70-kg man would be equivalent to that in 8 oz of red meat or 2 cups of beans. For a 56-kg woman, intake would be 6.25 oz of meat or slightly more than 1.5 cups of beans.	Reduce oil used in preparing soups to <1 tsp. Prepare frijoles cocidos (boiled beans) instead of frijoles refritos (refried beans). Prepare meats asadas (grilled) instead of fried. Chill and skim fat off broths and stocks when preparing caldos (soups). Use low-fat milk instead of whole milk and cream. Avoid high-fat cheeses using part–skim milk queso fresco instead. Bake corn tortilla chips to replace fried chips. Rather than frying tortillas, heat in foil in oven, in heavy pan for short time on each side, or in microwave. Restrict chorizo (sausage) and menudo (tripe soup) to special occasions. Drain fat from fried chorizo, and trim visible fat from meats. Avoid using lard in cooking. Use polyunsaturated oils or olive oil instead.

with Diabetes (*Continued*)

Carbohydrate	Alternative Sweeteners	Sodium	Alcohol
Use corn tortillas instead of flour tortillas. Make tortillas from scratch using whole-wheat flour and appropriate type of margarine. Include beans daily to maintain high levels of soluble dietary fiber consumption. Increase intake of fresh fruits and vegetables. Drink water or diet soda instead of sweetened soft drinks. If diabetes is controlled and body weight is reasonable, occasionally incorporate sweets, such as pan dulce. Account for calories in the total meal plan. Use no added sugar in licuados and aguas frescas.	If client frequently consumes sweetened carbonated soft drinks, replace with water and diet sodas. Use artificial sweeteners in coffee and atole (hot beverage thickened with cornstarch).	Taste food before using salt. Minimize consumption of salty snack foods, such as chips, chicharrones (fried pork rinds), and dips. Instead of salt, use lemon in beer or on fruits such as melon. Add flavor to foods using onion, garlic, cumin, oregano, cilantro, and other spices.	Beer is consumed most frequently. Choose "light" beer, and reduce frequency or quantity consumed if excessive.

(*Continued*)

Table 15.3 Nutrition Implications for Selected Populations

	Calories	Protein	Total Fat and Cholesterol
Navajo	Traditional Navajo food preparation and consumption favors fried foods, added fat, and frequent consumption of high-fat products. Amount and type of fat must be modified to decrease caloric intake and reduce obesity and its associated health risks.	Recommended amount should be individualized depending on intake, size, etc. Portion size should be emphasized. Most clients probably consume adequate protein. However, those who have very low incomes, are isolated, and/or elderly or physically challenged may not consume adequate amounts. Advise clients that dried beans and peas are low-fat sources of protein.	Use lower-fat cooking methods and less blood sausage. Choose lean mutton and other meats. Mutton is a popular staple and many Navajo feel that a fat sheep is a healthy sheep. Encourage them to trim off the fat before cooking. Spoon off and discard fat from commodity meats. Eat less high-fat meat, such as Spam, bologna, wieners, sausage, bacon, corned beef, and fried meats. Use small amounts of vegetable oil or fat-free broth when cooking instead of lard, fatback, pig's feet, and bacon grease. Eat fewer high-fat dairy products, such as commodity cheese, or mix commodity cheese with reduced-fat or nonfat cheeses. Control portion sizes. Eat cereal, bread, and tortillas more often than eggs for breakfast.
Soul and Traditional Southern	Traditional soul food favors fried foods, added fat, and frequent consumption of high-fat products. The amount and type of fat must be modified to decrease caloric intake and reduce obesity and its associated health risks.	Protein intake should be individualized. Portion size should be emphasized. Meatless main dishes are encouraged.	Intake of high-fat meats, such as chicken wings, bologna, sausage, and fried meats, should be avoided. Vegetable oil, skin-free smoked turkey necks, Liquid Smoke, margarine, and fat-free broth should replace lard, fatback, ham hocks, and bacon grease when seasoning vegetables. Encourage use of egg substitutes in recipes.

with Diabetes (*Continued*)

Carbohydrate	Alternative Sweeteners	Sodium	Alcohol
Emphasize the benefits of whole-wheat and whole-grain breads and cereals. Potatoes, beans, and corn should be incorporated into meal patterns. Encourage more vegetables (hominy) in stews and less meat. Make Navajo tacos with larger amounts of beans, lettuce, and tomatoes, smaller amounts of meat, and smaller pieces of fry bread. Eat more breads and cereals, such as blue corn mush, oatmeal, or a low-sugar, high-fiber dry cereal at breakfast. Make tortillas and other quick-bread items with whole-wheat flour replacing half the white flour. Encourage consumption of whole fruits instead of fruit juice and smaller portions of high-sugar foods.	Some clients may not have easy access to safe, good-tasting water. Encourage purchasing bottled or gallon water instead of soda or substituting diet for regular soda. Discuss non-sugar-sweetened versions of foods available, such as fruit-flavored gelatin and beverages. Some clients mistakenly believe that the risks from using artificial sweeteners are greater than risks from high blood glucose levels from intake of sugar.	Clients should eat high-salt items, such as bologna and Spam, in moderation.	High rates of alcohol abuse among Native Americans—including Navajos—warrant that special care be taken never to encourage alcohol consumption. All clients should be queried regarding their alcohol use and referred for appropriate counseling if there are indications of abuse. Alcohol intake often stimulates food intake, and most clients with diabetes should avoid excess food intake.
Emphasize benefits of whole-wheat and whole-grain breads and cereals. Encourage fresh fruits and vegetables instead of canned. Beans and peas, rice, sweet and white potatoes, and corn should be incorporated into meal patterns. Sweets, such as a small portion of pound cake or sweet potato pie, can occasionally be eaten.	Sugar-free soft drinks, ice cream, frozen yogurt, powdered drinks, hot beverages, Popsicles, yogurt, pudding, and gums made with alternative sweeteners can be incorporated into the meal plan.	Avoid frequent consumption of smoked, dried, or salt-cured meat products. Discourage use of salt and salty seasonings, such as meat tenderizer. Boiled peanuts should be avoided by those on a sodium-restricted diet. Prepared buttermilk and buttermilk biscuits have a significant sodium content.	Intake of home-distilled liquor and frozen sweetened drinks should be discouraged.

17. Diabetes Care and Education Practice Group of The American Dietetic Association: *Ethnic and Regional Food Practices: Alaska Native*. Chicago, IL and Alexandria, VA, The American Dietetic Association and the American Diabetes Association, 1993

18. Diabetes Care and Education Practice Group of The American Dietetic Association: *Ethnic and Regional Food Practices: Soul and Traditional Southern*. Chicago, IL and Alexandria, VA, The American Dietetic Association and the American Diabetes Association, 1995

19. Diabetes Care and Education Practice Group of The American Dietetic Association: *Ethnic and Regional Food Practices: Hmong American*. Chicago, IL and Alexandria, VA, The American Dietetic Association and the American Diabetes Association, 1992

20. Diabetes Care and Education Practice Group of The American Dietetic Association: *Ethnic and Regional Food Practices: Navajo*. Chicago, IL and Alexandria, VA, The American Dietetic Association and the American Diabetes Association, 1991

21. Diabetes Care and Education Practice Group of The American Dietetic Association: *Ethnic and Regional Food Practices: Jewish*. Chicago, IL and Alexandria, VA, The American Dietetic Association and the American Diabetes Association, 1989

Ms. Holzmeister is a pediatric nutritionist at Phoenix Children's Hospital, Phoenix, AZ.

Medical Nutrition Therapy and Diabetes Complications

16. Hypertension and Medical Nutrition Therapy

JUDITH WYLIE-ROSETT, EdD, RD

Highlights

- The Joint National Committee (JNC) on Prevention, Detection, Evaluation and Treatment of High Blood Pressure recommends a blood pressure goal of <130/85 mmHg in individuals with diabetes and proteinuria ≤1 g/day. When proteinuria is >1 g/day, the JNC recommends a blood pressure goal of <125/75 mmHg.
- Clinical trial data suggest that a weight loss of 4.5 kg (10 lb) can be as effective as first-level drugs in controlling blood pressure. Weight reduction can also lessen medication dosage and improve quality of life.
- On the basis of meta-analyses of controlled clinical trials involving sodium restriction, the JNC recommends reducing sodium intake to 2,400 mg/day to reduce blood pressure in individuals with hypertension. However, metabolic studies indicate that severe sodium restriction can increase lipid levels and biomarkers of insulin resistance.

INTRODUCTION

The 6th Joint National Committee (JNC) on Prevention, Detection, Evaluation and Treatment of High Blood Pressure defines hypertension as an elevated blood pressure with a systolic level of ≥140 mmHg and/or a diastolic level of ≥90 mmHg or use of antihypertensive medication (1). The JNC blood pressure classifications are listed in Table 16.1. A systolic blood pressure level <120 mmHg and a diastolic level <80 mmHg are considered optimal (1).

Table 16.1 Blood Pressure Classifications

Category	Blood Pressure (mmHg)		
	Systolic		Diastolic
Optimal	<120	and	<80
Normal	<130	and	<85
High-Normal	130–139	or	85–89
Hypertension			
Stage 1	140–159	or	90–99
Stage 2	160–179	or	100–109
Stage 3	≥180	or	N ≥ 110

When systolic and diastolic blood pressures fall into different categories, the higher category should be selected to classify the individual's blood pressure status. In addition to classifying stages of hypertension on the basis of average blood pressure levels, clinicians should specify presence or absence of target organ disease and additional risk factors. This specificity is important for risk classification and treatment. Optimal blood pressure with respect to cardiovascular risk is <120/80 mmHg. However, unusually low readings should be evaluated for clinical significance. Hypertension is based on the average of two or more readings taken at each of two or more visits after an initial screening. From the Joint National Committee on Prevention, Detection, Evaluation and Treatment of High Blood Pressure (1).

Estimates from the National Health and Nutrition Examination Survey (NHANES) III and the 1990 census indicate that as many as 50 million Americans have hypertension (1). The prevalence of hypertension increases to 60% or more of the population >60 years of age (1). Among Americans >60 years of age examined in NHANES III, 60% of non-Hispanic whites, 71% of non-Hispanic African Americans, and 61% of Mexican Americans had elevated blood pressure (1,2). Estimates of the prevalence of hypertension in individuals with diabetes range from 40 to 70%. In type 2 diabetes, essential hypertension often precedes the development of diabetes as a concomitant condition associated with the metabolic syndrome. Hypertension can also develop as the result of diabetic nephropathy. Irrespective of the etiology of hypertension in diabetes, it is considered a major factor in the development of the cardiovascular complications of diabetes.

Diabetes, other risk factors for cardiovascular disease, and evidence of end-organ damage elevate the hypertension risk strata as indicated in Table 16.2. Elevated blood pressure results in the following target-organ diseases: cardiac (evidence of coronary disease, left ventricular dysfunction, or cardiac failure), cerebrovascular (transient ischemic attack or stroke—also termed "brain attack" to convey the need for emergency medical treatment) (3), peripheral vascular (absence of one or more major pulses in the extremities, except the dorsalis pedis), renal (serum creatinine ≥1.5 mg/dl, ≥1+ proteinuria, microalbuminuria), retinal (hemorrhages or exudates) (1). The JNC recommends drug therapy for a less elevated blood pressure in individuals with diabetes or in other high-risk categories. Although the evidence regarding specific medication options is beyond the scope of this chapter, the JNC recommends that the blood pressure treatment goal be <130/85 mmHg in individuals with diabetes and proteinuria ≤1 g/day. When proteinuria is >1 g/day, a blood pressure goal of <125/75 mmHg is recommended. Clinical trial data indicate that angiotensin-converting enzyme (ACE) inhibitors are renoprotective (4) and are thus the medication of choice when diabetic proteinuria is present.

Over the past 2 decades, there has been a dramatic increase in the rates of awareness, treatment, and control of hypertension. NHANES I data (1971–1972) indicate a hypertension awareness rate of 51% and a blood pressure control rate of 10%. NHANES III phase 2 (1988–1991)

Table 16.2 Components of Cardiovascular Risk Stratification in Patients with Hypertension

Major Risk Factors
- Smoking
- Dyslipidemia
- Diabetes
- Age >60 years
- Sex (men and postmenopausal women)
- Family history of cardiovascular disease: women <65 years or men <55 years

Target Organ Damage/Clinical Cardiovascular Disease
- Heart diseases
  - −Left ventricular hypertrophy
  - −Angina or prior myocardial infarction
  - −Prior coronary revascularization
  - −Heart failure
  - −Stroke or transient ischemic attack
- Nephropathy
- Peripheral arterial disease
- Retinopathy

From the Joint National Committee on Prevention, Detection, Evaluation and Treatment of High Blood Pressure (1).

data indicate that 73% of all hypertensive individuals are aware of their diagnosis, that 55% are treated with antihypertensive medication, and that 29% have achieved blood pressure control to levels ≤140/90 mmHg (1). This improvement in awareness, treatment, and control was associated with a decrease in the age-adjusted mortality rate of nearly 60% for stroke and 53% for coronary heart disease (1).

Numerous randomized controlled clinical trials have provided strong evidence that lowering blood pressure reduces morbidity and mortality. A 1990 meta-analysis (using 9 major prospective studies and 14 randomized clinical trials) indicated that a 42% reduction in stroke and a 20–25% reduction in coronary heart disease were achievable from a 5- to 6-mmHg reduction in diastolic blood pressure (5,6). Reducing elevated isolated systolic blood pressure from a mean of 155 mmHg to a mean of 143 mmHg resulted in a 36% reduction in the stroke rate (7).

In the U.K. Prospective Diabetes Study (UKPDS), in individuals with type 2 diabetes, lowering blood pressure to a mean of 144/82 mmHg significantly reduced strokes, diabetes-related deaths, heart failure, microvascular complications, and visual loss (8,9). ACE inhibitors and beta-blockers were equally effective and safe to use. However, because of the low prevalence of nephropathy in the study subjects, it was unclear whether either drug exerted a protective effect on the progression of nephropathy. The results of a current randomized clinical trial will provide additional evidence that can be used to establish blood pressure management guidelines focusing on diabetes. Interim results from the randomized controlled clinical trial Appropriate Blood Pressure Control in Diabetes (ABCD) indicated that treatment with the ACE inhibitor enalapril resulted in lower rates of fatal and nonfatal coronary disease than did treatment with the calcium-channel blocker nisoldiprine in hypertensive patients with diabetes (10). Other end points of the 5-year ABCD Trial include glomerular filtration rate, urinary albumin excretion, left ventricular hypertrophy, retinopathy, and neuropathy. The ABCD study population includes 470 hypertensive individuals and 480 normotensive individuals, all of whom have type 2 diabetes, and its results are expected to provide guidance in the clinical management of diabetes and hypertension.

Pharmacological studies demonstrate the importance of reducing blood pressure in preventing stroke and coronary disease (1). However, the focus of this chapter is on medical nutrition therapy (MNT) as primary and adjunctive therapy for hypertension. Therefore, specific antihypertensive medication will be discussed only in relation to MNT nutrition therapy for diabetes.

The JNC (1) has reviewed research and has achieved consensus that the adverse effects of hypertension can be prevented by the following treatment: *1*) controlling blood pressure to a level ≤135/85 mmHg in individuals with diabetes (use of ACE inhibitors for diabetic nephropathy); *2*) modifying lifestyle to achieve blood pressure control and/or reduce overall cardiovascular risk; *3*) adding, increasing, or changing antihypertensive medications if blood pressure remains ≥140/90 mmHg for 3–6 months; and *4*) selecting antihypertensive therapy that does not worsen any concomitant disease or therapy.

Among individuals with diabetes, pharmacological therapy is recommended in the treatment of hypertension (1). Although lifestyle modification and MNT for hypertension and diabetes have not been directly addressed in randomized controlled clinical trials, the literature addressing lifestyle modification in hypertension treatment provides insights regarding diabetes.

HYPERTENSION TREATMENT AND MNT

The evidence for inclusion of MNT as a component of hypertension treatment guidelines for patients with diabetes is based on consideration of study designs, nutrition variables, subject characteristics, study lengths, study endpoints, and types of analyses. The 6th JNC (1) adapted the study classifications of Last and Abramson (11) in reviewing the strength of evidence for prevention and treatment of high blood pressure. The type of studies reviewed and the abbreviations used are from the 6th JNC (1). Because of the large number of studies, the evidence considered in evaluation of the efficacy of the MNT option is limited to randomized controlled trials and meta-analyses of such studies. The types of studies considered by the 6th JNC include:

1. Randomized controlled trials (Ra)
2. Meta-analyses (M)
3. Retrospective analyses, often termed case-control studies (Re)
4. Prospective follow-up, also known as cohort studies (F)
5. Cross-sectional population studies, also known as prevalence studies (X)
6. Previous review or position statement (Pr)
7. Clinical interventions—nonrandomized (C)

The extent to which studies can be generalized to the treatment of hypertension in diabetes depends on a number of factors. The study design and duration need to be sufficient to determine whether a lifestyle modification or nutrition therapy is practical, acceptable, and feasible for patients with diabetes and hypertension.

Data analyses need to address how a study intervention affects subjects with diabetes if the study is not focusing on diabetes per se. The number of study subjects with diabetes needs to be enough to ensure that there is sufficient statistical power to determine how the intervention interacts with diabetes and/or its treatment (i.e., whether the nutrition variables adversely affect diabetes control or whether diabetes alters the effects of the treatment on hypertension control or study endpoints). Analyses should determine whether treatment effects differ in subcategories of study subjects that may be related to the common concomitant conditions (obesity, dyslipidemia) or diabetic complications or the diabetes treatment(s).

Dietary Modifications

The JNC's recommendations for lifestyle modifications for hypertension prevention and management, which are outlined in Table 16.3, focus on the needs of the general population. Table 16.4 summarizes randomized clinical trials that address the effects of various dietary and nutrient modifications on blood pressure.

Weight reduction. Data from randomized clinical trials indicate that a comprehensive approach to lifestyle modification can be effective in lowering blood pressure to prevent the development of overt hypertension and in treating hypertension (12,13). Randomized clinical trials have also demonstrated that calorie restriction and weight loss can not only reduce blood pressure but also reduce left ventricular mass (14). Although one controlled trial failed to demonstrate any additive effect

---

Table 16.3 Lifestyle Modifications for Hypertension Prevention and Management

- Lose weight, if overweight
- Limit alcohol intake to no more than 1 oz (30 ml) of ethanol (e.g., 24 oz [720 ml] of beer, 10 oz [300 ml] of wine, or 2 oz [60 ml] of 100-proof whiskey) per day or 0.5 oz (15 ml) per day for women and lighter-weight people
- Increase aerobic physical activity (30–45 min) most days of the week
- Reduce sodium intake to no more than 100 mmol/day (2.4 g sodium/6 g NaCl)
- Maintain adequate intake of dietary potassium (~90 mmol/day)
- Maintain adequate intakes of dietary calcium and magnesium for general health
- Reduce intakes of dietary saturated fat and cholesterol for overall cardiovascular health
- Stop smoking

From the Joint National Committee on Prevention, Detection, Evaluation and Treatment of High Blood Pressure (1).

Table 16.4 Randomized Controlled Clinical Trials: Effects of Dietary Modification on Blood Pressure

Intervention	Results	Population	Duration	Reference
Dietary plan was designed to be "ideal" with 7–8 servings/day grains, 4–5 servings/day vegetables, 4–5 servings/day fruits, 2–3 servings/day low-fat dairy products, ≤2 servings/day meat, and 4–5 servings/week nuts or legumes.	BP decreased significantly in both hypertensive and nonhypertensive groups.	Eligibility criteria included sBP <160 and dBP 80–95 (n = 459).	8 weeks	12
Intervention goals included >4.5 kg weight loss, dietary Na <1,800 mg, modified-fat diet, <26 g alcohol, and exercise 30 min 3 times/week.	Hypertension conversion rate was 8.8% in lifestyle group compared with 19.2% in control group.	Participants were 10–49% over desirable body weight and had high-normal BP (n = 201).	5 years	13
Individualized dietary intervention was planned to achieve a 1,000 kcal deficit, with 15% of calories from protein, 30% from fat, and 55% from carbohydrate.	Dietary intervention resulted in a mean weight loss of 8.3 kg and a decrease in BP. Left ventricular mass decreased by 20% (16% adjusted for body surface area).	Eligibility criteria included BMI >26 and stage 1 or 2 hypertension (n = 41).	21 weeks	14
Study was to determine whether the effects of dietary and exercise intervention were additive compared with exercise training vs. diet.	All three intervention arms had similar effects on lowering BP.	Participants were sedentary, overweight, and had high normal BP or stage 1 or 2 hypertension (n = 55).	12 weeks	15
Hypocaloric or low-sodium diet was tested with drug therapy.	Weight-reduction and low-sodium groups had lower rates of cardiovascular events.	Eligibility criteria included age 60–80 years and dBP 95–110 mmHg (n = 875; 585 obese, 290 lean).	3 years	16

(Continued)

Table 16.4 Randomized Controlled Clinical Trials: Effects of Dietary Modification on Blood Pressure (Continued)

Intervention	Results	Population	Duration	Reference
Study used factorial design to evaluate nine diet-drug combinations. Interventions included low-Na, high-K diet, weight reduction, beta-blockers, and diuretics. Step up of drugs if BP was not controlled.	All interventions decreased BP; weight loss had similar effects to first-step drug dose but Na/K modification was less effective.	Eligibility criteria included being 110–160% of desirable body weight and stage 1 or 2 hypertension.	26 weeks	17–19
Phase 1 intervention arms included weight loss; Na reduction; and supplementation with Ca, Mg, K, or fish oil. Study results were used to select intervention for phase 2.	BP decreased with weight loss and Na restriction, but not with any of the supplements.	Participants were 35–54 years of age and had dBP 80–89 mmHg (n = 2,128).	18 months	20
Na-restriction controlled clinical trials were selected for a meta-analysis. Study inclusion criteria included having Na-restriction and control groups, monitoring by timed Na excretion, and using both sBP and dBP as outcomes measures.	Decrease for a 100 mmol/day decrease in Na was 3.7 mmHg for sBP (P > 0.001) and 1.0 mmHg for dBP (P < 0.001) in trials with hypertensive subjects. There were no significant changes in BP in trials with normotensive subjects.	Analysis of data from 56 randomized clinical trials (n = 1,131 hypertensive subjects; n = 2,374 normotensive subjects).	Varied	21
Controlled clinical trials that included a comparison of omega-3 fatty acid supplementation to no treatment were analyzed. Net BP change was calculated based on mean BP change in the control group minus change in the intervention group.	Diet supplementation with >3 g/day of omega PUFA reduced BP significantly for hypertensive but not normotensive subjects.	This meta-analysis of controlled clinical trials included 11 normotensive (n = 728) and 6 hypertensive (n = 291) trials.	Varied	31

Controlled clinical trials that included a Ca supplementation arm were included in the meta-analysis.	Ca supplement resulted in a 1.7-mmHg reduction in sBP and no effect on dBP.	Data from 28 active treatment arms from 22 studies were included (n = 1,231).	Varied	32
Controlled clinical trials that included a comparison of K supplementation to no treatment were analyzed. Findings of the trial were pooled after the results of each trial were weighted by the inverse of its variance.	Mean reduction in BP 3.1 and 2.0 mmHg for sBP and dBP, respectively. BP-lowering effect was greater in studies in which Na intake was high and/or dietary K intake was low.	This meta-analysis included 33 controlled clinical trials (n = 2,609).	Varied	33

BP, blood pressure; dBP, diastolic blood pressure; PUFA, polyunsaturated fatty acid; sBP, systolic blood pressure.

of combining exercise and dietary change in lowering blood pressure (15), weight loss per se lowers the dose requirement for blood pressure medication (16). The Trial of Antihypertensive Intervention and Management (TAIM) achieved a mean weight loss of 4.5 kg (10 lb) (17–19), and this level of weight loss was as effective as the first level of medication in controlling hypertension (19). The JNC also indicated that 4.5-kg (10-lb) weight loss can be effective in controlling stage 1 hypertension (1). Several clinical trials suggest that equivalent levels of blood pressure reduction can be achieved with as much as a 50% reduction in medication dosage when combined with weight-reduction intervention (19). The level of side effects was also reported to be lower (17).

Sodium restriction and electrolyte balance. The efficacy of sodium restriction and weight loss was demonstrated in phase 1 of the Trial of Hypertension Prevention (TOHP) (20). Modifying dietary intake to reduce sodium and increase potassium intake was more difficult to achieve than was reducing weight in overweight TAIM participants (17). Increasing dietary potassium intake was particularly difficult (18). However, maintaining a normal blood potassium level is important to prevent the adverse effects of diuretic therapy on blood glucose levels that may be the result of potassium depletion (1). Dietary or pharmacological intervention to maintain normal potassium levels can reduce insulin resistance and improve blood glucose levels.

Meta-analysis of sodium intervention studies indicates that sodium restriction has a blood pressure–lowering effect only in trials conducted in individuals with hypertension (21). This beneficial effect was not found in trials conducted in normotensive subjects (22). Table 16.5 lists studies that address questions related to the benefits and potential risks associated with sodium restriction in the management of diabetes. Sodium sensitivity appears to be higher in selected populations, such as individuals with diabetes and older adults (22). Although sodium sensitivity has been linked to diabetes, a controlled clinical trial found that glucose tolerance deteriorated and insulin levels were higher during sodium restriction, even in individuals identified as sodium sensitive (23). A small randomized trial of calcium-channel blockers found that the addition of a low-sodium diet did not have an independent effect on albumin excretion in patients with type 2 diabetes (24). In a study of patients with type 1 diabetes, nephropathy, and high-normal or hypertensive blood pressure levels, decreasing sodium from 200 mmol (4,600 mg) to 100 mmol (2,300 mg) achieved a slight reduction in blood pressure, and the blood pressure correlated with angiotensin II levels (25). In controlled intervention studies of nondiabetic subjects, sodium restriction resulted in higher lipid levels and increased insulin resistance in both normotensive and hypertensive subjects (26–28). Prospective epidemiological studies have linked lower urinary sodium excretion to higher myocardial infarc-

Table 16.3 Studies Addressing Sodium Sensitivity of Potential Risks Associated With Sodium Restriction

Study Methods	Design	Results	Population	Reference
Study consisted of 1-week feeding periods in random order to assess BP effects of high and low Na intake. Subjects were classified as salt sensitive if rise in MAP ≥5 mmHg on high Na intake, salt resistant if change was <5 mmHg, and counterregulators if MAP rose by 5 mmHg.	Ra	Overall MAP rose from 101.9 to 103.7 mmHg during salt load. Overall, 23.9% were salt sensitive, 50% were salt resistant, and 17.4% were counterregulators. Among those >45 years, 10 of 11 were salt sensitive.	Subjects were white, nonobese, aged 25–80 years, with essential hypertension ($n = 46$).	22
Study evaluated whether salt sensitivity was related to GTT response during low-Na diet (34 mmol Na) and high-Na diet (347 mmol Na). The effects of Na on glucose and insulin independent of Na sensitivity were also examined. AUC for glucose and insulin were calculated. Na sensitivity was calculated as the difference between BPs between the two Na periods.	Ra	AUC for both glucose and insulin during the GTT was lower during the high-Na period, and glucose and insulin responses were not related to the index for salt sensitivity.	Subjects had essential hypertension ($n = 31$).	23
Purpose of the study was to determine whether albumin excretion in patients treated with either of two long-acting Ca-channel blockers differed with 250-mmol Na or 50-mmol Na diet. The medication protocol altered to maintain BP <140/90 mmHg.	Ra	Albumin excretion level was reduced with the initiation of medication and was not altered by Na level as long as BP was maintained in the target range.	Subjects had type 2 diabetes, hypertension, renal insufficiency, macroalbuminuria, and were treated with furosemide ($n = 15$).	24
A 4-week double-blind intervention trial using Na supplementation compared the effects of Na intake of 90 mmol vs. 190 mmol on exchangeable body Na, fluid balance, and volume, and components of the renin-angiotensin-aldosterone system, arterial natriuretic peptide and catecholamines.	Ra	Diastolic BP was 3.9 mmHg and lower in the low-Na group. Na excretion correlated with blood volume, BP, angiotensin II, and renin levels.	Subjects had type 1 diabetes, nephropathy, and high-normal, or stage 1, hypertension.	25

(Continued)

Table 16.5 Studies Addressing Sodium Sensitivity or Potential Risks Associated with Sodium Restriction (*Continued*)

Study Methods	Design	Results	Population	Reference
Fasting serum lipids, glucose, insulin, and C-peptide levels were examined after 1-week dietary periods of 200-mmol or 20-mmol Na intake. Individuals were examined after either placebo or 2 mg of the α_1-adrenergic blocker doxazosin.	Ra	Increase of total and LDL cholesterol on low-Na diet was reduced by doxazosin. C-peptide level was lower on the low-salt diet with the placebo but similar with the doxazosin.	Subjects were healthy normotensive volunteers (n = 16).	26
Study evaluated 60- to 80-mmol Na intake in combination with either 100-mmol Na supplement or placebo. Lipid parameters were evaluated at the end of each 4-week dietary period.	Ra	Changes in Na excretion were not predictive of variability in BP. Low-Na period had the least favorable lipid profile.	Participants had hypertension controlled by Ca-channel blocker (n = 99).	27
Study tested the effects of 1-week normal dietary period (24 mmol Na) and low-sodium period (20 mmol Na) using a randomized crossover design.	Ra	Dietary salt restriction increased resistance to vasodilating effects of insulin. Vascular sensitivity to insulin was inversely correlated with MAP and plasma norepinephrine.	Participants were either normotensive (n = 5) or borderline hypertensive (n = 8).	28
Union workers with treated hypertension were evaluated to determine whether urinary Na excretion level was related to subsequent fatal MI.	F	MIs were inversely related to level of Na excretion during follow-up period with a mean of 3.8 years.	Hypertensive union workers in a BP treatment program (n = 2,937).	29
Baseline dietary data from NHANES I (1971–1975) participants were evaluated in relation to mortality data collected in 1992.	F	CVD mortality was inversely related to baseline Na intake in multivariate analysis.	Representative sample of U.S. population (n = 20,729).	30

AUC, area under the curve; BP, blood pressure; CVD, cardiovascular disease; GTT, glucose tolerance test; MAP, mean arterial pressure; MI, myocardial infarction.

tion rates in a cohort of treated hypertensive patients (29) and in a subsequent evaluation of the general population in NHANES I (30).

Dietary supplements. The TOHP study failed to demonstrate any benefits of supplemental use of fish oils, potassium, or calcium (20). Meta-analyses of controlled clinical trials of supplements fail to establish the efficacy of omega-3 fatty acid (31) or calcium supplementation (32). However, a meta-analysis did demonstrate a modest effect of potassium supplements on systolic blood pressure (33).

Dietary Approaches to Stop Hypertension (DASH) trial. The DASH trial is a multicenter randomized controlled trial to study dietary patterns rather than single nutrients. The 8-week results demonstrated a blood pressure–lowering effect of the dietary pattern that was high in fruits and vegetables, low in total and saturated fat and cholesterol, and high in whole grains, as well as being moderately low in sodium (3,000 mg) (12). Unique features of the DASH trial are the focus on dietary patterns, the study population, 67% of whom are from minority groups, and its potential for generalization to the population at large (34–36).

SUMMARY

The scientific evidence strongly supports controlling hypertension to prevent renal and other diabetic complications. In the UKPDS, ACE inhibitors and beta-blockers were equally effective and beneficial in treating hypertension. ACE inhibitors may be the medication of choice if albuminuria is present because they are renoprotective and because more recent evidence suggests that they may be cardioprotective as well. The final results of the ABCD Trial will be released shortly and will give evidence to judge the best medical treatment approach for individuals with diabetes and hypertension. Extrapolating from more general studies, weight reduction appears to be the treatment of choice for hypertension in diabetes. Sodium restriction appears to be effective in lowering blood pressure in sodium-sensitive individuals, but a severe sodium restriction can worsen lipids, insulin resistance, and possible cardiovascular risk.

The 6th JNC report (1) provides guidance for the prevention, diagnosis, and treatment of hypertension in individuals with diabetes and hypertension. The JNC recommendations indicate:

1. Blood pressure needs to be rigorously controlled to prevent renal and other cardiovascular complications of diabetes.
2. Medication is recommended for all individuals with diabetes who have hypertension.

3. The choice of medication varies with concomitant conditions. If albuminuria is present, ACE inhibitors are indicated.
4. Weight reduction can lessen medication dosage and improve quality of life.
5. There is growing evidence that counseling needs to focus on a food pattern that is low in sodium, low in total and saturated fat and cholesterol, and rich in fruit, vegetables, and whole grains rather than on simple nutrient modification.
6. Sodium restriction may reduce blood pressure, especially in those who are sodium sensitive. If severe sodium restriction is used in treatment, lipid levels and indicators of insulin resistance need to be carefully monitored.

Treatment recommendations are based on extrapolation of data from nondiabetic individuals as well as on the limited studies focusing on diabetes and hypertension.

REFERENCES

1. The 6th report of the Joint National Committee on prevention, detection, evaluation, and treatment of high blood pressure. *Arch Intern Med* 157:2413–2446, 1997

2. Burt VL, Cutler JA, Higgins M, Horan MJ, Labarthe D, Whelton P, Brown C, Roccella EJ: Trends in the prevalence, awareness, treatment and control of hypertension in the adult US population: data from the health examination surveys, 1960 to 1991. *Hypertension* 26:60–69, 1995

3. Camarata PJ, Heros RC, Latchaw RE: "Brain attack": the rationale for treating strokes as a medical emergency. *Neurosurgery* 34:144–157, 1994

4. Lewis EJ, Hunshiker LG, Bain RP, Rohde RE, the Collaborative Research Study Group: The effect of angiotensin-converting enzyme inhibition on diabetic nephropathy. *N Engl J Med* 329:1456–1462, 1993

5. Collins R, Peto R, MacMahon S, Hebert P, Fieback NH, Eberlein KA, Godwin J, Qizilbash N, Taylor JO, Hennekens CH: Blood pressure, stroke and coronary heart disease. 2. Short-term reduction in blood pressure: overview of randomised drug trial in their epidemiological context. *Lancet* 335:827–838, 1990

6. MacMahon S, Peto R, Cutler J, Collins R, Sorlie P, Neaton J, Abbott R, Godwin J, Dyer A, Stamler J: Blood pressure, stroke, and coronary heart disease. 1. prolonged differences in blood pressure: prospective observational studies corrected for the regression dilution bias. *Lancet* 335:765–774, 1990

7. SHEP Cooperative Research Group: Prevention of stroke by antihypertensive drug treatment in older persons with isolated systolic hypertension: final results of the Systolic Hypertension in the Elderly Program (SHEP). *J Am Med Assoc* 265:3255–3264, 1991

8. U.K. Prospective Diabetes Study Group: Tight blood pressure control and risk of macrovascular and microvascular complications in type 2 diabetes: UKPDS 38. *BMJ* 317:703–715, 1998

9. U.K. Prospective Diabetes Study Group: Efficacy of atenolol and captopril in reducing risk of macrovascular and microvascular complications in type 2 diabetes: UKPDS 39. *BMJ* 317:713–720, 1998

10. Estacio RO, Jeffers B, Hiatt WR, Biggerstaff SL, Gifford N, Schrier RW: The effect of nisoldiprine as compared with enalapril on cardiovascular outcomes in patients with non-insulin-dependent diabetes and hypertension. *N Engl J Med* 338:645–652, 1998

11. Last JM, Abramson JH (Eds.): *A Dictionary of Epidemiology.* 3rd ed. New York, Oxford University Press, 1995

12. Appel LJ, Moore TJ, Obarzanek E, Vollmer WM, Svetky LP, Sacks FM, Bray GA, Vogt TM, Cutler JA, Windhauser MM, Lin PH, Karanja N, the DASH Collaborative Research Group: A clinical trial of the effects of dietary pattern on blood pressure. *N Engl J Med* 336:1117–1124, 1997

13. Stamler R, Stamler J, Gosch FC, Civinelli J, Fishman J, McKeever P, McDonald A, Dyer AR: Primary prevention of hypertension by nutritional-hygienic means: final report of a randomized, controlled trial. *J Am Med Assoc* 262:1801–1807, 1989

14. MacMahon SW, Wilcken DEL, MacDonald GR: The effects of weight reduction of left ventricular mass. *N Engl J Med* 314:334–339, 1986

15. Trial of Hypertension Prevention Collaborative Research Group: The effects of weight loss and sodium reduction intervention on blood pressure and hypertension incidence in overweight people with high normal blood pressure: the Trials of Hypertension Prevention, phase II. *Arch Intern Med* 157:657–667, 1997

16. Whelton PK, Appel LJ, Espeland MA, Applegate WB, Ettinger WH Jr, Kostis JB, Kumanyika S, Lacy CR, Johnson KC, Folmar S,

Cutler JA, the TONE Collaborative Research Group: Sodium restriction and weight loss in the treatment of hypertension in older persons: a randomized controlled trial of nonpharmacologic interventions in the elderly. *JAMA* 279:839–846, 1998

17. Wassertheil-Smoller, Oberman A, Blaufox MD, Davis B, Langford H: The Trial of Antihypertensive Interventions and Management: final results with regard to blood pressure, cardiovascular risk and quality of life. *Am J Hypertens* 5:37–44, 1992

18. Wylie-Rosett J, Wassertheil-Smoller S, Blaufox MD, Blaufox MD, Davis BR, Langford HG, Oberman A, Jennings S, Hataway H, Stern J, Zimbaldi N: Trial of Antihypertensive Intervention and Management: greater efficacy with weight reduction than with a sodium-potassium intervention. *J Am Diet Assoc* 93:408–414, 1993

19. Wassertheil-Smoller S, Blaufox D, Oberman A, Langford HG, Davis BR, Wylie-Rosett J: Adequate weight loss alone and combined with drug therapy in the treatment of mild hypertension. *Arch Intern Med* 152:131–136, 1993

20. Trial of Hypertension Prevention Collaborative Research Group: The effects on nonpharmacological intervention on blood pressure of persons with high normal blood levels: results of the Trial of Hypertension Prevention Phase 1. *J Am Med Assoc* 267:1213–1220, 1992

21. Midgley JP, Matthew AG, Greenwood CM, Logan AG: Effect of reduced dietary sodium on blood pressure: a meta-analysis of randomized controlled trials. *J Am Med Assoc* 275:1590–1597, 1996

22. Overlack A, Ruppert M, Lkolloch R, Kraft K, Stumpe KO: Age is a major determinant of the divergent blood pressure responses to varying salt intake in essential hypertension. *Am J Hypertens* 8:829–836, 1995

23. Iwaoka T, Umeda T, Inoue J, Naomi S, Sasaki M, Fujimoto Y, Gui C, Ideguchi Y, Sato T: Dietary NaCl restriction deteriorated oral glucose tolerance in hypertensive patients with impairment of glucose tolerance. *Am J Hypertens* 7:460–463, 1994

24. Bakris GL, Smith A: Effects of sodium intake on albumin excretion in patients with diabetic nephropathy treated with long-acting calcium antagonists. *Ann Intern Med* 125:201–204, 1996

25. Mulhauser I, Prange K, Sawicki PT, Bender R, Dworschak A, Schaden W, Berger M: Effects of dietary sodium on blood pressure in IDDM patients with nephropathy. *Diabetologia* 39:212–219, 1996

26. Fleiser D, Nowack R, Allendorf-Ostwald N, Kohl B, Huginger A, Ritz E: Serum lipid changes on low salt diet: effects of alpha 1-adreneregic blockage. *Am J Hypertens* 6:320–324, 1993

27. McCarron DA, Weder AB, Egan BM, Krishna GG, Morris CD, Cohen M, Oparil S: Blood pressure and metabolic responses to moderate sodium restriction in isradipine-treated hypertensive patients. *Am J Hypertens* 10:68–76, 1997

28. Feldman RD, Logan AG, Schmidt ND: Dietary salt increased vascular insulin resistance. *Clin Pharm Ther* 60:444–451, 1996

29. Alderman MH, Madhavan S, Cohen H, Sealey JE, Laragh JH: Low urinary sodium is associated with greater risk of myocardial infarction among treated hypertensive men. *Hypertension* 25:1144–1152, 1995

30. Alderman MH, Cohen H, Madavan S: Dietary sodium intake and mortality: the National Health and Nutrition Examination Survey (NHANES I). *Lancet* 351:781–785, 1998

31. Appel LJ, Miller ER 3rd, Seider AJ, Welton PK: Does supplementation of diet with 'fish oil' reduce blood pressure? A meta-analysis of controlled clinical trials. *Arch Intern Med* 153:1429–1438, 1993

32. Allender PS, Cutler JA, Follman D, Cappuccio FP, Pryer J, Elliot P: Dietary calcium and blood pressure: a meta-analysis of randomized clinical trials. *Ann Intern Med* 124:825–831, 1996

33. Whelton PK, He J, Cutler JA, Brancati FL, Appel LJ, Follmann D, Klag MJ: Effects of oral potassium on blood pressure: meta-analysis of randomized controlled clinical trials. *J Am Med Assoc* 277:1624–1632, 1997

34. Sacks FM, Oberzanek E, Windhauser MM, Svetkey LP, Vollmer WM, McCullough M, Karanja N, Lin PH, Steele P, Proschan MA, et al.: Rationale and design of the Dietary Approaches to Stop Hypertension trial (DASH): a multicenter controlled-feeding study of dietary patterns to lower blood pressure. *Ann Epidemiol* 5:108–118, 1995

35. Blackburn GL: Functional foods in the prevention and treatment of disease: significance of the Dietary Approaches to Stop Hypertension study. *Am J Clin Nutr* 66:1067–1071, 1997

36. Zemel MB: Dietary patterns and hypertension: the DASH study (Dietary Approaches to Stop Hypertension). *Nutr Rev* 55:303–305, 1997

Dr. Wylie-Rosett is Professor of Epidemiology and Social Medicine and Director of the Demonstration and Education Division of the Diabetes Research and Training Center at Albert Einstein College of Medicine, Bronx, NY.

17. Nephropathy and Medical Nutrition Therapy

MADELYN L. WHEELER, MS, RD, FADA, CDE

Highlights

- A meta-analysis indicated that a low-protein diet (0.6–0.85 g protein/kg/day) in people with diabetes significantly slowed the increase in urinary albumin level or the decline in glomerular filtration rate or creatinine clearance, particularly in those with type 1 diabetes and macroalbuminuria; however, there are concerns about methodology and adherence in the studies involved.
- There has been no scientific conclusion on the value of plant versus animal protein, especially in patients with type 2 diabetes. However, in the limited studies reported, plant protein appears not to be harmful; therefore, it is reasonable to recommend the substitution of plant-based protein for animal-based protein.
- Further research is needed before definitive recommendations can be made about protein (amount or type) intake for people with micro- or macroalbuminuria.

INTRODUCTION

It is estimated that 20–30% of people with diabetes have microalbuminuria (20–200 µg/min or ~30–300 mg/day) and 20–30% have macroalbuminuria (>300 mg/day) (1). In individuals with either type 1 or type 2 diabetes, microalbuminuria predicts the development of macroalbuminuria and clinical nephropathy and is correlated with overall death rate and with death rates from cardiovascular disease. Currently recommended treatment focuses on methods that might reverse micro- or macroalbuminuria or slow the rate of decline: *1*) improved glucose control (reduction of hyperglycemia by oral agents, insulin, and/or diet) (2,3) and 2) reduction of blood pressure to ~130/70 mmHg by use of angiotensin-converting enzyme (ACE) inhibitors (4–6).

Diabetes medical nutrition therapy, particularly in terms of alteration of dietary protein, is also a potential method for slowing the development and/or rate of progression of diabetic renal disease. The following two general questions are related to this issue:

1. Does reduction in the amount of protein reduce risk and/or slow the progression of early diabetic nephropathy (micro- or macroalbuminuria)?
2. Does change in the type or source of protein (e.g., animal versus plant) reduce risk for or slow the progression of early diabetic nephropathy (micro- or macroalbuminuria)?

Note that the questions address microalbuminuria and macroalbuminuria but do not cover end-stage renal disease.

DIETARY PROTEIN

Food consumption data from the U.S. Department of Agriculture 1977–1978 and 1985 surveys indicate that 14–18% of total food energy intake is derived from protein. Foods of animal origin contribute ~65% of the protein, with the remaining 35% coming from plant protein (7). The Recommended Dietary Allowance for "reference" protein is 0.75 g/kg/day (rounded off to 0.8 g/kg/day) for adults, with reference protein defined as "highly digestible high-quality protein such as egg, meat, milk, or fish" (8). Clinically, however, this figure of 0.8 g/kg/day is usually assumed to include *both* animal and plant protein. An estimate of mean minimum daily protein requirement for healthy adults, based on Food and Agricultural Organization, World Health Organization, United Nations University (FAO/WHO/UNU) recommendations is 0.6 g/kg/day (9).

In a large cross-sectional study from Europe (10), the protein intake of 2,696 individuals with type 1 diabetes was assessed by 3-day food records and compared with albumin excretion rate (AER). Total protein intake for Europeans averaged 17.6% of energy (1.46 g/kg/day), with 12.2% of energy representing animal protein intake and 5.2% representing plant protein intake. Interestingly, in this study, individuals with macroalbuminuria had total and animal protein intakes significantly higher than did individuals with normoalbuminuria; however, there was no significant relationship for plant protein. Another cross-sectional study of adults with type 1 diabetes in Tasmania, using a food frequency questionnaire, determined that protein intake was 18.2% of energy for individuals with normoalbuminuria and 18.9% of energy for those with microalbuminuria (11). Finally, a cross-sectional study of individuals with type 2 diabetes in the U.S. indicated, based on 3-day food records, that those with normoalbuminuria ate 0.81 g protein/kg/day and those with microalbuminuria ate 0.79 g protein/kg/day (12).

There has been concern about the quality of plant protein (ability to support growth) compared with animal protein. Since 1919, the protein efficiency ratio method has been used to measure the protein quality of human foods. It measures the ability of a protein to support growth in rapidly growing rats. However, this method overestimates the value of some animal protein for *human* growth while underestimating the value of some plant proteins. In 1989, the FAO of the United Nations recommended (13) and in 1993 the Food and Drug Administration approved (14) the use of the protein digestibility–corrected amino acid score (PDCAAS), which is based on the human amino acid requirements of a 2- to 5-year-old child (not a rat) corrected for digestibility, as the method to evaluate the protein quality of human foods. (See Table 17.1 for PDCAAS scores for selected foods.) Using this method corrects many of the overestimates of quality for animal protein and underestimates for plant protein (15).

PROTEIN AMOUNT

Does reduction in the amount of protein reduce risk and/or slow the progression of early diabetic nephropathy (micro- or macroalbuminuria)? Several studies

Table 17.1 Protein Digestibility–Corrected Amino Acid Scores (PDCAAS) for Selected Foods

Product	PDCAAS Score
Casein	1.00
Egg white	1.00
Soybean protein concentrate	0.99
Beef	0.92
Soybean protein isolate	0.92
Chickpeas, canned	0.71
Pinto beans, canned	0.57
Rolled oats	0.57
Whole wheat	0.40

Adapted from FAO/WHO (13).

have been reported that involve individuals with diabetes, amount of protein, and early renal disease. Table 17.2 gives characteristics of studies of individuals with macroalbuminuria (16–21), and Table 17.3 gives characteristics of studies of individuals with microalbuminuria (17,22,23). Almost all studies involved subjects with type 1 diabetes and varied in length from 3 weeks to 3 years. Protein varied from a low of 0.6 g/kg/day for restricted-protein periods to 2 g/kg/day for control periods. All these studies either used a randomized, concurrent control design or were time-controlled studies with a nonrandomized crossover design. Five of the studies (16,18–20,22) were included in Pedrini's meta-analysis of protein restriction (24). In this meta-analysis, there were a total of 108 patients with type 1 diabetes, with a mean length of follow-up of 9–35 months. (See Tables 17.2 and 17.3.) Pedrini et al. (24) interpret their results to indicate that a low-protein diet (0.6–0.85 g/kg/day) can significantly slow the increase in urinary AER in individuals with normo- or microalbuminuria and the decline in glomerular filtration rate (GFR) or creatinine clearance in those individuals with diabetes and macroalbuminuria.

Issues/Concerns

The first concern is that there are several methodological issues that make Pedrini's conclusions less supportable. For example, different endpoints were used:

- The endpoint for the four studies of subjects with macroalbuminuria was a decrease in renal function (GFR/creatinine clearance >0.1 ml/min/month).
- For the study involving subjects with microalbuminuria, the endpoint was a change in microalbuminuria (an increase in AER of >10% from baseline).

In addition, the meta-analysis results were complicated by the fact that 9 of the 108 subjects were treated with ACE inhibitors, 6 in the low-protein groups. Finally, there was no consistency (and sometimes no description) of the source or type of protein for these low-protein diets.

Second, when considering all studies:

1. There was no consistency when the amount of protein was reduced. In three of the eight studies, the amount of plant protein remained about the same as that during the control period, whereas the amount of animal protein was decreased (19,21,22). In one study, the low-protein diet involved all plant protein supplemented with amino and keto acids (18). Two studies (16,23) made no mention of the source of protein in the diets, and another study

Table 17.2 Characteristics of Studies of Amount of Protein and Diabetic Macroalbuminuria

Study	Subjects	Follow-Up (months)	Prescribed Protein Intake (g/kg/day)	Significant Outcome Measures	Notes
Ciavarella et al. (16)*	7 type 1	4.5	0.71	AER ↓	Adherence measured by periodic diet interview and urinary urea nitrogen.
	9 type 1	11.7	1.44	AER ↑	Control period.
Yue et al. (17)	2 type 1 2 type 2	3	0.6	AER ↓ GFR, no change Creatinine clearance ↓	Protein is 0.6 g/kg ideal body wt. Diet tailored to suit individual; no distinction made between different sources of protein. Adherence measured by monthly diet assessment and urinary urea nitrogen.
		2 pre 2 post		Usual	Control periods.
Barsotti et al. (18)*†	8 type 1	16	1.2–1.4		Control period.
		17	0.25–0.6	AER ↓	All plant protein, supplemented with amino acids and ketoanalogs. Adherence measured by urinary urea nitrogen.
Walker et al. (19)*†	19 type 1	29	1.13		Control period.

		33	0.67	AER ↓ GFR, reduced rate of decline	20 g plant + 20 g animal protein/day; some urine protein losses replaced. Adherence measured every 1–2 months by comprehensive diet history and weighed food record; urinary urea nitrogen every 3 months.
Zeller et al. (20)*	20 type 1	35	0.6	AER ↓ GFR ↓ (vs. control diet)	70–80% protein of high biological value; urine protein losses replaced; reduced-phosphorus diet. All patients received regular counseling by study dietitian. Adherence measured by dietary history and urinary urea nitrogen each month for 3 months, and at least every 3 months thereafter.
	15 type 1	35	at least 1.0	AER ↑	Control period.
Raal et al. (21)	11 type 1	6	0.8 (actual 0.87)	AER ↓ GFR stabilization	Diets tailored to suit individual requirements. Reduced protein mainly due to a decrease in animal protein. Adherence measured using 1-month dietary recall and urinary urea nitrogen at start of study and 3 and 6 months later.
	11 type 1	6	>1.6 (actual 2.0)	AER, no change GFR ↓	Control period. Adherence measures same as above.

A decrease in albumin excretion rate (AER) is beneficial. With macroalbuminuria, reducing the rate of decline or stabilizing the glomerular filtration rate (GFR) is considered beneficial. *Study included in meta-analysis by Pedrini et al. (24); †crossover design.

Table 17.3 Characteristics of Studies of Amount of Protein and Diabetic Microalbuminuria

Study	Subjects	Follow-Up	Prescribed Protein Intake (g/kg/day)	Significant Outcome Measures	Notes
Yue et al. (17)	1 type 2	3 months	0.6	AER ↓ GFR, no change	See Table 17.2
Dullaart et al. (22)*	14 type 1	24 months	0.6 (0.79 actual)	AER ↓ GFR ↓	Represents a reduction of from 10% to 5% of energy as animal protein and from 7% to 6% as plant protein. Adherence measured by 1-week food recall at baseline and end of each year; protein intake assessed using urinary urea nitrogen.
	16 type 1	24 months	1.09	AER, no change GFR ↓	Control period. No change in percentage of energy from animal protein (11% to 10%) or plant protein (6%). Adherence measures same as above.
Pomerleau (23)†	12 type 2	3 weeks	2	AER, no change GFR, no change	Protein is 2 g/kg desirable wt; 0.8 g protein/kg from food and 1.2 g protein/kg from supplements (casein, gelatin, vegetable protein, yeast, and soy). Individualized 7-day-cycle menus used. Adherence measured by 3-day food records and urinary urea excretion at beginning, middle, and end of study.
		3 weeks	0.8	AER ↓ GFR ↓	Protein is 0.8 g/kg desirable wt, same as above except no supplements were used. Cycle menus used. Instruction and adherence measures same as above.

A decrease in albumin excretion rate (AER) is beneficial. With microalbuminuria, many people with diabetes have a higher than normal glomerular filtration rate (GFR), hyperfiltering; reduction to normal is beneficial. *Study included in meta-analysis by Pedrini et al. (24); †crossover design.

(17) made no distinction as to source. Only one study (20) indicated that in the restricted-protein part of the study, the protein was 70–80% high-biological protein. This begs the question, "Was it the decrease in amount or the change of source that produced the described outcome?"

2. Foods were prepared and eaten at home (i.e., unsupervised), and unfortunately, few described any education that might have been provided about what foods to eat or how to prepare them. Retrospective diet adherence was analyzed in some studies using an assessment method ("diet interview," food recall, weighed food record). A few studies did not mention assessment of adherence with food intake at all. In all studies, 24-h urine samples were collected periodically to calculate protein intake from the urinary urea nitrogen (25).

The third concern is that other than two short-term studies with small numbers of subjects (17,23), no studies of this nature have been reported in individuals with type 2 diabetes.

Fourth, there is concern that protein restriction may be detrimental (e.g., may produce malnutrition or muscle wasting) in the progression of diabetic nephropathy. This is based on the fact that there is an increase in protein degradation and essential amino acid oxidation accompanying severe insulin deficiency in type 1 diabetes (26,27). However, Brodsky et al. (28) concluded that type 1 diabetic subjects adapt normally to dietary protein restriction (0.6 g/kg/day) and that "undernutrition" during this moderate protein depravation probably occurs during episodes of poor glycemic control. In people with type 2 diabetes who are normoalbuminuric, Gougeon et al. (29) found that whole-body protein metabolism is elevated in hyperglycemia but can be improved with exogenous insulin doses sufficient to restore normoglycemia.

Finally, when meal plans for reduced protein are calculated, the protein from *both* plant and animal sources traditionally makes up the total figure. To provide more "high biological" protein, the plant protein amount is reduced, most often by using protein-free starch products (such as pasta, flour, and rice). This makes everyday meal planning difficult, expensive, and often less than palatable.

Possible Mechanisms

It has been hypothesized that higher-protein diets may show detrimental effects on renal function because of increased glucagon production and/or increased specific amino acids. For example, Rudberg et al. (30) showed that the increase in GFR on a diet where 20% of energy is from protein (compared with 10% of energy from protein) was significantly correlated with the increase in glucagon and the branched-chain amino acids isoleucine and valine; AER was unchanged and was corre-lated with IGF-1 (insulin-like growth factor 1) (30).

PROTEIN TYPE

Does change in the type or source of protein (e.g., animal versus plant) reduce risk for or slow the progression of early diabetic nephropathy (micro- or macroalbu-minuria)? Interest in type of protein and its possible effect on early renal disease has been generated by a small number of studies one meal in length and by three short-term crossover studies (see Table 17.4). These studies show, in general, that plant-based protein, when eaten in amounts comparable with animal-based protein, may have beneficial effects on reduction of hyperfiltration and AER. Nakamura and colleagues (31–34) have studied the acute (3-h) response to a number of different protein foods in individuals with type 2 diabetes. They found, for example, that the GFR of individuals with type 2 diabetes who were normoalbuminuric increased significantly when tuna was eaten, but did not increase when bean curd (tofu), egg white, or cheese was eaten.

Jibani et al. (35) studied the effects of a predominantly vegetable diet in eight patients with type 1 diabetes and microalbuminuria. After 8 weeks on their usual diets (baseline daily protein intake was 60% ani-mal), subjects followed a predominantly vegetarian diet for an additional 8 weeks (protein intake approximated the usual diet, but 30% was ani-mal protein and the rest was vegetable protein). After the predominantly vegetarian diet, subjects were followed for an additional 8 weeks on their baseline diets. AER fell significantly from the end of the first 8 weeks of the usual diet (baseline) to the end of the intervention diet, but returned to baseline values after the second 8 weeks of the usual diet. Unfortu-nately, during the test diet period, *total* protein was reduced to 0.4 g/kg body wt (a 28% reduction from the usual diet). Because of the small num-ber of subjects in the study, the authors were not able to determine whether the reduction in total protein intake rather than the reduction in the intake of protein of animal origin was predominantly responsible for the fall in fractional albumin clearance.

Kontessis et al. (36) compared the renal, metabolic, and hormonal responses to protein of animal or vegetable origin (4 weeks each) in nine normotensive nonproteinemic subjects with type 1 diabetes. GFR and renal plasma flow were significantly lower on the vegetable-protein com-pared with the animal-protein diets, and renal vascular resistance was higher.

Pecis's study design is interesting because one of the comparisons was 3 weeks of a "usual" diet (1.4 g protein/kg/day) rich in red meat with 3 weeks of a "usual" diet (1.2 g protein/kg/day) with the majority of meat

Table 17.4 Characteristics of Studies of Type of Protein Involving Diabetic Subjects

Study	Subjects	Follow-Up	Protein Source	AER	Outcome Measures	Notes
Barsotti (18) (See Table 17.2)						
Nakamura et al. (31)	20 type 2	1 meal (3 h)	Tuna fish, 1 g/kg	Normal	GFR ↑	No significant change in AER for any challenge.
			Same as above	Micro	GFR ↓	
			Same as above	Macro	GFR, no change	
			Bean curd, 1 g/kg	Normal	GFR, no change	
			Same as above	Micro	GFR, no change	
			Same as above	Macro	GFR, no change	
Nakamura and colleagues (32–34)	6 type 2	1 meal (3 h)	Tuna fish, 0.7 g/kg	Normal	GFR ↑	No significant change in AER for any challenge.
			Boiled egg white, 0.7 g/kg	Normal	GFR, no change	
			Boiled egg white, 1.4 g/kg	Normal	GFR, no change	

(Continued)

Table 17.4 Characteristics of Studies of Type of Protein Involving Diabetic Subjects (*Continued*)

Study	Subjects	Follow-Up	Protein Source	AER	Outcome Measures	Notes
Nakamura and colleagues (*continued*)			Cheese, 0.7 g/kg	Normal	GFR, no change	
			Tofu, 0.7 g/kg	Normal	GFR, no change	
Jibani et al. (35)*	8 type 1	8 weeks	70% animal, 30% plant	Micro		Control period. No adherence measures described.
		8 weeks	30% animal, 70% plant	Micro	AER ↓ GFR, no change	Total protein intake not comparable with control period (reduced by 0.4 kg).
Kontessis et al. (36)*	9 type 1	4 weeks	70% animal, 30% plant (1.1 g/kg/day)	Normal		Control period. Adherence measured by 3-day weighed diet each period and urinary urea nitrogen.
		4 weeks	100% plant (0.95 g/kg/day)	Normal	AER ↓ GFR ↓	Adherence measures same as above.
Pecis et al. (37)*	15 type 1	3 weeks	79% of meat protein as beef, 21% as chicken (1.4 g/kg/day)	Normal		Control period. Adherence measured by periodic urinary urea nitrogen measurement and weekly diet check.

| 3 weeks | 100% plant and milk (0.5 g/kg/day) | Normal | GFR ↓ | 7% calories as protein. Adherence measures same as above. |
| 3 weeks | 85% of meat protein as chicken, 15% as fish (1.2 g/kg/day) | Normal | GFR ↓ | Adherence measures same as above. |

A decrease in albumin excretion rate (AER) or normalization of glomerular filtration rate (GFR) is beneficial. *Crossover design.

protein as chicken plus a little fish (no red meat) (37). Compared with the red meat diet, the chicken/fish diet reduced GFR significantly in individuals with type 1 diabetes and normoalbuminuria, particularly those who were hyperfiltering.

Issues/Concerns

First, the studies (longer than one meal) using plant-based protein in individuals who have type 1 diabetes have been short-term (3–8 weeks) and have included small numbers of subjects (8–15 subjects), and one (35) did not account for differences in amounts of protein in comparable diets.

Second, except for Nakamura's 3-h protein challenges, food intake adherence issues were the same as in the studies involving amount of protein. Subjects prepared and ate their meals at home (unsupervised). None of the studies discussed education or instruction about what foods to eat or how to prepare or purchase them. One study did not discuss adherence at all (35); the other two acknowledged periodic retrospective diet assessment and 24-h urine collections for protein analyses.

Third, no studies have been conducted in individuals who have type 2 diabetes. Finally, quality of plant protein does not appear to be an issue, as indicated by high PDCAAS scores of many plant proteins, especially soy products (see Table 17.1).

Possible Mechanisms

Several possible mechanisms have been hypothesized for the beneficial effects of plant compared with animal protein. For example,

- Different hormonal responses: Fioretto et al. (38) have postulated that individuals with type 1 diabetes (and normoalbuminuria) have, on average, an impaired renal hemodynamic response to a meat meal that is due to a relative failure in glucagon rise and in turn to stimulation of renal prostaglandin synthesis.
- Different plasma amino acid levels: Glycine, alanine, and arginine are amino acids involved in renal hemodynamics, and they induce a rise in plasma glucagon and GFR (39). They appear to be found in decreasing amounts in red meat < tuna < bean curd. And Nakamura et al. (31) noted that the branched-chain amino acids (valine, leucine, isoleucine) are found in higher levels in bean curd than in tuna.

SUMMARY

Improved blood glucose control and reduction of hypertension by use of ACE inhibitors can slow the development and rate of progression of renal disease. Studies involving a reduced amount of protein (0.6–0.8 g/kg/day), compared with usual amounts, have generally shown a benefit for individuals with type 1 diabetes, particularly for macroalbuminuria (improved AER or GFR). Unfortunately, the *sources* of protein in these studies were not standardized. It is not known if eating reduced or even usual amounts of protein mainly from plant sources may be beneficial. Little or no discussion has been provided about instruction for home meal planning and food preparation, and adherence has been checked infrequently and retrospectively.

Because of the above issues (particularly the questions raised about plant versus animal protein) and because of previously mentioned methodological problems, specific recommendations about amount of protein and diabetes cannot be made at this time. Dietary protein restriction to <0.8 g/kg/day might be recommended to selected diabetic patients, such as those who have a progressive increase in proteinuria despite good glycemic control and the use of ACE inhibitors. However, quality-of-life issues would need to be considered when adding one more restriction (protein) to an already complicated treatment regimen. And the question remains: Should the reduction of protein to 0.6–0.8 g/kg/day be in *total* protein (animal plus plant) or just animal protein?

While it has not been shown scientifically that substituting plant-based protein for animal-based protein reduces risk for the development or progression of diabetic renal disease, exchanging some or all of daily animal-based protein for plant-based protein, particularly at normal rather than reduced intake, is not harmful and could be recommended. In addition to possible renal benefit, it would most likely reduce total and saturated fat intake and increase fiber intake (three recommendations to decrease risk of cardiovascular disease).

Longer-term controlled clinical trials where food intake of subjects is carefully monitored are needed to determine whether certain types of protein (plant versus animal protein, different plant proteins, different animal proteins) have a beneficial effect on reducing risk or slowing progression of early diabetic renal disease. After there is scientific evidence in the area of source of protein, perhaps further determinations can be made about amount of protein (animal, plant, as well as total protein).

REFERENCES

1. National Diabetes Data Group: *Diabetes in America*. 2nd ed. Washington, DC, U.S. Govt. Printing Office, 1995 (DHHS publ. no. NIH 95-1468), p. 6

2. The Diabetes Control and Complications Trial Research Group: The effect of intensive treatment of diabetes on the development

and progression of long-term complications in insulin-dependent diabetes mellitus. *N Engl J Med* 329:977–986, 1993

3. Vasquez B, Flock EV, Savage PJ, Nagulesparan M, Bennion LJ, Baird HR, Bennett PH: Sustained reduction of proteinuria in type 2 (non-insulin-dependent) diabetes following diet-induced reduction of hyperglycaemia. *Diabetologia* 26:127–133, 1984

4. Viberti G, Mogensen CE, Groop LC, Pauls JF: Effect of captopril on progression to clinical proteinuria in patients with insulin-dependent diabetes mellitus and microalbuminuria. *JAMA* 271:275–279, 1994

5. Lewis EJ, Hunsicker LG, Bain RP, Rohde RD: The effect of angiotensin-converting-enzyme inhibition on diabetic nephropathy. *N Engl J Med* 329:1456–1462, 1993

6. Ahmad J, Siddiqui MA, Ahmad H: Effective postponement of diabetic nephropathy with enalapril in normotensive type 2 diabetic patients with microalbuminuria. *Diabetes Care* 20:1576–1581, 1997

7. Food and Nutrition Board: *Recommended Dietary Allowances.* 10th ed. Washington, DC, National Academy Press, 1989, p. 68

8. Food and Nutrition Board: *Recommended Dietary Allowances.* 10th ed. Washington, DC, National Academy Press, 1989, pp. 58–59

9. FAO/WHO/UNU: *Energy and Protein Requirements.* Geneva, World Health Organization, 1985 (Tech. Rep. Ser., no. 724)

10. Toeller M, Buyken A, Heitkamp G, Brämswig S, Mann J, Milne R, Gries FA, Keen H, the EURODIAB IDDM Complications Study Group: Protein intake and urinary albumin excretion rates in the EURODIAB IDDM complications study. *Diabetologia* 40:1219–1226, 1997

11. Riley MD, Dwyer T: Microalbuminuria is positively associated with usual dietary saturated fat intake and negatively associated with usual dietary protein intake in people with insulin-dependent diabetes mellitus. *Am J Clin Nutr* 67:50–57, 1998

12. Summerson JH, Bell RA, Konen JC: Dietary protein intake, clinical proteinuria, and microalbuminuria in non-insulin-dependent diabetes mellitus. *J Renal Nutr* 6:89–93, 1996

13. FAO/WHO: *Protein Quality Evaluation.* New York, United Nations, 1991 (FAO Food and Nutrition Paper 51)

14. Food labeling: protein quality (21 CFR 1, 101). *Federal Register* 58:2103–2106, 1993

15. Young VR, Pellett PL: Plant proteins in relation to human protein and amino acid nutrition. *Am J Clin Nutr* 59 (Suppl.):1203S–1212S, 1994

16. Ciavarella A, DiMizio G, Stefoni S, Borgnino LC, Vannini P: Reduced albuminuria after dietary protein restriction in insulin-dependent diabetic patients with clinical nephropathy. *Diabetes Care* 10:407–413, 1987

17. Yue DK, O'Dea J, Stewart P, Conigrave AD, Hosking M, Tsang J, Hall B, Dale N, Turtle JR: Proteinuria and renal function in diabetic patients fed a diet moderately restricted in protein. *Am J Clin Nutr* 48:230–234, 1988

18. Barsotti G, Ciardella F, Morelli E, Cupisti A, Mantovanelli A, Giovannetti S: Nutritional treatment of renal failure in type 1 diabetic nephropathy. *Clin Nephrol* 29:280–287, 1988

19. Walker JD, Bending JJ, Dodds RA, Mattock MB, Murrells TJ, Keen H, Viberti GC: Restriction of dietary protein and progression of renal failure in diabetic nephropathy. *Lancet* ii:1411–1415, 1989

20. Zeller K, Whittaker E, Sullivan L, Raskin P, Jacobson HR: Effect of restricting dietary protein on the progression of renal failure in patients with insulin-dependent diabetes mellitus. *N Engl J Med* 324:78–84, 1991

21. Raal FJ, Kalk WJ, Lawson M, Esser JD, Buys R, Fourie L, Panz VR: Effect of moderate dietary protein restriction on the progression of overt diabetic nephropathy: a 6-mo prospective study. *Am J Clin Nutr* 60:579–585, 1994

22. Dullaart RPF, Beusekamp BJ, Meijer S, van Doormaal JJ, Sluiter WJ: Long-term effects of protein-restricted diet on albuminuria and renal function in IDDM patients without clinical nephropathy and hypertension. *Diabetes Care* 16:483–492, 1993

23. Pomerleau J, Verdy M, Garrel DR, Nadeau MH: Effect of protein intake on glycaemic control and renal function in type 2 (non-insulin-dependent) diabetes mellitus. *Diabetologia* 36:829–834, 1993

24. Pedrini MT, Levey AS, Lau J, Chalmers TC, Wang PH: The effect of dietary protein restriction on the progression of diabetic and nondiabetic renal diseases: a meta-analysis. *Ann Intern Med* 124:627–632, 1996

25. Maroni BJ, Steinman TI, Mitch WE: A method for estimating nitrogen intake of patients with chronic renal failure. *Kidney Int* 27:58–65, 1985

26. Nair K, Ford G, Halliday D: Effect of insulin treatment on in vivo whole body leucine kinetics and oxygen consumption in insulin-deprived type 1 diabetic patients. *Metab Clin Exp* 36:491–495, 1987

27. Umpleby AM, Boroujerdi MA, Brown PM, Carson ER, Sonksen PH: The effect of metabolic control on leucine metabolism in type 1 (insulin-dependent) diabetic patients. *Diabetologia* 29:131–141, 1986

28. Brodsky IG, Devlin JT: Effects of dietary protein restriction on regional amino acid metabolism in insulin-dependent diabetes mellitus. *Am J Physiol* 270:E148–E157, 1996

29. Gougeon R, Pencharz PB, Sigal RJ: Effect of glycemic control on the kinetics of whole-body protein metabolism in obese subjects with non-insulin-dependent diabetes mellitus during iso- and hypoenergetic feeding. *Am J Clin Nutr* 65:861–870, 1997

30. Rudberg S, Dahlqvist G, Aperia A, Lindblad BS, Efendic S, Skottner, Persson B: Indications that branched chain amino acids, in addition to glucagon, affect the glomerular filtration rate after a high protein diet in insulin-dependent diabetes. *Diabetes Res* 16:101–109, 1991

31. Nakamura H, Takasawa M, Kasahara S, Tsuda A, Momotsu T, Ito S, Shibata A: Effects of acute protein loads of different sources on renal function of patients with diabetic nephropathy. *Tohoku J Exp Med* 159:153–162, 1989

32. Nakamura H, Yamazaki M, Chiba Y, Tamura N, Momotsu T, Ito S, Shibata A, Kamoi K, Yamaji T: Glomerular filtration response to acute loading with protein from different sources in healthy volunteers and diabetic patients. *Tohoku J Exp Med* 162:269–278, 1990

33. Nakamura H, Yamazaki M, Chiba Y, Tani N, Momotsu T, Kamoi K, Ito S, Yamaji T, Shibata A: Acute loading with proteins from different sources in healthy volunteers and diabetic patients. *J Diabetic Complications* 5:140–142, 1991

34. Nakamura H, Ebe N, Ito S, Shibata A: Renal effects of different types of protein in healthy volunteer subjects and diabetic patients. *Diabetes Care* 16:1071–1075, 1993

35. Jibani MM, Bloodworth LL, Foden E, Griffiths KD, Galpin OP: Predominantly vegetarian diet in patients with incipient and early clinical diabetic nephropathy: effects on albumin excretion rate and nutritional status. *Diabetic Med* 8:949–953, 1991

36. Kontessis PS, Trevisan R, Bossinakou I, Roussi D, Sarika L, Stipsanelli K, Iliopoulou E, Grigorakis S, Papantoniou A, Souvatzoglou

A: Renal, metabolic, and hormonal responses to proteins of different origin in normotensive, nonproteinuric type 1 diabetic patients. *Diabetes Care* 18:1233–1240, 1995

37. Pecis M, deAzevedo MJ, Gross JL: Chicken and fish diet reduces glomerular hyperfiltration in IDDM patients. *Diabetes Care* 17:665–672, 1994

38. Fioretto P, Trevisan R, Valerio A, Avogaro A, Borsato M, Doria A, Semplicini A, Sacerdoti D, Jones S, Bognetti E, Viberti GC, Nosadini R: Impaired renal response to a meat meal in insulin-dependent diabetes: role of glucagon and prostaglandins. *Am J Physiol* 258:F675–F683, 1990

39. Ando A, Kawata T, Hara Y, Yaegashi M, Arai J, Sugino N: Effects of dietary protein intake on renal function in humans. *Kidney Int* 36:S64–S67, 1989

Ms. Wheeler is Coordinator, Research Dietetics, with Indiana University School of Medicine's Diabetes Research and Training Center in Indianapolis, IN.

18. Diabetic Gastropathy and Medical Nutrition Therapy

Madelyn L. Wheeler, MS, RD, FADA, CDE

Highlights

- Treatments suggested for diabetic gastropathy include optimization of glycemic control, dietary modifications, various pharmacological options, and surgery.
- While there is no scientific evidence for effective treatment by dietary modification in diabetic gastropathy, professional judgment and clinical practice indicate the efficacy of small frequent meals, low fat content of foods, and use of liquid or blenderized meals.

INTRODUCTION

Diabetic gastropathy (also known as *gastroparesis diabeticorum* or *diabetic gastroparesis*) is characterized by abnormally delayed emptying of foods, particularly solid foods, from the stomach (1). From published clinical and epidemiological studies, there is little indication that people with diabetes are at much higher risk of this than the general population (2). Typically, the symptoms of diabetic gastropathy are similar to those of gastric outlet obstruction: nausea and vomiting, early satiety, bloating, and abdominal pain. This condition is usually attributed to autonomic neuropathy and abnormalities of gut hormones such as motilin and gastrin; however, other mechanisms suggested include hyperglycemia, abnormal levels of electrolytes, and altered secretion of insulin and glucagon (3). Treatments suggested for gastroparesis include

- glycemic control optimization, particularly because hyperglycemia appears to slow the rate of gastric emptying (4–6)

- dietary modifications (1,3,7–9) such as
  - small frequent meals
  - low fat content
  - low fiber content
  - use of food with soft consistency; replacing solid with liquid meals
- various pharmacological options (10), such as cholinergic drugs, dopamine antagonists (11), and motilin-receptor agonists (12)
- surgical treatment: jejeunostomy enteral feeding; gastrectomy

DIETARY MODIFICATION

No controlled trial of treatment by dietary modifications either in the management of symptoms of diabetic gastropathy or in the improvement of glycemic control in individuals who have diabetic gastropathy has been reported. Therefore, recommendations have been made based on professional judgment and clinical practice, and the specific dietary recommendations often provided to patients with diabetic gastroparesis have not changed substantially since Kassander's description in 1958 (1). They appear to be based on logical interpretation of gastric physiology (13,14) and interpolation from gastrointestinal studies of other disease states or from research involving healthy individuals.

Small Frequent Meals

There is concern that patients who complain of early satiety and bloating may reduce the quantity and frequency of food intake and that their nutritional status can become compromised, particularly in terms of energy and essential vitamins and minerals (15,16). Having frequent, small meals, nutritionally balanced for the whole day, may be better tolerated and would lessen the possibility of impaired nutritional status.

Low Fat Content

Fat appears to be the most potent inhibitor of gastric emptying; with the longest chain fatty acids having the greatest delay in emptying (8,14). Reducing the amount of fat may produce less delay in gastric emptying.

Low Fiber Content

The main concern with lowering fiber content appears to be that combining fibrous vegetables and poorly digestible solids with limited gastric motility may provide a predisposition for bezoar formation (9). Also, it has been thought that soluble fibers may act as gastric motility inhibitors; however, Leatherdale (17) found no change in emptying pattern when people with type 2 diabetes and a later and slower-than-normal phase of gastric emptying were given a guar supplement (17). Therefore, it appears that lowering fiber content may be a questionable recommendation, given that the average daily fiber intake in the U.S. is only about 10–13 g/day.

Replacing Solid with Liquid/Blenderized Meals

In diabetic gastropathy, liquid/blenderized meals appear to be digested normally (7); however, hypertonic formulas should be avoided because they can further delay gastric emptying (18).

OTHER CONSIDERATIONS

It has been suggested that because exercise appears to increase solid-meal gastric emptying rates in healthy individuals (19), it might do the same in people with diabetic gastropathy. Although the results of one small report in this area were inconclusive (20), postprandial exercise (such as walking) is an excellent recommendation for anyone, with or without diabetic gastropathy.

Finally, adjustment of insulin doses and timing so that there is a better match with the delayed nutrient absorption and postprandial rise in glucose levels should also be considered. For example, regular insulin could be given after a meal rather than before because duration of regular insulin may be longer and without a defined peak in individuals with diabetic gastropathy (21).

SUMMARY

Treatments to be considered for diabetic gastropathy include optimization of glycemic control, dietary modifications (particularly small frequent meals of low fat content and liquid/blenderized consistency), pharmacological options, and surgery. Controlled clinical trials evaluating the relationships among dietary intake, food choices, gastrointestinal symptoms, and gastric motility are needed to provide scientific evidence for the efficacy of dietary modification.

REFERENCES

1. Kassander P: Asymptomatic gastric retention in diabetics (gastroparesis diabeticorum). *Ann Intern Med* 48:797–812, 1958

2. Everhart JE: Digestive diseases and diabetes. In *Diabetes in America.* 2nd ed. Harris MI, Cowie CC, Stern MP, Boyko EJ, Reiber GE, Bennett PH, Eds. Washington, DC, U.S. Govt. Printing Office, 1995 (NIH publ. no. 95-1468), pp. 457–483

3. Nilsson P: Diabetic gastroparesis: a review. *J Diabetes Complications* 10:113–122, 1996

4. Horowitz M, Maddox AF, Wishart JM, Harding PE, Chatterton BE, Shearman DJC: Relationships between oesophageal transit and solid and liquid gastric emptying in diabetes mellitus. *Eur J Nucl Med* 18:229–234, 1991

5. Barnett JL, Owyang C: Serum glucose concentration as a modulator of interdigestive gastric motility. *Gastroenterology* 94:739–744, 1988

6. Fraser RJ, Horowitz M, Maddox AF, Harding PE, Chatterton BE, Dent J: Hyperglycaemia slows gastric emptying in type I (insulin-dependent) diabetes mellitus. *Diabetologia* 33:675–680, 1990

7. Cronin B: Nutritional concerns in gastrointestinal neuropathy. *Diabetes Educ* 18:531–535, 1992

8. Gentry P, Miller PF: Nutritional considerations in a patient with gastroparesis. *Diabetes Educ* 15:374–376, 1989

9. Parrish CR: Gastrointestinal issues in persons with diabetes. In *Handbook of Diabetes Medical Nutrition Therapy.* Powers MA, Ed. Gaithersburg MD, Aspen, 1996, pp. 618–637

10. Horowitz M, Wishart JM, Jones KL, Hebbard GS: Gastric emptying in diabetes: an overview. *Diabetic Med* 13 (Suppl. 5):S16–S22, 1996

11. Melga P, Giusti R, Mansi C, Sciaba L, Ciuchi E, Prando R: Chronic administration of levosulpiride and glycemic control in IDDM patients with gastroparesis. *Diabetes Care* 20:55–58, 1997

12. Ishii M, Baba T, Nakamura T, Takebe K, Kasai F: Erythromycin derivative improves gastric emptying and insulin requirement in diabetic patients with gastroparesis. *Diabetes Care* 20:1134–1137, 1997

13. Macdonald IA: Physiological regulation of gastric emptying and glucose absorption. *Diabetic Med* 13 (Suppl. 5):S11–S15, 1996

14. Thomas JE: Mechanics and regulation of gastric emptying. *Physiol Rev* 37:453–474, 1957

15. Goldberg KB, Lasichak A, Rock CL: Dietary adequacy in patients with diabetic gastroparesis. *J Am Diet Assoc* 97:420–422, 1997

16. Ogorek CP, Davidson L, Fisher RS, Krevsky B: Idiopathic gastroparesis is associated with a multiplicity of severe dietary deficiencies. *Am J Gastroenterol* 86:423–428, 1991

17. Leatherdale BA, Green DJ, Harding LK, Griffin D, Bailey CJ: Guar and gastric emptying in non-insulin dependent diabetes. *Acta Diabetol Lat* 19:339–343, 1982

18. Bury KD, Jambunathan G: Effects of elemental diets on gastric emptying and gastric secretion in man. *Am J Surg* 127:59–64, 1974

19. Moore JG, Datz FL, Christian PE: Exercise increases solid meal gastric emptying rates in men. *Dig Dis Sci* 35:428–432, 1990

20. Lipp RW, Schnedl WJ, Hammer HF: Does postprandial walking influence delayed gastric emptying in patients with long-standing IDDM? (Letter). *Diabetes Care* 19:1306, 1996

21. Ishii M, Onuma T, Nakamura T, Baba T, Kasai F, Takebe K: Altered postprandial insulin requirement in IDDM patients with gastroparesis. *Diabetes Care* 17:901–903, 1994

Ms. Wheeler is Coordinator, Research Dietetics, with Indiana University School of Medicine's Diabetes Research and Training Center in Indianapolis, IN.

19. Nutrition Support and Diabetes

M. MOLLY MCMAHON, MD

Highlights

- For the hospitalized patient with diabetes who requires parenteral or enteral nutrition, the nutritional assessment, indications for nutrition support, estimate of nutritional needs, and guidelines for metabolic monitoring are similar to those of the nondiabetic patient.
- Once it has been determined that nutrition support is necessary, the optimal route for nutrient delivery should be determined. The enteral route is preferred for nutrient delivery if the gastrointestinal tract is functional.
- A major goal of glucose management is to avoid the extremes of hyper- and hypoglycemia. For stressed hospitalized patients, a reasonable aim is to maintain glucose levels between 100 and 200 mg/dl (5.6 and 11.1 mmol/l).
- Careful monitoring of vital signs, hemodynamic data, weight, fluid balance, plasma glucose and electrolytes, and acid-base status is essential.

INTRODUCTION

Because of the prevalence of diabetes and the comorbidity of the disease, most physicians and health care providers will manage hospitalized diabetic patients receiving nutrition support. In addition to discussing nutrition support for this group of patients, this chapter will review new information regarding adverse effects of hyperglycemia on immune function.

The homeostatic mechanisms that maintain euglycemia in the postabsorptive state and buffer the postprandial glycemic excursion in nondiabetic subjects are impaired in patients with diabetes. These patients have both preprandial and postprandial hyperglycemia due to excessive hepatic glucose release, impaired glucose uptake, and decreased insulin secretion and/or action.

Severe stress can cause hyperglycemia in patients without an antecedent diagnosis of diabetes. Severe stress (as during a serious illness) is accompanied by significant increases in plasma concentrations of counterregulatory hormones (that is, glucagon, epinephrine, cortisol, and growth hormone) that increase hepatic glucose release and decrease peripheral glucose uptake. Stress causes an even greater derangement in glucose metabolism in patients with diabetes because they cannot increase insulin secretion as a compensatory response. The exaggerated glucose response following a stress-dose counterregulatory hormone infusion in healthy subjects with diabetes in comparison with nondiabetic subjects is one explanation for the deterioration in glucose control that occurs in stressed diabetic patients. Cytokines may also profoundly affect carbohydrate metabolism. Typically, the interleukins cause hyperglycemia. Endotoxin can cause hyperglycemia or hypoglycemia.

GLUCOSE GOALS

A major goal in the care of the hospitalized patient is to avoid the extremes of hyperglycemia and hypoglycemia. A reasonable aim is to maintain glucose levels between 100 and 200 mg/dl (5.6 and 11.1 mmol/l). Avoidance or minimization of hyperglycemia in hospitalized patients is important. The health care provider should attempt to identify the cause(s) of hyperglycemia. Illness or infection, overfeeding (nutrition support, dextrose-containing crystalloid, dextrose absorption during peritoneal dialysis, and medications formulated in lipid emulsion, such as propofol), medications (e.g., corticosteroids, sympathomimetic infusion, cyclosporine), insufficient insulin, and/or volume depletion can cause hyperglycemia. Because unexplained hyperglycemia may be a harbinger of infection, the central catheter should always be considered a potential source of infection.

During a short time period, hyperglycemia can adversely affect fluid balance and immune function. As the filtered load of glucose increases, it eventually exceeds tubular reabsorptive capacity. As a result, glucose remains in the tubular lumen and acts as an osmotic diuretic, increasing the urinary loss of electrolytes and water. Impaired polymorphonuclear function in diabetic patients has long been recognized. In vitro studies document that hyperglycemia is associated with abnormalities in granulocyte adhesion, chemotaxis, phagocytosis, and intracellular killing (1–4). Most studies report that phagocytosis can be corrected or substantially improved with control of blood glucose (1,3). Respiratory burst function and superoxide anion production are impaired in patients with type 2 diabetes and are improved by glucose control. Respiratory burst is a critical element in the activation of microbicidal systems because this burst of oxidative metabolism generates toxic products of oxygen (5). A significant reduction in the respiratory burst also occurs in neutrophils of healthy nondiabetic subjects following exposure to glucose concentrations >200 mg/dl (>11.1 mmol/l). Hyperglycemia also adversely affects complement function (2). The opsonic function of complement is impaired because glucose binds to the biochemically active site of complement, thereby inhibiting complement attachment to the microbial surface. A recent study reported that increased cytosolic calcium levels in polymorphonuclear leukocytes of diabetic patients adversely affect immune function. Increased cytosolic calcium in leukocytes of diabetic patients was directly correlated with glucose values and was associated with decreased phagocytosis (6). Three months of oral hypoglycemic agent therapy resulted in improved glucose control, a reduction in cytosolic calcium levels, and a significant improvement in phagocytosis. Lastly, an association between hyperglycemia and infection with *Candida albicans* has long been recognized. *C. albicans* expresses a surface protein that is homologous with the α-chain of the neutrophil receptor for complement. There is an abrupt increase in protein expression during hyperglycemia. This protein impairs phagocytosis of the yeast by binding to complement and inhibits adhesion of the yeast to endothelial surfaces. This mechanism may explain, in part, the increased incidence of *Candida* infections in diabetic patients.

An obvious follow-up question is, "Are there clinical studies documenting adverse effects of hyperglycemia?" A growing body of clinical evidence has linked hyperglycemia to nosocomial infection in stressed hospitalized patients:

1. The rate of central catheter–related infections was approximately five times higher in diabetic patients receiving central parenteral nutrition than in nondiabetic patients receiving the same nutrition (B.R. Bistrian, personal communication).
2. As discussed earlier, hyperglycemia was the most common risk factor for *Candida* infection (2).
3. A recent meta-analysis summarizing results from prospective randomized trials comparing parenteral with enteral nutrition in critically ill patients reported that significantly fewer enterally fed patients (compared with parenterally fed patients) experienced septic complications (16% vs. 35%, respectively). While the authors concluded that the route of administration of nutrients was the key factor in the observed differences, hyperglycemia may have been an additional variable responsible for the increased infection rate. The average glucose at the conclusion of the study

was 230 mg/dl (12.8 mmol/l) in the parenterally fed patients, compared with a mean of 130 mg/dl (7.2 mmol/l) in the enterally fed group (7).

4. The recently designed Veterans Affairs Trial was designed to test the hypothesis that perioperative parenteral nutrition decreases the incidence of serious complications following major abdominal or thoracic surgical procedures in malnourished patients. Although there was a reduction in noninfectious complications in the patients receiving parenteral nutrition, infectious complications were 2.2 times more common (8). Nutritionists would not refute the conclusion that only malnourished patients should receive preoperative support; however, it is important to point out that the higher infection rate observed in patients receiving parenteral nutrition may have resulted in part from severe hyperglycemia. Serum glucose >200 mg/dl (>11.1 mmol/l) occurred in 20% of patients receiving parenteral nutrition and in 1% of the control group. Patients receiving parenteral nutrition were also allowed to eat, and the combined caloric intake averaged ~45 kcal/kg body wt, which significantly exceeds requirements. Such overfeeding can lead to hyperglycemia.

5. A higher incidence of mediastinitis was found in diabetic patients (compared with nondiabetic patients) following coronary artery bypass graft surgery (9).

6. A recent study suggests that hyperglycemia itself is an independent risk factor for the development of infection. Investigators monitoring perioperative glucose control in 100 previously uninfected diabetic patients undergoing elective surgery and the subsequent development of postoperative infection found that hyperglycemia (glucose levels in excess of 220 mg/dl [12.2 mmol/l]) on postoperative day 1 was associated with a higher rate of infection. There was no difference between the two groups in type or duration of diabetes, patient age, percentage of ideal body weight, recent weight loss in excess of 10%, percentage of patients with preoperative length of stay longer than 1 day, or surgical wound classification (10).

Hyperglycemia has also been associated with a higher mortality in diabetic compared with nondiabetic patients following acute myocardial infarction (11). Improved outcome was observed in diabetic patients who, following myocardial infarction, were treated with intravenous insulin infusion during the hospitalization or with glucose-insulin infusion during the hospitalization followed by multiple daily insulin injection programs.

Avoidance or minimization of hypoglycemia is also important. Identifying neuroglycopenic and adrenergic symptoms of hypoglycemia is difficult in severely ill patients who are sedated or dependent on mechanical ventilation. In addition, patients with long-standing diabetes may have hypoglycemic unawareness, a loss of the ability to recognize the warning symptoms of hypoglycemia. The physician should always attempt to identify the factor or factors responsible for hypoglycemia. Potential causes include unanticipated discontinuation of nutrition support, resolution of severe stress, discontinuation or decreased doses of corticosteroids or sympathomimetic agents, renal dysfunction, severe hepatitis, sepsis, and diabetic gastroparesis.

NUTRITIONAL ASSESSMENT

Nutritional assessment, indications for nutritional support, and estimate of nutritional needs for critically ill diabetic patients are similar to those of nondiabetic patients. However, diabetes can affect the entire gastrointestinal tract. Significant diabetic gastroparesis is typically observed in patients with type 1 diabetes. This diagnosis should be strongly suspected if patients experience bloating, early satiety, nausea, and postprandial vomiting (especially of partially digested food retained from earlier meals). It is important to accurately diagnose diabetic gastroparesis to avoid attributing the gastrointestinal symptoms to tube feeding alone or to other factors capable of affecting gut motility. Review of the patient's medication list is important to determine if any of the prescribed medications may delay gastric emptying. These medications include α_2-adrenergic agonists, anticholinergic agents (tricyclic antidepressants, antihistamines), beta blockers, calcium-channel blockers, and narcotics. Acute hyperglycemia can decrease gastric emptying. Constipation, diarrhea, and fecal incontinence may also develop with long-standing diabetes.

Protein catabolism (with eventual depletion of body protein) can be a consequence of starvation or severe illness. In the classic sense, malnutrition results from starvation. Nevertheless, either severe illness or illness superimposed on starvation is by far the more common cause of protein catabolism in hospitalized patients.

Interpretation of the nutritional assessment of critically ill patients is enhanced by an understanding of the cytokine and hormonal milieu of sickness. Anorexia is common in patients with severe illness. Cytokine infusion has been shown to cause a significant reduction in food intake. It is important to recognize that illness and cytokines cause an acute decrease in plasma albumin. This decrease can be attributed to altered capillary permeability (allowing albumin to move from the intravascular to the extravascular space) and to an increase in catabolism. In addition, cytokines can downregulate the albumin gene and thereby decrease the rate of messenger RNA translation. Therefore, during severe illness, hypoalbuminemia is an excellent marker of the stress response but a poor marker of nutritional status. The importance of hypoalbuminemia is supported by studies reporting that hypoalbuminemia at hospital admission is associated with increased morbidity and mortality rates. Finally, although weight is often a key anthropometric marker, the weight of hospitalized patients must be carefully interpreted. Many critically ill patients have increased total body water and salt due to the underlying illness (e.g., malnutrition or cardiac, renal, or hepatic disease), the treatment (e.g., crystalloid or colloid infusion), or the hormonal milieu of critical illness and refeeding. Thus, weight loss alone is not a requisite for initiation of nutrition support.

In general, a recent (previous 3- to 6-month interval) weight loss in excess of 10% from usual weight necessitates a more thorough nutritional assessment. A recent unintentional weight loss of 10–20% of usual weight suggests moderate protein-calorie malnutrition, and a loss of >20% usually indicates severe malnutrition. In addition to the magnitude of recent weight loss, the presence or absence of clinical markers of stress and the anticipated time that the patient will be unable to eat determines the need for nutrition intervention. Usually, a weight loss of up to 10% of body weight is well tolerated, and in the absence of significant stress, the provision of dextrose-containing crystalloid solutions and electrolytes alone is adequate for as long as 7–10 days. Studies that demonstrated a beneficial influence of nutrition support on clinical outcome administered nutrition for a minimum of 1 week (12,13). No data have been established that nutrition support of briefer duration is of clinical benefit.

Avoidance of overfeeding is important because an excess of calories can exacerbate hyperglycemia. The daily energy expenditure of a hospitalized patient can be estimated by using a formula, such as the Harris-Benedict equation, by providing a certain number of kilocalories per kilogram of body weight, or by indirect calorimetry. During the past decade, numerous studies have shown that the actual energy expenditure of most hospitalized patients is between 100 and 120% of caloric expenditure predicted by the Harris-Benedict equation (Table 19.1) (14,15). No consensus exists about nutritional requirements of obese patients, and data are limited. Certain investigators have recommend that in obese patients, the weight used to estimate caloric requirements be the weight halfway between the ideal and current weight. We recommend providing ~75% of basal caloric requirements calculated on the basis of the obese weight. Outcome studies are needed to resolve this controversy.

In general, the malnourished patient with normal renal and hepatic function should receive 1.0 to 1.5 g protein/kg body wt; the higher end of the range being for more stressed patients. Studies report that no greater sparing of protein occurs when exogenous protein is provided in amounts exceeding 1.5 g/kg/day (16). Intravenous fat emulsion should be limited to ~30% of the total calories and provided continuously. Most complica-

Table 19.1 Guidelines for Calorie, Protein, and Lipid Requirements

Calories	Basal calories by using the HB equation* to HB plus 20%
Protein	1.0–1.5 g/kg body wt
Lipids	30% of total calories over 24 h

Indirect calorimetric measurement of daily caloric needs can be considered for the following groups of patients: severely stressed patients (e.g., closed head injury, multiple trauma, severe burn), volume-overloaded patients in whom the "dry weight" estimate is uncertain, nutritionally supported patients in whom weaning from mechanical ventilation is difficult, or in patients requiring home parenteral nutrition. Guidelines for protein assume normal hepatic and renal function.

*HB (Harris-Benedict) equation:
Men $66.5 + (13.8 \times$ wt, kg$) + (5.0 \times$ ht, cm$) - (6.8 \times$ age, years$)$
Women $65.5 + (9.6 \times$ wt, kg$) + (1.8 \times$ ht, cm$) - (4.7 \times$ age, years$)$

tions (that is, impairment of the reticulothelial system clearance and immune function) related to the use of intravenous fat occur at higher infusion rates.

The enteral route, rather than the parenteral, is the preferred route for delivery of nutrition if the gastrointestinal tract is functioning. Advantages of enteral nutrition include its lower cost, its avoidance of central catheter–related complications, its more physiological route, and its trophic effect on gastrointestinal cells.

MANAGEMENT DURING PARENTERAL NUTRITION

Many approaches can be used to achieve glucose control and to avoid the extremes of hypoglycemia and hyperglycemia in diabetic patients receiving nutrition support. Our approach has worked to meet the needs of the institution in which many physicians prescribe the nutrition (17). (McMahon et al. [18] provides another model for management.)

- Dextrose in the parenteral nutrition (PN) is limited to ~200 g on the first day of nutrition.
- The majority of diabetic patients will require insulin coverage when glucose is infused. For patients previously treated with insulin or oral hypoglycemic agents or for patients with fasting glucose values consistently >200 mg/dl, it is our practice to initially place 0.1 U regular insulin per gram of dextrose (e.g., 15 U/liter D 15% [150 g/l]). In our experience, this ratio of

insulin to dextrose is unlikely to be associated with hypoglycemia and thus minimizes the need to waste a bag of PN.

* It is our practice initially to measure reflectance meter glucose values frequently and to administer supplemental subcutaneous regular insulin according to a subcutaneous insulin algorithm (Table 19.2). Once glycemic control is acceptable, an alteration in the frequency of glucose monitoring may be appropriate.

* If over a 24-h period glucose values consistently exceed 200 mg/dl (11.1 mmol/l), the PN insulin is increased each day by 0.05 U regular insulin per gram of dextrose to a maximum of 0.2 U insulin per gram of dextrose. If the plasma glucose remains >200 mg/dl (>11.1 mmol/l) with insulin coverage of 0.2 U per gram of PN dextrose and adherence to the subcutaneous insulin algorithm, initiation of an intravenous insulin infusion should be considered. Our group has implemented the use of an order form to standardize the insulin infusion (Table 19.3).

* In general, the PN dextrose load should not be increased until the glucose values of the previous 24-h period are consistently <200 mg/dl (<11.1 mmol/l).

* Insulin in the PN should be proportionally increased or decreased when the PN dextrose content is increased or decreased.

* The incidence of symptomatic hypoglycemia after discontinuation of PN is uncommon provided that the patient has not received excessive calories. However, if the patient has a serum creatinine >2.0 mg/dl or if the PN admixture contains >0.2 U insulin per gram of dextrose, the glucose concentration should be monitored closely during the first hour after discontinuation of PN. If the patient develops hypoglycemia, parenteral dextrose should be administered (Table 19.4). A

Table 19.2 Guidelines for Subcutaneous Regular Insulin Supplementation

Glucose (mg/dl)	Subcutaneous Regular Insulin Dose (U)
200–250	2–3
251–300	4–6
301–350	6–9
>350	8–12

Adjustment of this algorithm may be required for differences in patient weight, response to insulin, and treatment goals. Insulin should not be administered more often than every 4–6 h.

Table 19.3 Intravenous Insulin Infusion Algorithm and Guidelines

Glucose (mg/dl)	IV Infusion Rate (ml/h)	Insulin Infusion Rate (U/h)
>400	8	8
351–400	6	6
301–350	4	4
250–300	3	3
200–249	2.5	2.5
150–199	2	2
120–149	1.5	1.5
100–119	1	1
70–99	0	0
<70	0	0

- Glucose goals should be defined for each patient. In stressed patients, a glucose goal range of 100–200 mg/dl is appropriate. This infusion algorithm is designed for the average 70-kg patient and may require modification for smaller or larger patients. This infusion is not appropriate for treatment of diabetic ketoacidosis or hyperosmolar states.
- Glucose should be measured hourly until glucose concentrations have stabilized in patient's goal glucose range for 4 h. Frequency of testing may then be decreased to every 2 h, and once glucose control remains stable, to every 4 h.
- If hyperglycemia persists, this algorithm may be increased by 50% increments for each glucose range >200 mg/dl. Risk of hypoglycemia may be greater if algorithm is increased for glucose values <200 mg/dl.
- In patients treated with insulin, plasma potassium, magnesium, and phosphorus concentrations may decrease rapidly and should be monitored.
- At time of conversion from intravenous to subcutaneous insulin therapy, intravenous infusion should be continued for 2–3 h following administration of first subcutaneous insulin dose.

substantial (50%) reduction of insulin in the following day's PN admixture should decrease the incidence of recurrent hypoglycemia. Similar reductions in the PN insulin should also be made if there is a significant decrease in the mean glucose concentration over a 24-h period to values below the goal range.

MANAGEMENT DURING ENTERAL NUTRITION

While subcutaneous insulin administration usually prevents hyperglycemia in patients receiving enteral calories, glycemic control may be difficult to achieve. Until the patient has been shown to tolerate tube

---

Table 19.4 Treatment of Hypoglycemia in Hospitalized Adult Patients with Diabetes on Insulin or Oral Agents

I. Symptomatic hypoglycemia should be treated as follows:
   A. If patient is able to swallow safely, provide oral administration of glucose. Patient should ingest ~15 g carbohydrate. Examples:
      1. 2 sugar packets/cubes or
      2. 15 g glucose tablets/gel or
      3. 1/2 cup (4 oz) fruit juice
   B. If patient is not able to take oral feeding safely or is NPO for any reason, do the following:
      1. If intravenous access is available, administer 1/2 ampoule (12.5 g) D50W intravenously.
      2. If no intravenous access is present, administer 1 mg glucagon by subcutaneous or intramuscular injection. Following glucagon treatment, for those patients who are not NPO, provide a snack to prevent subsequent hypoglycemia.
   C. Contact the service responsible for the patient's diabetes management.
II. For treatment of asymptomatic hypoglycemia (glucose ≤60 mg/dl), follow steps A through C above.
III. Glycemic monitoring following treatment:
   Obtain capillary glucose determination in 15 min. If glucose is not >80 mg/dl, repeat treatment outlined above. Recheck glucose value in 15 min. Repeat further treatment (and glucose checks at 15-min intervals) until glucose is >80 mg/dl.

---

feeding, intermediate-acting insulin should be used with caution. Short-acting insulin is preferred, to minimize the risk of hypoglycemia that could result from the continued absorption of insulin from longer-acting insulin preparations following unexpected discontinuation of tube feeding. Once the tube-feeding infusion rate has reached 30–40 ml/h, the use of intermediate-acting insulin generally is safe.

- If tube feedings are to be administered during the day, we frequently begin by providing one-half of the patient's preadmission morning insulin dose as intermediate-acting insulin. Increases in the tube feeding infusion rate should be avoided until adequate glucose control has been achieved. Intermediate-acting insulin should be given in the evening if the tube feeding is administered during the night. Twice-daily administration of intermediate-acting insulin may be required if the tube feedings are administered continuously over 24 h.
- If the feedings are infused by gravity administration, the glucose level should be checked immediately before the feeding is initiated and no sooner than 4 h following the end of the prior

feeding. While some patients receiving this form of feeding can be managed with intermediate-acting insulin alone, others will need combined treatment with intermediate- and short-acting insulins.

* The tube-feeding rate should not be altered until appropriate adjustments have been made in the insulin dose(s).
* Gastroparesis may make tube-feeding tolerance more difficult. In our experience, the majority of patients with diabetic gastroparesis tolerate jejunal feedings when iso-osmolar formulas are started at a low rate (e.g., 20 ml/h) and advanced slowly (e.g., 10–20 ml/h increment increase every 12 h) to the goal infusion rate. Selected patients require gastric decompression. Glucose control can affect gastric emptying, and delayed gastric emptying may make regulation of glucose control difficult. Hyperglycemia may further delay gastric emptying, while hypoglycemia may result in patients treated with insulin or oral hypoglycemic agents not absorbing food normally because of a delay in gastric emptying.
* Unexpected discontinuation of tube feeding may cause hypoglycemia in patients who are treated with subcutaneous injections of insulin. Glucose levels should be carefully monitored to determine whether intravenous infusion of a dextrose-containing solution is necessary to prevent subsequent hypoglycemia.
* Oral hypoglycemic agents can be used to treat hyperglycemia in medically stable patients with well-controlled type 2 diabetes and normal renal and hepatic function, and they may be administered by feeding tube. We do not recommend the use of metformin in hospitalized patients, because lactic acidosis may occur with renal, cardiac, or hepatic dysfunction.
* In patients with unstable diabetes and significant hyperglycemia, an intravenous insulin infusion may be necessary.

The recent availability of enteral formulas lower in carbohydrate and higher in fat content than standard formulas has prompted studies comparing glycemic responses. While initial studies suggested that the glycemic response to the lower carbohydrate product was blunted compared with that to standard formulas, a follow-up study reported that the glycemic response was variable in each patient (19). The clinical significance of these studies is unclear because the subjects ingested very small amounts of formula over a few hours, a very different pattern than that of continuous tube feeding or gravity administration of feeding. The high fat content could impair gastric emptying in patients with gastroparesis. With regard to fiber content, the current American Diabetes Association position statement on nutrition (20) states that although selected soluble fibers are capable of delaying glucose absorption from the small intestine, the effect of dietary fiber on glycemic control is probably insignificant. Therefore, the fiber intake recommendations for individuals with diabetes are probably the same as for the general hospitalized population. During hospitalization, avoidance of overfeeding is likely more important than is the use of a specific enteral formula. Outcome studies will be necessary to address this issue.

METABOLIC MONITORING

Careful metabolic monitoring is critical to ensure safe use of nutritional support in the diabetic patient. Accurate recording of daily weight and fluid balance is essential. An admission glycated hemoglobin measurement is useful to estimate recent glucose control and to design a diabetes management program following hospital discharge. In addition to the usual monitoring required for nondiabetic patients receiving nutrition support, attention should be focused on the effects of hyperinsulinemia on fluid balance and electrolytes and on triglyceride levels. With an acute increase in plasma insulin, renal sodium excretion decreases, which may lead to salt and water retention. Hyperinsulinemia may also decrease plasma levels of potassium, magnesium, and phosphorus. Hyperinsulinemia shifts potassium and magnesium into skeletal muscle and hepatic cells. Glucose- and insulin-stimulated glycolysis stimulate the cellular uptake and utilization of phosphorus for the phosphorylation of glucose and fructose and for the synthesis of adenosine triphosphate. Therefore, serum potassium, magnesium, and phosphorus concentrations should be monitored until the levels are stable. For patients with known hypertriglyceridemia, a triglyceride level should be checked before and during fat emulsion administration. For patients with pancreatitis, with poorly controlled diabetes, or on medications formulated in fat emulsion, triglyceride level should be checked before initiating fat emulsion. In general, fat emulsion should be reduced or avoided if triglycerides exceed 400 mg/dl.

OUTCOME

Well-designed prospective randomized trials will be needed to determine the risks, costs, and benefits of achieving glucose control and of providing nutrition support to malnourished diabetic patients.

REFERENCES

1. Alexiewicz JM, Kumar D, Smogorzewski M, Klin M, Massry SG: Polymorphonuclear leukocytes in noninsulin-dependent diabetes

mellitus: abnormalities in metabolism and function. *Ann Intern Med* 123:919–924, 1995

2. Hostetter M: Perspectives in diabetes: handicaps to host defense: effects of hyperglycemia on C3 and *Candida albicans. Diabetes* 39:271–275, 1990

3. MacRury SM, Gemmell CG, Paterson KR, MacCuish AC: Changes in phagocytic function with glycemic control in diabetic patients. *J Clin Pathol* 42:1143–1147, 1989

4. McMahon M, Bistrian BR: Host defenses and susceptibility to infection in patients with diabetes mellitus. *Infect Dis Clin North Am* 9:1–9, 1995

5. Ortmeyer J, Mohsenin V: Glucose suppresses superoxide generation in normal neutrophils: interference in phospholipase D activation. *Am J Physiol* 264:C402–C410, 1993

6. Alexiewicz JM, Kumar D, Smogorzewski M, Klin M, Massry SG: Polymorphonuclear leukocytes in non-insulin-dependent diabetes mellitus: abnormalities in metabolism and function. *Ann Intern Med* 123:919–924, 1995

7. Moore FA, Feliciano DV, Andrassy RJ, McArdle AH, Booth FV, Morgenstein-Wagner TB, Kellum JM Jr, Welling RE, Moore EE: Early enteral feeding, compared with parenteral, reduces post-operative septic complications: the results of a meta-analysis. *Ann Surg* 216:172–183, 1992

8. The Veterans Affairs Total Parenteral Nutrition Cooperative Study Group: Perioperative total parenteral nutrition in surgical patients. *N Engl J Med* 325:525–532, 1993

9. Wallace LK, Starr NJ, Leventhal MJ, Estafanous FG: Hyper-glycemia on ICU admission after CABG is associated with increased risk of mediastinitis or wound infection (Abstract). *Anesthesiology* 85:A286, 1996

10. Pomposelli JJ, Baxter JK 3rd, Babineau TJ, Pomfret EA, Driscoll DF, Forse RA, Bistrian BR: Early postoperative glucose control predicts nosocomial infection rate in diabetic patients. *JPEN* 22:77–81, 1998

11. Malmberg K, Ryden L, Efendic S, Herlitz J, Nicol P, Waldenstrom A, Wedel H, Welin L: Randomized trial of insulin-glucose infusion followed by subcutaneous insulin treatment in diabetic patients with acute myocardial infarction (DIGAMI Study): effects on mortality at 1 year. *J Am Coll Cardiol* 26:57–65, 1995

12. Müller JM, Keller HW, Brenner V, Walter M, Holzmüller W: Indications and effects of preoperative parenteral nutrition. *World J Surg* 10:53–63, 1986

13. Heatly RV, Williams RHP, Lewis MH: Pre-operative intravenous feeding: a controlled trial. *Postgrad Med J* 55:541–545, 1979

14. McMahon M, Farnell MB, Murray MJ: Nutrition support of critically ill patients. *Mayo Clin Proc* 68:911–920, 1993

15. Hunter DC, Jaksic T, Lewis D, Benotti PN, Blackburn GL, Bistrian BR: Resting energy expenditure in the critically ill: estimations versus measurement. *Br J Surg* 75:875–878, 1988

16. Shaw JHF, Wildbore M, Wolfe RR: Whole body protein kinetics in severely septic patients. *Ann Surg* 205:288–294, 1987

17. McMahon M, Rizza RA: Nutritional support in hospitalized patients with diabetes mellitus. *Mayo Clin Proc* 71:587–594, 1996

18. McMahon M, Manji N, Driscoll DF, Bistrian BR: Parenteral nutrition in patients with diabetes mellitus: theoretical and practical considerations. *JPEN* 13:545–553, 1989

19. Peters AL, Davidson MB: Effects of various enteral feeding products on postprandial blood glucose response in patients with type 1 diabetes. *JPEN* 16:69–74, 1991

20. American Diabetes Association: Nutrition recommendations and principles for people with diabetes mellitus (Position Statement). *Diabetes Care* 21 (Suppl. 1):S32–S35, 1998

Dr. McMahon is Director of Clinical Nutrition and Consultant, Division of Endocrinology, Metabolism, Nutrition, and Internal Medicine at the Mayo Clinic, Rochester, MN.

Nutrition and Lifestyle

20. Lifestyle and the Prevention of Diabetes

Rena R. Wing, PhD

Highlights

- Intervention studies evaluating the effects of diet and exercise (separately or in combination) on conversion from impaired glucose tolerance to diabetes provide support for the benefits of lifestyle interventions. However, methodological limitations prevent definite conclusions.
- Research studies suggest that even modest behavior changes may have a large impact on risk reduction, and diet plus exercise is the most effective approach to long-term weight control. This suggests combination therapy is most appropriate for the prevention of diabetes.
- Although conclusive data are not available, encouraging individuals to lose modest amounts of weight (~5–10%) and to increase physical activity (500–1,000 kcal/week) may be sufficient to reduce risk of diabetes while improving overall health and reducing risk of cardiovascular disease and mortality.

INTRODUCTION

The prevalence of type 2 diabetes is increasing dramatically worldwide. Although genetic factors clearly contribute to the development of type 2 diabetes, lifestyle factors are the major determinant of this worldwide increase. Data from migrating populations, such as Chinese and Japanese, and comparisons of urban and rural populations dramatically illustrate the importance of lifestyle factors in the development of diabetes (1–3). Given the importance of lifestyle factors, type 2 diabetes would appear to be at least in part a preventable disease. Evidence to support this comes

351

from a wide variety of studies, including epidemiological studies of the risk factors for diabetes (4–9) and experimental studies examining the effects of diet, exercise, or weight loss on glycemic control or insulin sensitivity (10–14). Several studies have directly assessed the effects of lifestyle interventions in individuals at high risk of developing type 2 diabetes on the development of this disease. The purpose of this chapter is to review these intervention studies in detail and to provide related guidelines for clinical practice. Before doing so, however, the epidemiological data on lifestyle factors related to diabetes will be briefly reviewed as background for these intervention trials.

EPIDEMIOLOGICAL EVIDENCE

Obesity, body fat distribution, physical activity, and dietary intake are among the factors that have been examined in relation to the development of type 2 diabetes. Epidemiological studies addressing these factors have been carefully reviewed by Hamman (15) and by Manson and Spelsberg (16), with extensive charts and tables summarizing all of the relevant studies; the interested reader should consult these references. The present chapter provides an overview of these epidemiological studies, focusing on the prospective studies because they provide the strongest evidence.

Obesity and Body Fat Distribution

Obesity has long been recognized as an important lifestyle risk factor for diabetes. In prospective studies of the effect of obesity on the development of type 2 diabetes (6,9,17), the age-adjusted risk for those in the highest weight category compared with those in the lowest weight category ranges from 1.43 to 60.9. The duration of obesity also appears to be an important risk factor for diabetes (18). Manson and Spelsberg (16) estimate that maintaining desirable weight (BMI $\leq$22.4 kg/m^2 in women and $\leq$22.7 kg/m^2 in men), compared with being obese (BMI $\geq$27.3 kg/m^2 in women and $\geq$27.8 kg/m^2 in men), would result in a 50–75% reduction in risk of type 2 diabetes.

Independent of overall body fat, there is also an increased risk of developing diabetes in those who have more central adiposity. Using waist-to-hip ratio as a measure of central adiposity, prospective studies have shown increased risk of diabetes in men (19) and women (20) with more central adiposity.

Physical Activity

Several prospective studies of physical activity and type 2 diabetes have been conducted (Table 20.1). In one study of ~6,000 men followed

Table 20.1 Prospective Studies of Physical Activity and Risk of Developing Diabetes

Measure	RR (CI)
Leisure-time physical activity (kcal/week)*	
<500	1.00
500–999	0.94
1,000–1,499	0.79
1,500–1,999	0.78
2,000–2,499	0.68
2,500–2,999	0.90
3,000–3,499	0.86
≥3,500	0.52
Frequency of vigorous activity in men (times/week)†	
0	1.00
1	0.77 (0.55–1.07)
2–4	0.62 (0.46–0.82)
≥5	0.58 (0.40–0.84)
Frequency of vigorous activity in women (times/week)‡	
0	1.00
1	0.74 (0.6–0.91)
2	0.55 (0.44–0.68)
3	0.73 (0.59–0.90)
4+	0.63 (0.53–0.75)

CI, confidence interval; RR, relative risk. *Data from Helmrich et al. (21). †Data from Manson et al. (5). ‡Data from Manson et al. (4).

for 14 years (21), the risk of developing diabetes was decreased 6% for every 500 kcal increase in leisure-time physical activity. Two other studies assessed activity by asking about frequency of vigorous activity (sufficient to produce sweat). These studies, one following >87,000 women for 8 years (4) and the other following >21,000 men for 5 years (5), both showed that increases in frequency of vigorous activity significantly reduced the risk of type 2 diabetes. The effect persisted after adjusting for BMI. However, the benefits of exercise were shown to be particularly apparent in the overweight (5) and in those at greatest risk for diabetes (21). Based on these studies, Manson and Spelsberg (16) conclude that a 30–50% reduction in risk would be associated with regular or vigorous exercise versus a sedentary lifestyle.

Note that increasing exercise would contribute to reduced risk of diabetes not only directly, as discussed in the studies above, but also indirectly through an effect of exercise on body weight. A large number of studies have shown that physical activity is associated with decreased obesity and better long-term maintenance of weight loss (22,23).

Diet

Fewer prospective studies of the effect of diet on the development of diabetes are available, and results are far less consistent. None of these studies have shown a relationship between sucrose, fiber, or carbohydrate intake and risk of diabetes. In studies with Seventh Day Adventists (24), vegetarian diets have been associated with decreased risk of diabetes, and in the Nurses Health Study, higher intakes of vegetable fat, magnesium, potassium, and calcium were all associated with decreased risk (25). Several studies have suggested that fat intake increases the risk of diabetes; in one such study (26), a sixfold excess risk of conversion from impaired glucose tolerance (IGT) to type 2 diabetes was observed for every 40-g increase in fat intake.

The benefits of lowering fat intake in preventing diabetes may also be mediated indirectly, through the effects of dietary fat on body weight. Again, results here are somewhat inconsistent, but lowering fat intake appears to have at least a short-term effect on body weight (27,28).

INTERVENTION STUDIES

Based on this epidemiological literature and the large number of studies showing benefits of lifestyle intervention on insulin resistance, glucose tolerance, and obesity (29–32), several intervention studies have evaluated the effect of diet and exercise on conversion from IGT to diabetes (Table 20.2). Individuals with IGT are usually selected for these studies because they are at particularly high risk of developing diabetes (33). Diet and exercise have been evaluated singly and in combination. Each of these studies will be described in detail.

Lifestyle Intervention Program, New Zealand

Evidence suggesting the benefit of lifestyle intervention is found in a small study conducted in New Zealand by Bourn et al. (34). In this study, subjects with IGT (*n* = 32) were required to demonstrate IGT, as defined by World Health Organization (WHO) criteria, in two out of three oral glucose tolerance tests (OGTTs). The fact that these subjects had persistent elevations in glucose makes it unlikely that they would revert to normal glucose tolerance in the absence of intervention. However, the absence of a control group in this study makes interpretation of the results quite difficult.

The description of the intervention offered these participants is limited, but the following information is provided: Subjects received dietary advice and completed food diaries and another OGTT every 3 months. Between each measure, subjects received at least one phone call for support and information. The diet focused on increasing complex carbohy-

Table 20.2 Intervention Studies Using Lifestyle Approaches to Prevent Diabetes

Author (Reference)	Subjects	Glucose Levels	Design	Treatment Groups	Follow-Up (years)	Incidence of Diabetes (%)
Bourn et al. (34)	32 IGT 22 (69%) completed	Fasting <140 mg/dl 2-h <200 mg/dl	No control group	Diet + Exercise Diet: complex carbohydrate 50–55% kcal; fat <30%; fiber 20 g/1,000 kcal; ↑ P:S fat ratio; ↓ sugars; weight loss Exercise: ≥30 min on 3 days/week, or ~450 kcal	2 3 (n = 19)	23 16
Page et al. (36)	Treatment group: 23 IGT 18 (78%) at 6 months 17 (74%) at 2 years Control group: 8 IGT 7 (88%) at 6 months 6 (75%) at 2 years	Fasting >100 mg/dl 2-h >140 mg/dl	Randomized 2:1 to intervention vs. control group	Diet + Exercise Diet: carbohydrate >55% of kcal; fat <20%; P:S ratio >1.0; fiber = 20 g/1,000 kcal; weight loss encouraged Exercise: ≥20 min on 3 days/week, or ~300 kcal Control No intervention	2	18 No data
Eriksson and Lindgärde (37)	Treatment group: 181 IGT 161 (89%) completed	Fasting ≤120 mg/dl 2-h 126–199 mg/dl	No random assignment	Diet + Exercise Diet: ↓ sugar; ↓ calories; ↓ fiber; ↑ unsaturated fat	5	10.6

(Continued)

Table 20.2 Intervention Studies Using Lifestyle Approaches to Prevent Diabetes (Continued)

Author (Reference)	Subjects	Glucose Levels	Design	Treatment Groups	Follow-Up (years)	Incidence of Diabetes (%)
	Control group: 79 IGT 56 (71%) completed			Exercise: 2 supervised exercise sessions/week (60 min each); ~600 kcal/week		28.6
				Control: no intervention		
Pan et al. (39)	557 IGT 530 (95%) completed	Fasting <140 mg/dl 2-h 140–199 mg/dl	Randomized by clinic	Diet: 25–30 kcal/kg; 55–65% carbohydrate, 25–30% fat for nonobese; obese told to limit calories	6	43.8
				Exercise: increase by 100 kcal/day (700 kcal/week)		41.1
				Diet + Exercise: combination		46.0
				Control: no intervention		67.7
Wing et al. (40)	154 obese, FH+ (90 with IGT) 129 (84%) completed	Fasting <140 mg/dl 2-h <200 mg/dl	Randomized	Diet: low-calorie (800–1,200 for weeks 1–8; then 1,200–1,500) low-fat (20% fat)	2	30.3
				Exercise: 1,500 kcal/week of moderate intensity exercise (brisk walking), 5 days/week of exercise		14.0
				Diet + Exercise: combination		15.6
				Control: subjects given manual to use on their own		7.0

P:S, polyunsaturated-to-saturated.

drates to 50–55% of calories, increasing dietary fiber (especially soluble fiber) toward 20 g/1,000 kcal, decreasing fat to 20% of calories, increasing polyunsaturated-to-saturated fat ratio, and limiting intake of extrinsic sugars. The author stated that since many participants were overweight, calorie reduction was also encouraged.

Subjects were recommended to exercise for at least 30 min 3 days/week, and activities such as walking and low-impact aerobics were encouraged. A 1 h/week supervised exercise session was also available.

The results of this study are difficult to present because in some cases data from subjects with IGT were combined with data from a group of individuals with 2 diabetes who also participated. Moreover, the sample size decreased over the study period; thus, data at baseline and at 2 years come from different subjects, and change scores are not provided. It is apparent that behavior changes were greatest at 3 months. Changes in women were still apparent at 24 months, whereas many of the behavior changes were no longer apparent in men. In women, energy intake decreased from 1,490 kcal/day at baseline to 1,214 kcal/day at 24 months, fat intake decreased from 38% of calories to 30% of calories, and fiber increased from 12 g/1,000 kcal to 16 g/1,000 kcal. In men, energy intake was ~1,870 kcal/day at baseline and 2 years, and 37% of calories were from fat at both times; however, fiber intake increased from 11 g/1,000 kcal to 13 g/1,000 kcal. The physical activity goal was met by 14% of the subjects with IGT at baseline and by 20–30% during the lifestyle intervention.

Subjects with IGT experienced a 2.6-kg weight loss in the first 3 months of the program, but then regained to their baseline weight. Improvements in fasting glucose, 2-h glucose, and lipids were seen at 3–12 months, but they were not sustained. Glycated hemoglobin (HbA_1) and 2-h glucose remained below baseline levels over the 2 years. At the end of the 2-year study, 9 of the 22 (41%) subjects had normal glucose tolerance, 36% still had IGT, and 23% had worsened to diabetes.

Recently, a 3-year follow-up of these subjects was published (35). Nineteen of the 22 subjects were retested. Of these 19, 10 (53%) had normal tolerance (47% of these same 19 subjects had normal tolerance at 2 years), 6 still had IGT, and 3 (16%) had diabetes. Although there is no control group with which to compare these results, the large number of individuals who had persistent IGT at baseline but then reverted to normal tolerance over 3 years suggests that the lifestyle intervention had a positive impact on the course of the disease.

Page et al.: Healthy Lifestyle Intervention

A shorter period of lifestyle intervention was used by Page et al. (36) in their study of "healthy living." A total of 31 subjects with IGT were randomly assigned to a 6-month diet-and-exercise intervention ($n = 23$)

or a control group (n = 8). IGT was defined on the basis of two CIGMA (continuous infusion of glucose with model assessments) tests. Subjects with fasting glucose >100 mg/dl or a 60-min glucose of >167 mg/dl (which is equivalent to a 2-h OGTT level of 140 mg/dl) met criteria for IGT.

The "healthy-living" group received dietary advice from a dietitian aimed at increasing fiber to 20 g/1,000 kcal, increasing carbohydrate to 55% of total intake, and decreasing fat to 20%, with a polyunsaturated-to-saturated fat ratio of 1.0. Weight loss was encouraged to a target BMI of ≤25 kg/m². Although information is not provided on the frequency of contact, home visits to discuss dietary changes with the spouse are mentioned. Exercise was prescribed individually. In general, the goal was a minimum of 20 min of exercise three times per week; free supervised exercise sessions were available to the subjects.

Subjects who completed this 6-month intervention (n = 18) had an increase in VO_2 max from 2.5 l/min to 2.7 l/min and a decrease in BMI from 26 to 25 kg/m². Systolic blood pressure, LDL cholesterol, and total cholesterol decreased in the intervention group, but showed little change in the control group.

There was no further intervention after 6 months, but at 2 years, 17 of the subjects who received the intervention and 6 control subjects were reexamined. BMI had returned to baseline in the intervention subjects. A similar number of intervention and control subjects had maintained some weight loss (two control; seven intervention) and were participating in at least 1 h/week of vigorous activity (four subjects in each condition). The only metabolic parameter that showed sustained improvement in the intervention subjects was LDL cholesterol. Fasting glucose increased from 99 to 108 mg/dl in the healthy-living group, and three of the subjects (18%) developed diabetes. The proportion of control subjects who developed diabetes is not stated.

Subsequent analyses compared those who had adopted a healthier lifestyle at 2 years (were exercising and had no weight gain; n = 13) with those who had gained weight and had not increased their exercise (n = 10). These analyses, which collapsed across the initial randomized groups, showed that those subjects who developed a healthy lifestyle had a decrease in BMI of 1 unit, while the others had an increase of 1 unit. Fasting and 2-h glucose remained unchanged in the former but increased in the latter. Data on the percentage of each group who developed diabetes were not provided.

The Malmö Feasibility Study

Another study to determine whether lifestyle intervention could prevent conversion from IGT to type 2 diabetes was conducted in Malmö, Sweden (37). A group of 260 individuals with IGT (fasting glucose

≤120 mg/dl and 2-h value 126–199 mg/dl) were invited to participate in a diabetes prevention program. A total of 181 agreed to participate, 161 of whom completed the 5-year study. The 79 subjects with IGT who were not enrolled in the treatment formed a nonrandomized control group.

The intervention included diet and exercise, with some subjects beginning with diet and others with exercise (38). Although there is little information provided on this intervention, the dietary advice (fewer plain sugar products, more fiber and unsaturated fat, and overall reduction in calorie intake) was given initially by a physician and a dietitian, with monthly contacts arranged. The exercise program included two supervised sessions (60 min each) with various activities (calisthenics, walking-jogging, soccer, and badminton). Some subjects, however, chose to follow the exercise protocol on their own, without participating in group sessions.

Over the 5-year study, estimated maximal oxygen uptake (milliliters per minute per kilogram) increased by 10% in the lifestyle intervention group, while it decreased by 4.9% in the control group. BMI decreased by 2.3% in treated subjects (approximately –2 kg) and increased by 0.5% in control subjects. Changes in weight were greatest at 1 year, but 71% maintained some weight reduction over the 5 years.

Diabetes developed in 10.6% of the intervention subjects compared with 28.6% of the control subjects; the relative risk of developing diabetes in intervention versus control subjects was 0.37 (confidence interval 0.20–0.68). Improvements in glucose tolerance were correlated with weight reduction ($r = 0.19$, $P < 0.02$) and increased fitness ($r = 0.22$, $P < 0.02$). Both changes contributed equally to the reduction in risk of diabetes.

The lifestyle intervention also led to greater decreases in triglyceride levels than in the control group and to greater decreases in 2-h insulin levels. Improvements in blood pressure were comparable in the two groups, but more participants in the control condition than intervention subjects required antihypertensive medication.

Da Qing Study

The strongest evidence of the benefits of lifestyle intervention is found in the Da Qing IGT and Diabetes Study (39). In this study, 110,660 men and women from 22 health care clinics in Da Qing, China, were screened for IGT and type 2 diabetes. Of these, 577 were found to have IGT and agreed to participate in the intervention study. Of the 577, 530 were followed for 6 years or until diabetes developed.

Subjects were randomized by clinic to one of four treatment groups. In clinics assigned to the diet-only condition, participants with a BMI <25 kg/m^2 were prescribed a diet of 25–30 kcal/kg body wt, with 65% carbohydrate, 10–15% protein, and 25–30% fat. Subjects were encouraged to increase consumption of vegetables and to limit their intake of simple sugars and alcohol. Heavier subjects were instructed to limit calories to achieve a 0.5–1.0 kg/month weight loss until reaching a BMI of 23 kg/m². Dietary instruction was provided through individualized counseling by physicians and group counseling sessions held weekly for 1 month, monthly for 3 months, and then quarterly for the remainder of the study.

Subjects in the exercise-only condition also attended counseling sessions weekly for 1 month, monthly for 3 months, and then quarterly, but they exercised on their own, with individual selection of specific activities. Individuals over age 50 were instructed to increase their exercise by 1 unit/day; healthier individuals under age 50 were encouraged to try to achieve a 2 unit/day increase. Examples of exercise "units" included 30 min of mild exercise (e.g., slow walking, shopping, house cleaning), 20 min of moderate activity (e.g., faster walking, cycling, doing heavy laundry), 10 min of strenuous activity (slow running, climbing stairs, disco dancing for the elderly), or 5 min of very strenuous activity (e.g., jumping rope, playing basketball, swimming). Thus, a unit of activity appeared to be ~90–100 kcal for a 150-lb person, and the exercise goal would be to increase activity by 700 kcal/week.

Subjects in the diet-plus-exercise condition received instructions on both of the lifestyle approaches and attended sessions on the same contact schedule.

Subjects in the control group were given general information about IGT, diet, and exercise, but attended no classes.

The changes in behavior over the 6-year study were modest and in most cases did not differ between treatment conditions. Calorie intake decreased by 99 kcal/day in the control group, 96 kcal/day in the exercise-only group, 126 kcal/day in the diet-only group, and 242 kcal/day in the diet-plus-exercise group, with no significant differences between conditions. Likewise, no differences were seen in macronutrient distribution, with 1–2% increases in fat intake and 1–2% decreases in carbohydrate intake in all four conditions. The only behavior changes that differed across conditions were for exercise. The exercise-only and diet-plus-exercise groups increased exercise by 0.6 unit/day and 0.8 unit/day, respectively, whereas the other groups reported little or no increases. There were no significant differences in weight change between conditions. In subjects with a BMI ≥25, BMI decreased by 0.9–1.6 kg/m², whereas in those with BMI <25, BMI increases of 0.2–0.8 kg/m² were experienced.

Despite these relatively limited behavior changes, the results in terms of preventing diabetes were quite dramatic. Over the 6 years, the cumulative incidence of diabetes defined by WHO criteria was 67.7% in the control group, compared with 43.8% in the diet-only group, 41.1% in the exercise-only group, and 46% in the diet-plus-exercise group. The effect of treatment was observed in both lean and overweight individuals. The effects of diet and exercise were comparable, and no greater benefit was seen when these two approaches were combined.

The Family History Study by Wing and Colleagues

All of the studies reviewed above selected subjects with IGT for their study population. Although such subjects are at particularly high risk of developing diabetes, conducting screenings to identify these subjects is an expensive undertaking. Therefore, Wing et al. (40) chose to study overweight subjects with a family history of diabetes (one or both biological parents), who could thus identify themselves as being at risk for diabetes. Previous studies have shown high rates of diabetes in overweight individuals with diabetic parents (9). Such individuals may also be highly motivated to change their behavior to prevent diabetes.

A total of 154 subjects entered the study. Although the only glucose criteria for entering was absence of diabetes (fasting glucose <140 mg/dl and 2-h value <200 mg/dl), 90 (54%) of those entering the study met criteria for IGT. Subjects were randomly assigned to a diet, exercise, diet-plus-exercise, or control group and followed over 2 years.

The control group received a behavioral weight control manual but was given no further treatment contact. The other groups attended meetings weekly for 6 months and biweekly for the next 6 months, and they participated in two 6-week refresher courses in year 2. Treatment meetings were conducted in groups of ~15–20 subjects co-led by a team of therapists, including a behavior therapist and a dietitian, an exercise physiologist, or both. The diet condition began with 7 weeks of an intensive, structured diet (800–1,000 kcal/day, 20% fat) and then moved to a more flexible, 1,200–1,500 kcal regimen with <20% fat. Subjects monitored their calorie and fat intakes weekly for 6 months and then periodically throughout the 2 years. The focus of the treatment was on behavioral strategies to help participants make long-term changes in their eating behaviors.

The exercise group was instructed to gradually increase their activity to 1,500 kcal/week, with activities such as 3 miles of brisk walking completed 5 days/week. To help participants achieve these exercise goals, two supervised sessions per week were held for the first 10 weeks of the program. Later in the program, a walk followed each of the treatment meetings. Subjects monitored their own exercise and received training in behavioral strategies to maintain these changes long-term. The diet-and-exercise program consisted of both regimens described above, with less time devoted to each topic.

The benefits of the intervention were observed primarily at 6 months and then decreased over time. At 6 months, the two diet groups had each decreased their calorie intake by ~600 kcal/day and their fat intake by

5–10%, while the exercise groups reported much smaller dietary changes. The exercise groups increased their exercise expenditure by 657 kcal/week (exercise alone) and 1,028 kcal/week (diet-plus-exercise). Estimated VO_2 max improved in both of the exercise groups and also in the diet-only condition, probably because of weight loss. Over the first 6 months, the diet group lost 9.1 kg and the diet-plus-exercise group lost 10.1 kg. In contrast, the exercise-only group lost 2.1 kg, and the control group lost 1.5 kg. As a result of their substantial weight loss, the two diet groups also experienced significant decreases in fasting glucose, insulin, lipid, and blood pressure.

Unfortunately, neither the behavior changes nor the physiological changes persisted at 2 years. No significant differences between groups were seen for self-reported exercise, fitness, or dietary fat intake at 2 years. Likewise, weight losses did not differ by treatment group (weight changes of +1.0 to –2.5 kg).

There was a trend ($P = 0.08$) for difference between conditions in the proportion of subjects who developed diabetes; surprisingly, the risk of developing diabetes was greatest in the diet-only condition (30.3%) and lowest in the control group (7%). The rates of conversion from IGT to type 2 diabetes were also examined in the subset of individuals with IGT at baseline (data not presented in original manuscript). Again, the highest conversion rates were in the diet-only group (39%), and the lowest were in the control group (11%); the difference between groups approached significance ($P = 0.06$).

Secondary analyses, collapsing across treatment conditions, showed a highly significant effect of weight loss from baseline to 2 years on development of diabetes. Subjects who lost 4.5 kg over this interval had ~30% reduction in risk of developing diabetes. Estimated VO_2 max at 2 years was also related to risk of developing diabetes, but after adjusting for IGT and weight loss, it did not contribute independently to predicting development of diabetes. The benefits of a 4.5-kg weight loss were seen both in subjects with IGT and in subjects with normal glucose tolerance at baseline.

CONCLUSIONS FROM RESEARCH STUDIES

The studies cited above provide support for the benefits of lifestyle intervention. However, there are clear methodological limitations in these studies that prevent definite conclusions. Most importantly, only three of these studies were randomized trials (36,39,40). Several other points should be noted about these studies. The rate of development of diabetes in the control groups differed greatly across studies. In the Da Qing study (39), 11% per year developed diabetes; in the Malmö study (37), 5.7% per year developed diabetes; and among IGT subjects in the Wing study (40), 5.5% per year developed diabetes. The lower entry glucose level in the Malmö study may explain the low incidence in this study, but the Da Qing study used criteria comparable to those described by Wing for the IGT subjects. Thus, some of the difference between studies may reflect differences in the conversion rates of the control groups.

In all of these studies, the greatest behavior changes occurred initially (between 3 and 12 months), with a gradual return to baseline. By the end of the studies, the behavior changes were minimal. Despite this, substantial decreases in the incidence of diabetes were seen. These results suggest that even modest behavior changes may have a large impact on risk reduction. For example, Wing et al. (40) found that a sustained weight loss of only 4.5 kg reduced risk by 30%.

It is not clear from these studies whether diet, exercise, or a combination is the most effective approach. In the Malmö study (37), both an increase in VO₂ max and a decrease in weight were significantly related to the risk of developing diabetes, and the impact of these two changes appeared comparable. Pan et al. (39) found nonsignificant differences among diet, exercise, and the combination. Wing et al. (40) found a somewhat poorer outcome in the diet-only condition, but it is unclear whether this is an anomaly due to the small sample size or a true finding. In spite of these inconsistencies, the large number of studies in the weight-loss literature that have found diet plus exercise to be the most effective approach to long-term weight control (22) suggests that the combination intervention would be most appropriate for future studies and clinical practice.

The evidence from these specific intervention studies and the large background of epidemiological literature suggest the benefit of lifestyle intervention for prevention of diabetes. Based on these findings, the National Institutes of Health, National Institute of Diabetes and Digestive and Kidney Diseases has launched a 27-center randomized controlled trial (the Diabetes Prevention Program, or DPP) to investigate the effects of lifestyle intervention and pharmacological intervention on prevention of diabetes in those at high risk by virtue of having IGT (41). The lifestyle intervention focuses on changing both diet and exercise; the behavioral goals are to lose ≥7% of body weight, to increase exercise to ≥150 min/week of moderate-intensity activity (equivalent to ~700 kcal/week), and to sustain these changes throughout the 6-year trial. This study will provide the strongest evidence regarding the benefits of lifestyle intervention for individuals at risk for diabetes.

CLINICAL APPLICATIONS

As noted above, the literature reviewed in this chapter does not allow for firm conclusions regarding the effect of lifestyle intervention on prevention of diabetes. Such data will, however, be provided by the DPP. In the meantime, how should clinicians advise individuals at high risk for diabetes? Despite the lack of conclusive data, encouraging such individuals to lose weight and to increase their physical activity would appear to be extremely appropriate. Such general recommendations are useful in improving overall health and in reducing risks of cardiovascular disease and mortality.

Unfortunately, specific recommendations for the reduction of diabetes risk are more difficult to generate. How much weight loss is needed? What should the dose and intensity of exercise be? What type of diet would be recommended? Clinical trials to address those specific questions would require very large sample sizes and long follow-up intervals and consequently will probably never be conducted. However, based on literature available at this time and on the intervention studies that have been conducted, it would appear that modest weight losses of ~5–10% of body weight and modest increases in activity of 500–1,000 kcal/week may be sufficient to reduce the risk of diabetes. Such changes would also help to lower blood pressure and to improve lipids and insulin sensitivity. Thus, clinicians should emphasize these modest behavior changes for individuals at risk for diabetes.

REFERENCES

1. Zimmet PZ, McCarty DJ, deCourten MP: The global epidemiology of non-insulin-dependent diabetes mellitus and the metabolic syndrome. *J Diabetes Complications* 11:60–68, 1997

2. Fujimoto WY, Leonetti DL, Kinyoun JL, Newell-Morris L, Shuman WP, Stolov WC, Wahl PW: Prevalence of diabetes mellitus and impaired glucose tolerance among second generation Japanese American men. *Diabetes* 36:721–729, 1987

3. Ravussin E, Valencia ME, Esparza J, Bennett PH, Schulz LO: Effects of a traditional lifestyle on obesity in Pima Indians. *Diabetes Care* 17:1067–1074, 1994

4. Manson JE, Rimm EB, Stampfer MJ, Colditz GA, Willett WC, Krolewski AS, Rosner B, Hennekens CH, Speizer FE: Physical activity and incidence of non-insulin-dependent diabetes mellitus in women. *Lancet* 338:774–778, 1991

5. Manson JE, Nathan DM, Krolewski AS, Stampfer MJ, Willett WC, Hennekens CH: A prospective study of exercise and incidence of diabetes among US male physicians. *JAMA* 268:63–67, 1992

6. Colditz GA, Willett WC, Stampfer MJ, Manson JE, Hennekens CH, Arky RA, Speizer FE: Weight as a risk factor for clinical diabetes in women. *Am J Epidemiol* 132:501–513, 1990

7. Colditz GA, Willett WC, Rotnitzky A, Manson JE: Weight gain as a risk factor for clinical diabetes mellitus in women. *Ann Intern Med* 122:481–486, 1995

8. West KM: *Epidemiology of Diabetes and Its Vascular Lesions*. New York, Elsevier, 1978

9. Knowler WC, Pettitt DJ, Savage PJ, Bennett PH: Diabetes incidence in Pima Indians: contributions of obesity and parental diabetes. *Am J Epidemiol* 113:144–156, 1981

10. Long SD, O'Brien K, MacDonald KG, Leggett-Frazier N, Swanson MS, Pories WJ, Caro JF: Weight loss prevents the progression of impaired glucose tolerance to type II diabetes: a longitudinal interventional study. *Diabetes Care* 17:372–375, 1993

11. O'Dea K: Marked improvement in carbohydrate and lipid metabolism in diabetic Australian aborigines after temporary reversion to traditional lifestyle. *Diabetes* 33:596–603, 1984

12. Olefsky J, Reaven GM, Farquhar JW: Effects of weight reduction on obesity: studies of lipid and carbohydrate metabolism in normal and hyperlipoproteinemic subjects. *J Clin Invest* 53:64–77, 1974

13. Schneider SH, Amorosa LF, Khachadurian AK, Ruderman NB: Studies on the mechanism of improved glucose control during regular exercise in type 2 (non-insulin-dependent) diabetes. *Diabetologia* 26:355–360, 1984

14. Ruderman NB, Ganda OP, Johansen K: The effect of physical training on glucose tolerance and plasma lipids in maturity-onset diabetes. *Diabetes* 28:89–92, 1979

15. Hamman RF: Genetic and environmental determinants of non-insulin-dependent diabetes mellitus (NIDDM). *Diabetes Metab Rev* 8:287–338, 1992

16. Manson JE, Spelsberg A: Primary prevention of non-insulin-dependent diabetes mellitus. *Am J Prev Med* 10:172–184, 1994

17. Ohlson LO, Larsson B, Bjorntorp P, Eriksson H, Svardsudd K, Welin L, Tibblin G, Wilhelmsen L: Risk factors for type 2 (non-insulin-dependent) diabetes mellitus: thirteen and one-half years of follow-up of the participants in a study of Swedish men born in 1913. *Diabetologia* 31:798–805, 1988

18. Everhart JE, Pettitt DJ, Bennett PH, Knowler WC: Duration of obesity increases the incidence of NIDDM. *Diabetes* 41:235–240, 1992

19. Ohlson LO, Larsson B, Svardsudd K, Welin L, Eriksson H, Wilhelmsen L, Bjorntorp P, Tibblin G: The influence of body fat distribution on the incidence of diabetes mellitus. *Diabetes* 34:1055–1058, 1985

20. Lundgren H, Bengtsson C, Blohme G, Lapidus L, Sjostrom L: Adiposity and adipose tissue distribution in relation to incidence of diabetes in women: results from a prospective population study in Gothenburg, Sweden. *Int J Obes* 13:413–423, 1989

21. Helmrich SP, Ragland DR, Leung RW, Paffenbarger RS: Physical activity and reduced occurrence of non-insulin-dependent diabetes mellitus. *N Engl J Med* 325:147–152, 1991

22. Pronk NP, Wing RR: Physical activity and long-term maintenance of weight loss. *Obesity Res* 2:587–599, 1994

23. PiSunyer FX: The effects of increased physical activity on food intake, metabolic rate, and health risks in obese individuals. In *Treatment of the Seriously Obese Patient.* Wadden TA, Van Itallie TB, Eds. New York, Guilford, 1992, pp. 190–210

24. Snowdon DA, Phillips RL: Does a vegetarian diet reduce the occurrence of diabetes? *Am J Public Health* 75:507–512, 1985

25. Colditz GA, Manson JE, Stampfer MJ, Rosner B, Willett WC, Speizer FE: Diet and risk of clinical diabetes in women. *Am J Clin Nutr* 55:1018–1023, 1992

26. Marshall JA, Shetterly S, Hoag S, Hamman RF: Dietary fat predicts conversion from impaired glucose tolerance to NIDDM: The San Luis Valley Diabetes Study. *Diabetes Care* 17:50–56, 1994

27. Jeffery RW, Hellerstedt WL, French SA, Baxter JE: A randomized trial of counseling for fat restriction versus calorie restriction in the treatment of obesity. *Int J Obesity* 19:132–137, 1995

28. Insull W, Henderson MM, Prentice RL, Thompson DJ, Clifford C, Goldman S, Gorbach S, Moskowitz M, Thompson R, Woods M: Results of a randomized feasibility study of a low-fat diet. *Arch Intern Med* 150:421–427, 1990

29. Goldstein DJ: Beneficial health effects of modest weight loss. *Int J Obesity* 16:397–416, 1992

30. Kanders BS, Blackburn GL: Reducing primary risk factors by therapeutic weight loss. In *Treatment of the Seriously Obese Patient.*

Wadden TA, Van Itallie TB, Eds. New York, Guilford, 1992, pp. 213–230

31. Wing RR, Koeske R, Epstein LH, Nowalk MP, Gooding W, Becker D: Long-term effects of modest weight loss in type II diabetic patients. *Arch Intern Med* 147:1749–1753, 1987

32. Wing RR, Jeffery RW: Effect of modest weight loss on changes in cardiovascular risk factors: are there differences between men and women or between weight loss and maintenance? *Int J Obesity* 19:67–73, 1995

33. Edelstein SL, Knowler WC, Bain RP, Andres R, Barrett-Connor EL, Dowse GK, Haffner SM, Pettitt DJ, Sorkin JD, Muller DC, Collins VR, Hamman RF: Predictors of progression from impaired glucose tolerance to NIDDM: an analysis of six prospective studies. *Diabetes* 46:701–710, 1997

34. Bourn DM, Mann JI, McSkimming BJ, Waldron MA, Wishart JD: Impaired glucose tolerance and NIDDM: does a lifestyle intervention program have an effect? *Diabetes Care* 17:1311–1319, 1994

35. Bourn DM, Mann JI: The 3-yr follow-up of subjects with impaired glucose tolerance or non-insulin-dependent diabetes mellitus in a diet and exercise intervention programme. *Diabetes Nutr Metab* 9:240–246, 1996

36. Page RCL, Harnden KE, Cook JTE, Turner RC: Can lifestyles of subjects with impaired glucose tolerance be changed? A feasibility study. *Diabetic Med* 9:562–566, 1992

37. Eriksson KF, Lindgärde F: Prevention of type 2 (non-insulin-dependent) diabetes mellitus by diet and physical exercise. *Diabetologia* 34:891–898, 1991

38. Saltin B, Lindgärde F, Houston M, Horlin R, Nygaard E, Gad P: Physical training and glucose tolerance in middle-aged men with chemical diabetes. *Diabetes* 28:30–32, 1979

39. Pan XR, Li GW, Hu YH, Wang JX, Yang WY, An ZX, Hu ZX, Lin J, Xiao JZ, Cao HB, Liu PA, Jiang XG, Jiang YY, Wang JP, Zheng H, Zhang H, Bennett PH, Howard BV: Effects of diet and exercise in preventing NIDDM in people with impaired glucose tolerance. *Diabetes Care* 20:537–544, 1997

40. Wing RR, Venditti EM, Jakicic JM, Polley BA, Lang W: Lifestyle intervention in overweight individuals with a family history of diabetes. *Diabetes Care* 21:350–359, 1998

41. Diabetes Prevention Program Research Group: The Diabetes
    Prevention Program (DPP) (Abstract). *Diabetes* 46 (Suppl. 1):138A,
    1997

Dr. Wing is Professor of Psychiatry, Psychology and Epidemiology, and
Director of the Obesity/Nutrition Research Center, Western Psychiatric
Institute and Clinic, University of Pittsburgh Medical Center, Pittsburgh, PA.

21. Counseling and Education Strategies for Improved Adherence to Nutrition Therapy

MELINDA DOWNIE MARYNIUK, RD, MED, CDE, FADA

Highlights

- A patient-centered, or empowerment, approach to nutrition therapy for diabetes involves developing a nutrition plan based on the patient's usual eating habits and lifestyle and negotiating a medical management plan that will achieve good glucose control with an acceptable degree of change.
- Assessment beyond food intake alone facilitates problem solving. Blood glucose monitoring records are essential to evaluate the impact of food changes, activity, and other lifestyle factors or the need for additional changes in medical therapy, i.e., oral medications and/or insulin.
- Follow-up visits are essential to evaluate the effectiveness of therapeutic interventions.
- Successful nutrition therapy is a process of problem solving, adjustment, and readjustment.

INTRODUCTION

Adherence to nutrition and meal planning principles is one of the most challenging aspects of diabetes care (1–3). Having extensive knowledge about nutrition will not ensure that people with diabetes will follow healthful meal plans. Numerous studies have found that knowledge is not or is only weakly associated with positive outcomes related to lifestyle change (4–6). A critical role of the health care provider delivering medical nutrition therapy (MNT) and education is not only to impart information, but also to do it in a way that uses a variety of counseling and educational strategies that improve adherence.

369

To improve our effectiveness, we must think about our philosophy or beliefs about how people change. Is our patient care philosophy or approach to care traditional or patient-centered? The assumptions we have about how, when, and why people change behavior will influence our ability to serve our patients as much as or even more than the information we provide them (7).

A patient-centered or empowerment approach to care is based on the firm understanding that diabetes is a self-managed disease where the patient is 100% in charge and responsible for his or her own care. In the traditional approach, the provider takes that responsibility. Traditional dietary instruction involves calculating a structured diet from a physician's order, and the dietitian's role is to teach, persuade, and/or motivate patients to follow the nutritional recommendations. This approach has frustrated both health care providers, who complain that most patients do not adhere, and people with diabetes, who complain that traditional diet prescriptions are unrealistic and impossible to follow long term. Alternatively, the empowerment approach involves developing a nutrition plan based on the patient's usual eating habits and lifestyle and negotiating a medical management plan that will achieve good control with an acceptable degree of change. The health care provider spends time understanding the common lifestyle factors that may influence dietary adherence, such as negative emotions, feelings of deprivation, family support, or eating out (8). Behavioral strategies and problem-solving skills that help patients achieve and sustain successes in daily life are taught. This approach of empowerment training for patients may also result in improved glycemic control, as demonstrated by Anderson et al. (9).

In reality, diabetes MNT is often a blend of both patient-centered and traditional approaches. Behavioral scientists from the Diabetes Control and Complications Trial (DCCT) suggest that the excellent adherence and outcomes achieved from that study were due to a more patient-centered approach (10). Review the chart in Table 21.1 to gain a better understanding of your personal philosophy of patient care.

In several meta-analyses, diabetes education has been shown to be effective. Brown (11) found the largest beneficial effect of education on knowledge and self-care behavior. A subsequent meta-analysis by Brown et al. (12) examining the effectiveness of different strategies for promoting weight loss in type 2 diabetes found that diet changes alone had the largest statistically significant impact on weight loss and metabolic control. Padgett et al. (13) found a beneficial effect of education that used a combination of instructional and behavioral strategies, social learning, and diet instruction in improving knowledge and glycemic control. Clement (14) concluded in his technical review of over 100 studies in diabetes self-management education that three elements appeared critical for the success of self-management education:

1. The intervention must make extensive use of behavior change strategies.
2. The intervention must be appropriately matched to the needs and abilities of the patient.
3. The personnel must work closely with the patient's health care provider as part of an integrated team.

Therefore, it is not a question of whether or not diabetes education and MNT work, but of how to make both work better.

A variety of research reports have looked at how adherence to diabetes MNT can be improved. The design of controlled clinical trials to assess the effectiveness of MNT faces several obstacles. Most importantly, to deny MNT to a control group would be unethical. Some key research papers, as well as several technical reviews and meta-analyses, are summarized in Table 21.2.

From this literature, six counseling and educational strategies are derived that are likely to result in improved adherence to MNT. These

Table 21.1 Comparison of Traditional and Empowerment Viewpoints Regarding Diabetes Medical Nutrition Therapy

Traditional Viewpoint	Patient-Centered Viewpoint
Food choices affect physical health, including diabetes management.	Food choices affect psychosocial quality of life as well as physical health.
The dietitian is the expert in nutrition and is therefore in charge of developing a meal plan based on assessed needs.	The dietitian is the expert in nutrition and patients are the experts about themselves and their life circumstances.
The focus is on metabolic goals, such as weight and blood glucose levels. The dietitian provides instruction on an appropriate meal plan and teaches clients how to follow it.	Desired metabolic outcomes shape behavior-change plans but are not in themselves behaviors that clients can control. The focus is on behavioral goals, i.e., specific action steps that clients can control.
The dietitian feels effective and successful when clients follow nutrition recommendations.	The dietitian teaches behavior-change skills so that clients can achieve their own nutritional goals. The dietitian feels effective and successful when clients become skilled at making informed choices and solving problems.

From Anderson and Arnold (7).

Table 21.2 Summary of Key Research and Meta-Analysis Studies Related to Nutrition Self-Management Education for Diabetes

Author (Reference)	Study Objective	Sample Characteristics	Key Finding/Lessons Learned
Anderson et al. (9)	To evaluate the effect of an empowerment training program on diabetes control	Randomized, controlled group trial; outpatient	Patients who participate in empowerment training have improved blood glucose control.
Ary et al. (3)	To assess reasons for nonadherence to a diabetes regimen	208 adults (24 type 1, 184 type 2), outpatient	Subjects reported adhering least well to dietary and physical activity components of the regimen. The most common reasons for dietary nonadherence were the situational factors of eating out at restaurants and inappropriate food offers from others.
Boehm et al. (34)	To determine how the components of psychosocial adjustment to diabetes predict adherence to nutrition recommendations	117 type 2 adults, outpatient	Social support from family and friends is important in promoting adherence to nutrition behaviors, but receiving more support than desired negatively effects these behaviors.
Brown (11)	To study the effect of patient education on specific outcome variables	Meta-analysis, 82 studies	Study included an expanded sample of studies and psychological outcome variables that were added to the previously studied variables of patient knowledge, self-care behaviors, and metabolic control. Findings lend support to the effectiveness of diabetes patient education in improving patient outcomes.
Brown et al. (12)	To examine effectiveness of different strategies for promoting weight loss in type 2 diabetes	Meta-analysis	Diet alone had the largest statistically significant impact on weight loss and metabolic control. The combination strategy of diet and behavioral therapy plus exercise had a small effect on body weight, but a very significant impact on glycated hemoglobin.

Reference	Sample	Objective	Results
Campbell et al. (28)	70 type 2 adults, outpatient	To determine the effectiveness of a more intensive approach to education	Patients who participated in an intensive group education program that used techniques of extended time (13 h nutrition education vs. 5 h), simplified information, repetition, and a cognitive motivational approach had better outcomes than patients who attended a conventional program.
Delehanty and Halford (27)	687 type 1 participants in DCCT	To identify diet behaviors most associated with improved HbA_{1c}	The four nutrition behaviors associated with clinically significant reductions in HbA_{1c} are • Adherence to prescribed meal and snack plan • Adjustment of insulin dose in response to meal size • Prompt treatment of hyperglycemia (less food or more insulin) • Avoidance of overtreatment of hypoglycemia
Franz et al. (17)	179 type 2 adults, outpatient	To determine effectiveness of MNT provided by RDs using NPGs for type 2 diabetes	Small changes in lifestyle lead to very significant improvements in glucose control. By 6 weeks to 3 months it was known whether MNT had lead to target glucose goals, and if it had not, recommendations were made for changes in medical therapy, e.g., medications and/or insulin. From 3 to 6 months there is a slight increase in glucose levels, suggesting that ongoing interventions are important.
Franz et al. (18)	179 type 2 adults, outpatient	To determine if MNT is cost-effective	When dietitians acted on the outcomes from MNT and made recommendations for changes in medical therapy, intensive nutrition care following NPGs was cost-effective.

(Continued)

Table 21.2 Summary of Key Research and Meta-Analysis Studies Related to Nutrition Self-Management Education for Diabetes (*Continued*)

Author (Reference)	Study Objective	Sample Characteristics	Key Finding/Lessons Learned
Greenfield et al. (30)	To assess effect of training patients to be more active participants in their care	59 adults, outpatient	Training patients with diabetes to be more assertive with their health care providers by asking more questions, expressing opinions, and bringing up topics of concern led to improvements in glycated hemoglobin.
Hayaki and Brownell (29)	To summarize research examining group vs. individual interventions	Summary article of research	Group interventions may be at least as effective as individual interventions, presumably because of the social support created by groups.
Johnson and Valera (16)	To determine effectiveness of MNT by RDs	21 type 2 adults, outpatient	A quality-assurance audit indicated that 16 (76%) of the entire patient sample showed improved glycemic control with MNT provided by an RD; the mean number of nutrition counseling visits was 4.64 in a 6.4-month period.
Kavanagh et al. (33)	To predict adherence to diabetes treatment regimens and sustained diabetes control	63 adults, outpatient	Self-efficacy is a significant predictor of later adherence.
Kulkarni et al. (19)	To determine effect of using NPGs on dietitian behavior and patient outcomes in type 1 diabetes	54 type 1 adults, outpatient	Dietitians who followed NPGs spent more time with patients, were more likely to conduct a nutrition assessment, and paid more attention to glycemic control goals. NPG patients achieved a greater reduction in HbA_{1c} than did usual-care patients (−1.00 vs. −0.33).

Reference	Objective	Study design	Findings
Padgett et al. (13)	To evaluate the effects of educational and psychosocial interventions on diabetes	Meta-analysis, 93 studies	In a review that tested the effect of eight types of interventions (including didactic education, diet instruction, self-monitoring instruction, exercise instruction, and relaxation training in 7,451 patients), diet instruction showed the strongest and relaxation training the weakest effect.
Page et al. (26)	To evaluate retention after diabetes education	24 type 1 pediatric patients, outpatient	A diabetes team must work together to limit the number of recommendations made to a patient at each visit to maximize the probability that the most important recommendations are communicated and remembered.
Schundt et al. (8)	To identify and describe usual kinds of eating situations that adults with diabetes would find challenging	26 adults (12 type 1, 14 type 2), outpatient	Twelve types of problem situations were identified. An individual's ability to cope with these obstacles should be assessed so that treatment can be individualized. Sample problem situations include negative emotions, eating out, and resisting temptation.
Travis (23)	To identify factors that influence patients' use of diet regimens	75 type 2 adults, outpatient	Patients who received education explaining why their diet should be controlled were more likely to follow their meal plan than those who did not receive education. Also, those who had follow-up counseling adhered to their meal plan more frequently.

MNT, medical nutrition therapy; NPG, nutrition practice guideline.

strategies are summarized in Table 21.3 and are elaborated upon more fully in the rest of this chapter.

Team-Up with a Registered Dietitian

The dietitian is recognized as the professional most qualified to provide MNT (15). The standards of care published by the American Diabetes Association state that individualized nutrition recommendations and instructions should be done by a registered dietitian familiar with the components of diabetes MNT (1). Johnson and Valera (16) conducted a quality-assurance-audit study of clinical outcomes on 21 patients with type 2 diabetes and found that 76% of the sample showed improved glycemic control with MNT provided by a registered dietitian. Because not all dietitians are equally trained and knowledgeable in current recommendations of diabetes MNT, nutrition practice guidelines (NPGs) have been developed by The American Dietetic Association to help ensure that all patients have access to comprehensive, quality care. It has been shown that the patients of dietitians who follow NPGs achieve better outcomes than do those who receive standard therapy from dietitians (17–19). Therefore, the first step for improving adherence to MNT recommendations and for enhancing outcomes is to ensure that patients have access to the most qualified providers. The dietitian who is also a certified diabetes educator (CDE) has diabetes-specific training and will more likely be familiar with state-of-the-art resources such as NPGs.

Follow NPGs

NPGs provide a framework for comprehensive and outcome-focused interventions (20). The NPGs are based on a four-step process of care: assessment, goal setting, intervention, and evaluation. In a field test evaluation of NPGs for type 2 diabetes, the outcomes of patients receiving

---

Table 21.3 Counseling and Educational Strategies for Improved Adherence to Medical Nutrition Therapy

Strategies	References
1. Team-up with a registered dietitian	1, 15
2. Follow nutrition practice guidelines	16–18, 21–23
3. Plan interventions based on the patient's readiness to change	24
4. Set priorities	25–27
5. Use effective teaching and communication skills	28–30
6. Focus on behavior change/problem solving skills	10, 31–35

care from dietitians who followed NPGs were compared with the outcomes of patients receiving basic or usual nutrition care. Blood glucose levels had improved in both groups at the 3- and 6-month follow-ups, and a trend toward greater improvement was noted among patients treated according to the NPGs (17). Another research study of this same group demonstrated that MNT was also a cost-effective intervention (18). Similarly, in a field test study of the type 1 guidelines, levels of HbA_{1c} improved at 3 months in 88% of NPG patients as compared with 53% of usual-care patients (19).

A brief review of the four-step process of MNT follows, highlighting counseling and educational strategies for improving adherence.

Assessment. The assessment phase involves gathering important information that will help clarify therapeutic goals. Typical elements of assessment include reviewing the patient's usual eating habits, lifestyle influences on food intake, past nutrition education, and factors that may influence his or her readiness to change and adopt new behaviors.

Detailed assessments beyond food intake alone are required to facilitate problem solving and to help patients match insulin delivery to changes in food intake, activity, and other lifestyle factors. Using blood glucose records to evaluate the impact of foods eaten can be very useful. When dietitians extend their assessments beyond food intake, they redefine their relationships with their patients. In the process, dietitians are less likely to be perceived as food police and more likely to be viewed as important advocates of diabetes control (21).

From the experience of the DCCT, behavioral scientists suggest specific elements that should be reviewed in the assessment to support behavioral change. These include values and personal agenda, details of daily living, social support systems and whether family and friends may obstruct or enable change, and beliefs and understanding about diabetes and nutrition held not only by the patient but also by family members (10).

Assessment information may be gathered in a variety of ways, including forms completed by the patient before the visit, reviews of medical records, and interviews with the patient and referring physician. Given the limited time that may be available for nutrition intervention, the focus should be on assessing and identifying what the patient perceives to be the primary problem. It is an important skill of an experienced clinician or educator to focus the assessment quickly on the key priorities that will result in improved outcomes and to continue to collect additional assessment data at subsequent visits.

Goal setting. The health care provider and the patient should collaboratively determine short- and long-term nutritional goals and medical targets, as well as behavioral goals designed to meet those targets. If patients know what is expected of them and what specific targets they should strive to achieve, they will be more likely to meet those goals. Patients should know that their target glycated hemoglobin level may not necessarily be the "ideal" but that it is one that is realistic for them to achieve. For patients with type 2 diabetes, it is better to emphasize a glucose target rather than a target weight loss, which may be perceived as too difficult to achieve.

Behavioral goals are those specific steps a patient can take that result in progress toward a target outcome. These are steps over which the patient has some control. For example, a goal would not be a 20-lb weight loss or a 2-point drop in glycated hemoglobin, but instead a goal could be to snack on only one cookie at night or to take a 1-mile walk 5 days/week. Achieving these goals may move the patient closer to the targeted outcomes of improved glycated hemoglobin and weight. An important role of the health care provider is to break down the behavioral changes that may be required for improved health and diabetes control into small, realistic steps that the patient may be able to accomplish. Adherence will improve when the patient can realize small successes. If the therapeutic objective is to increase dietary fiber and decrease fat, a realistic recommendation might be to "add one serving of vegetables to the meal plan each day." Telling the patient to "eat more high-fiber foods" is less specific and therefore less likely to have a measurable impact.

To facilitate goal setting, an important question to ask at an initial assessment for a nutrition consultation is "Why are you here, and what can I help you with?" Writing down the agreed upon goals in the form of a contract helps serve as a reminder to the patient. As part of the education documentation form, patients can complete the following sentence, "I agree to. . . ." Also, it is more productive to focus on actions the patient can start taking rather than on actions that need to be stopped.

An important part of goal setting is to continuously review and reevaluate the goals. If goals are set with a patient but their progress is not reviewed at subsequent visits, the patient will be less likely to work toward future goals.

Intervention. Intervention refers to the health care professional's activities that enable, facilitate, or support the patient's diabetes management plan. Based on the assessment and goals, the health care provider will select a meal planning approach and teaching tools that will best meet the patient's needs. The meal plan could be a simple set of written instructions to alter eating times and to substitute one food for another; it could be an adaptation of the USDA Food Guide Pyramid for making healthful choices; or it could be more detailed, offering sample menus, carbohydrate counting guidelines, or exchange lists. Given the wide range of meal planning options and teaching tools available, health care providers can enhance adherence by selecting the one best suited for the patient's needs (22).

Evaluation. A detailed assessment, an individualized meal plan, and one-on-one instruction are of little value unless there is opportunity to evaluate the impact of the self-care plan and make modifications as necessary. At a follow-up visit, the educator evaluates progress in any of the behavioral goals, which would in turn lead to improvements in specific clinical outcomes such as glycated hemoglobin, weight loss, or lipid control.

To meet target goals, follow-up visits are essential to evaluate the effectiveness of therapeutic interventions. Follow-up also allows the opportunity for repetition of key information taught at previous visits. Research has shown that better outcomes and adherence are associated with follow-up care (17,19,23).

Plan Interventions Based on the Patient's Readiness to Change

To successfully guide patients through changing nutrition behaviors, the health care provider needs to understand where the patient is in the process of change. Ruggiero and Prochaska (24) have been studying the process of how individuals go through specific stages in the process of changing behaviors. The five stages include *1*) precontemplation, not thinking about making changes; *2*) contemplation, considering a change in the foreseeable future; *3*) preparation, seriously considering a change in the near future; *4*) action, in the process of changing behavior; and *5*) maintenance, continued change for an extended period. People go through each of these stages for changes to be made and maintained. Progression through the stages is not linear; most individuals relapse and recycle back through earlier stages.

The health care provider must assess the patient's stage or readiness to change to match the therapeutic recommendations. Mismatching stages can take several forms. It may result from pushing for action too early, before a patient is committed, or it could mean talking too long about change with a patient who is already ready to jump in and take action. Success in making changes should be measured not only when the patient achieves the action phase, but when he or she moves from the first to the second or the second to the third stage.

Applying this to nutrition and/or food strategies, the counselor could ask the patient if he has been thinking about making some food and/or exercise changes to improve glucose control. The patient may say, "No, not really," indicating a precontemplation stage; "Yes, as a matter of fact, I have been thinking a lot about it" (contemplation); or "Yes, funny you should ask, I just bought some new sneakers because I want to start walking regularly" (preparation). Talking to the person in the precontemplation stage about low-fat cooking ideas will be less effective than will having a discussion about benefits and barriers to improved glucose control. A discussion about this topic will help move him toward the contemplation stage. The counselor can measure success not only by the number of patients who have been moved to action or maintenance, but also by the patients who have moved from precontemplation to contemplation or from contemplation to preparation.

Set Priorities

Enthusiastic nutrition educators may proudly boast of the many long hours it takes to teach a patient all there is to know about MNT. However, they should usually be redirected to teach the smallest amount possible to do the job. Identify the one or two points that may need to be taught or the one or two behaviors that could be changed to have a meaningful impact on outcomes. Keep in mind how difficult following a meal plan can be. In a study of dietetic students who attempted to comply with a calorie-controlled diabetic meal plan for 1 week, only one student indicated she was able to adhere for the entire period (25). In another study, at the end of a clinic visit where patients had contact with several team members who each had made an effort to simplify instruction, patients still only recalled two of the seven recommendations that were made (26).

Research from the DCCT found that the four nutrition behaviors associated with clinically significant reductions in glycated hemoglobin were *1)* adherence to a prescribed meal plan, *2)* adjustment of insulin dose in response to meal size, *3)* prompt treatment of hyperglycemia, and *4)* avoidance of overtreatment of hypoglycemia (27). Nutrition counselors should focus on these behaviors because they are the ones most associated with improved clinical outcomes.

Use Effective Communication Skills

The nutrition health care provider must be a good counselor, teacher, listener, and facilitator. Effective communication skills are essential in gaining the patient's trust and ensure that the patient not only listens to the recommendations, but also participates in making decisions and developing the treatment plan. Training in active listening skills can help health care providers better hear what their patients are really saying and thus develop more meaningful treatment strategies. To encourage a frank and honest dialog, it is particularly important not to be judgmental about food choices or lifestyle habits that may be discussed. The location and setting of the nutrition counseling can also have an impact on the effectiveness of communication, and this raises several discussion points.

Very little teaching, other than of the most basic survival skills, can usually take place in an inpatient setting. However, adherence to MNT delivered in the hospital setting is likely to be good because the patient is usually motivated by whatever reason put him/her in the hospital in the first place. Because of time limitations and the often compromised attention span of patients in a hospital setting, dietitians need to make concise, simple recommendations. On the other hand, the reason for hospitalization could seriously interfere with the patient's interest in and attention to nutrition information.

A more realistic debate than the inpatient-versus-outpatient argument relates to the effectiveness of one-on-one versus group counseling. Largely because of economic forces, many diabetes education programs are being asked to see more patients with fewer staff, thereby necessitating the use of group education. Well-designed groups that take a patient-centered approach can be at least as effective as individual instruction (28,29). Patients with type 2 diabetes who have attended group training sessions report increased social support, increased sense of control over their disease, improved glucose control, and improved glycated hemoglobin levels (28). Furthermore, patients benefit from being able to learn from one another in a group setting.

Patients who are more actively involved in their health care will have better outcomes. This means ensuring that a patient can demonstrate a new skill or, at minimum, can discuss the application of a new behavior. Research has shown that patients with diabetes who are trained to be more assertive (by asking more questions, expressing opinions, and bringing up topics of concern), who express more positive and negative emotions, and who are more adept at eliciting information from their doctors experience better metabolic control (30). Nutrition counselors should encourage their patients to be assertive in this way.

Use of the right educational tools can also help the patient make changes. During the assessment, determine which of the available mediums the patient would benefit from most: written material, video, or computer-assisted instruction. No matter which method is selected, the tools should not be used without input before and after by the health care provider. A written tool should always be individualized. The nutrition counselor should use colored pens to add favorite foods, special instructions, or a personalized meal plan to a preprinted teaching tool. If a patient is instructed to watch a videotape or complete a computerized instruction program, a follow-up discussion to assess understanding and application is essential. The wide variety of nutrition education tools now available makes it easier to select the right tool without overwhelming the patient with unnecessary or irrelevant information (22).

Focus on Behavior Change

The importance of behavior-change strategies in diabetes self-management received heightened attention as a result of the DCCT. One of the key lessons learned was that health care professionals must resist the temptation to label patients as noncompliant and accept instead that almost all patients can improve their glycemic control when given appropriate assistance (10).

Foreyt and Goodrick (31) have identified several strategies for enhancing behavior change that can be applied to nutrition therapy. They are

- Self-monitoring—recording food intake in a diary to increase awareness
- Stimulus control—modifying environmental cues that trigger eating
- Contingency management—using a system of contrasts and rewards
- Cognitive behavioral strategies—changing thinking patterns related to target behaviors

In addition, Foreyt and Goodrick identified several strategies for maintaining behavior change. These include

- Participation in regular exercise
- Social support from family, friends, work groups, self-help groups, etc.
- Relapse-prevention training
- Continued support and follow-up

As part of the assessment process, the health care provider uses cognitive behavioral strategies to address motivations, beliefs, attitudes, coping skills, and environmental support. Two important beliefs to listen for are that patients *1*) consider diabetes to be serious and *2*) believe that their own actions can make a difference. Patients who hold these beliefs are more likely to engage in effective self-management behaviors than are those who do not have these beliefs (32). Research has shown that a person's self-efficacy, self-confidence in making and maintaining a change, is a significant predictor of later adherence (33). It is essential that support from family and friends be provided in the right balance; the right amount is important to promoting adherence, but more than the desired amount negatively effects these behaviors (34).

Successful MNT involves an ongoing process of problem solving, adjustment, and readjustment. Patients must be taught how to anticipate and deal with the wide variety of decisions they will face on a daily basis. A key objective for the nutrition counselor is simply to discuss problem solving skills and decision making strategies.

Because most people face decisions about food intake at least three times a day, the whole process of adherence can seem overwhelming. Schlundt et al. (35) suggest a realistic message that health care providers should be communicating to patients when it comes to behavioral guidelines for successful dietary self-management:

- Be consistent. The more predictable the timing, composition, and size of meals, the less decision making and adjustment is required.
- When you can't be consistent, be close.
- When you aren't close, make adjustments.
- Be prepared, plan ahead.
- Avoid "all or none" thinking.

CONCLUSION

In this era of health care, we need to continuously ask, "Are we making a difference?" As we pay more attention to outcomes of care, and not just processes, we realize that simply delivering information (like a meal plan) is not enough to ensure action. Patients must also be given the resources to help make the behavioral changes necessary to ensure the effectiveness of MNT. Nutrition therapy that is designed around a patient-centered framework may be more time-consuming and intellectually challenging, but its chances for success are much higher.

At the Joslin Diabetes Center, a bronze "Victory Medal" is awarded to people who have lived successfully with insulin-dependent diabetes for 50 years. The medal depicts three horses. In 1929, Elliott Joslin wrote (36):

> I look upon the diabetic as a charioteer and his chariot is drawn by three steeds named Diet, Insulin and Exercise. It takes will to drive one horse, intelligence to manage a team of two, but a man must be a very good teamster who can get all three to pull together.

Even 70 years ago, the importance of the person with diabetes being in the driver's seat to make the day-to-day decisions was recognized. Successful MNT will be that which uses a team approach respecting the patient's role as driver, follows recognized practice guidelines, is aimed at the patient's readiness to change, is priority focused, and teaches problem solving and behavior change skills using effective communication techniques.

REFERENCES

1. American Diabetes Association: Standards of medical care for patients with diabetes mellitus (Position Statement). *Diabetes Care* 21 (Suppl. 1):S23–S31, 1998

2. Lockwood D, Prey M, Galadish N, Hiss R: The biggest problem in diabetes. *Diabetes Educ* 12:30–33, 1986

3. Ary DV, Toobert D, Wilson W, Glasgow RE: Patient perspective on factors contributing to nonadherence to diabetes regimen. *Diabetes Care* 9:168–172, 1986

4. Benny LJ, Dunn SM: Knowledge improvement and metabolic control in diabetes education: approaching the limits? *Patient Educ Counsel* 16:217–229, 1990

5. Dunn SM: Rethinking the models and modes of diabetes education. *Patient Educ Counsel* 16:281–286, 1990

6. Glasgow RE, Osteen VL: Evaluating diabetes education: are we measuring the right outcomes? *Diabetes Care* 15:1423–1432, 1992

7. Anderson R, Arnold MS: From philosophy to practice. In *Diabetes Medical Nutrition Therapy*. Holler HJ, Pastors JG, Eds. Chicago, IL, The American Dietetic Association, 1997, pp. 95–97

8. Schundt DG, Rea MR, Kline SS, Pichert JW: Situational obstacles to dietary adherence for adults with diabetes. *J Am Diet Assoc* 94:874–876, 1994

9. Anderson RM, Funnell MM, Butler PM, Arnold MS, Fitzgerald JJ, Feste CC: Patient empowerment: results of a randomized controlled trial. *Diabetes Care* 18:943–949, 1995

10. Lorenz RA, Jannaasch K, Bubb J, Kramer J, Davis D, Lipps J, Jacobson A, Schlundt D: Changing behavior: practical lessons learned from the Diabetes Control and Complications Trial. *Diabetes Care* 19:648–652, 1996

11. Brown SA: Studies of educational interventions and outcomes in diabetic adults: a meta-analysis revisited. *Patient Educ Counsel* 16:189–215, 1990

12. Brown SA, Upchurch S, Anding R, Winter M, Ramirez G: Promoting weight loss in type II diabetes. *Diabetes Care* 19:613–624, 1996

13. Padgett D, Mumford E, Hynes M, Carter R: Meta-analysis of the effects of educational and psychosocial interventions on management of diabetes mellitus. *J Clin Epidemiol* 41:1007–1030, 1988

14. Clement S: Diabetes self-management. *Diabetes Care* 18:1204–1214, 1995

15. Task Force on the Clarification of Roles and Responsibilities in Providing Diabetes Self-Management Education: Report on the American Diabetes Association's Task Force on the Clarification of

Roles and Responsibilities in Providing Diabetes Self-Management Education. *Diabetes Spectrum* 10:155–158, 1997

16. Johnson E, Valera S: Medical nutrition therapy in non-insulin-dependent diabetes mellitus improves clinical outcome. *J Am Diet Assoc* 95:700–701, 1995

17. Franz MJ, Monk A, Barry B, McClain K, Weaver T, Cooper N, Upham P, Bergenstal R, Mazze R: Effectiveness of medical nutrition therapy provided by dietitians in management of non-insulin dependent diabetes mellitus: a randomized, controlled clinical trial. *J Am Diet Assoc* 95:1009–1017, 1995

18. Franz MJ, Splett PL, Monk A, Barry B, McClain K, Weaver T, Upham P, Bergenstal R, Mazze RS. Cost-effectiveness of medical nutrition therapy provided by dietitians for persons with non-insulin dependent diabetes. *J Am Diet Assoc* 95:1018–1024, 1995

19. Kulkarni K, Castle G, Gregory R, Holmes A, Leontos C, Powers M, Snetselaar L, Splett P, Wylie-Rosett J: Nutrition practice guide-lines for type 1 diabetes mellitus positively affect dietitian practices and patient outcomes. *J Am Diet Assoc* 98:62–70, 1998

20. The American Dietetic Association: *Nutrition Practice Guidelines for Type I and Type II Diabetes Mellitus.* Chicago, IL, The American Dietetic Association, 1996

21. Delehanty LM: Clinical significance of medical nutrition therapy in achieving diabetes outcomes and the importance of the process. *J Am Diet Assoc* 98:28–34, 1998

22. Wheeler ML, Barrier P, Broussard B, Daly A, Holler H, Holz-meister LA, Pastors JG, Schreiner B, Warshaw H: New diabetes nutrition care resources. *J Am Diet Assoc* 95:975, 1995

23. Travis T: Patient perceptions of factors that affect adherence to dietary regimens for diabetes mellitus. *Diabetes Educ* 23:152–156, 1997

24. Ruggiero L, Prochaska JO: Readiness for change: application of the transtheoretical model to diabetes. *Diabetes Spectrum* 6:21–60, 1993

25. Cotugna N, Vickery CE: Diabetic diet compliance: student dietitians reverse roles. *Diabetes Educ* 16:123–126, 1990

26. Page P, Verstraete DG, Robb JR, Etzwiler DD: Patient recall of self-care recommendations in diabetes. *Diabetes Care* 4:96–98, 1981

27. Delehanty L, Halford BN: The role of diet behaviors in achieving improved glycemic control in intensively treated patients in the DCCT. *Diabetes Care* 16:1453–1458, 1993

28. Campbell LV, Barth R, Gosper JK, Jupp JJ, Simons LA, Chisholm DJ: Impact of intensive educational approach to dietary change in NIDDM. *Diabetes Care* 13:841–847, 1990

29. Hayaki J, Brownell K: Behaviour change in practice: group approaches. *Int J Obesity* 20 (Suppl. 1):S27–S30, 1996

30. Greenfield S, Kaplan SH, Ware JE, Yano EM, Frank HJL: Patient participation in medical care: effects on blood sugar control and quality of life in diabetes. *J Gen Intern Med* 3:448–457, 1988

31. Foreyt JP, Goodrick K: Evidence for success of behavior modification in weight loss and control. *Ann Int Med* 119:698–701, 1993

32. Glasgow RE, Eakin EG: Dealing with diabetes self-management. In *Practical Psychology for Diabetes Clinicians*. Anderson BJ, Rubin RR, Eds. Alexandria, VA, American Diabetes Association, 1996, pp. 53–62

33. Kavanagh DJ, Gooley S, Wilson PH: Prediction of adherence and control in diabetes. *J Behav Med* 16:509–522, 1993

34. Boehm S, Schlenk EA, Funnell MM, Powers H, Ronis DL: Predictors of adherence to nutrition recommendations in people with NIDDM. *Diabetes Educ* 23:157–165, 1997

35. Schlundt DG, Pichert JW, Gregory B, Davis D: Eating and diabetes: a patient-centered approach. In *Practical Psychology for Diabetes Clinicians*. Anderson BJ, Rubin RR, Eds. Alexandria, VA, American Diabetes Association, 1996, pp. 63–72

36. Joslin EPJ: *Joslin Diabetes Manual*. Philadelphia, Lea & Febiger, 1929

Ms. Maryniuk is a program manager in the Affiliated Centers Division of the Joslin Diabetes Center, Boston, MA.

Index